MONSEN AND BAER

Memories of Perfume

Special Features:

The Perfumes of Lucien Lelong
- AND -
Masterpieces of Today

Perfume Bottle Auction VIII

May 16, 1998.

Auction:
Arlington Park Hilton Conference Center
3400 West Euclid Ave.
Arlington Heights, IL 60005 USA

Auctioneer: Michael DeFina

Auction Preview: All lots will be available for viewing
and inspection from 10:00 AM to 5:00 PM on Saturday, May 16, 1998.
Sale will begin at 5:00 PM, May 16, 1998.

Monsen and Baer
Box 529
Vienna, VA 22183 USA
(703) 938-2129 Fax (703) 242-1357

ISBN #0-9636102-8-7

Copyright 1998 © Monsen and Baer, all rights reserved.
*None of the photographs and text in this book may be reproduced by any means
including hardcopy, electronic and in cyberspace
unless the expressed permission of Monsen and Baer has been obtained in writing.*

Memories of Perfume

Table of Contents

Contents	p 2
Preface	pp 3
Conditions of Sale	pp 3-4
Bibliography on the Collection of Perfume	p 5
Books for Sale	p 6
New Books Available from Monsen and Baer	p 6
Monsen and Baer Publications	p 7

The Perfumes of Lucien Lelong - Les Parfums Lucien Lelong
    Randall B. Monsen — pp 8-35

Masterpieces of Today - Chefs-d'Oeuvre d'Aujourd'hui
    Christie Mayer Lefkowith — pp 36-46

MONSEN AND BAER PERFUME BOTTLE AUCTION VIII

Individual Lot Photographs and Descriptions	pp 47-128
Miniatures, Samples, First Sizes	pp 47-63
Factices, Memorabilia, Perfume Lamps	pp 63-68
Crown-Top - Porcelain - Decorative Perfume Bottles	pp 68-71
Atomizers and DeVilbiss	pp 71-77
Nineteenth and Early Twentieth Century Decorative Scent Bottles	pp 77-83
Art Glass - Baccarat - Richard - Sabino - Steuben	pp 83-91
Commercial Perfume Bottles	pp 92-109
French Masters of Perfume Bottle Design:	
Lalique, Daillet, Viard, Gaillard, Dépinoix, Jollivet	pp 109-118
Czechoslovakian Crystal Perfume Bottles	pp 118-128

Preface

To our fellow collectors in this country and abroad, greetings and good wishes! This is the eighth fully catalogued auction of perfume bottles to be held in the United States--the only auction of its kind in the United States devoted solely to perfume bottles and memorabilia of the fragrance industry--and this auction serves to support the International Perfume Bottle Association in that it is held during the annual IPBA Convention, and that a portion of the proceeds of the auction will be donated to that organization. If you are a serious collector of perfume bottles, you should become a member of the IPBA, the International Perfume Bottle Association. The IPBA publishes a wonderful Quarterly, a Membership Directory, and organizes an outstanding annual Convention. We will happily send membership information to all who request it.

Our two most recent books, *The Beauty of Perfume* [1996] and *The Legacies of Perfume* [1997], were both very well-received by the international audience of collectors. This year, we have produced a third hard-cover book, *Memories of Perfume,* containing descriptions of all the lots in the auction as well as two research articles for collectors. As we have done since the beginning, we also include translations of these articles in French and German; we are indebted to Peter Dechent and Thomas Cory [for the German translations], Christiane Angeli and Thomas Higonnet [for the French translations]. The photographs and descriptions of lots serve the obvious and primary function of information for the auction sale, but beyond that, they also have an archival function that collectors in the United States and abroad are coming to value highly. Eventually [possibly in the year 2000] we will provide a comprehensive index of all lots sold. Our overall goal is to provide the collector with a resource of documentation that can be used over and over again. The new book format provides a more durable object for collectors to use and re-use. The goal here goes beyond merely selling perfume bottles, though of course we wish to do that and to do it well. In a very real sense, we want to produce for collectors something that we, as collectors ourselves, would value and find useful--something we would want to own. Our sincere wish is that other collectors use it, learn from it, and enjoy it. *What we have said in the past bears repeating here: Knowledge–and the sharing of it–enhances the pleasure of collecting.*

Knowledge should be shared, but the source of it should always be properly acknowledged. Today, however, among those who write about perfume, the source of information is sometimes not acknowledged. The Monsen and Baer catalogues-eight volumes-now contain in total 663 pages of documentation and valuable research, with data, original research by many authors, and names and pictures of thousands upon thousands of perfumes. It is unfortunate that while many writers use our catalogues as a source of information, some nonetheless find themselves unable to provide a reference to our books and catalogues in their bibliographies and lists of references, thus concealing where the information was obtained. This contravenes centuries of accepted practice among scholars and researchers, and it reflects poorly upon those who do it.

We are quite convinced that collectors of the rather near future will look back longingly and wistfully upon this sale and will recognize that it was in fact an opportunity to acquire incredibly desirable perfume bottles at advantageous prices. Our hope is that each collector of today will also recognize this opportunity to acquire a wonderful perfume bottle for their collection.

If you have a truly wonderful perfume bottle that you would consider selling, then our 1999 auction, to be held near Washington, DC, on May 15, 1999, may be the perfect venue to do so. For those who would like to consign bottles for the 1999 auction, please contact us soon after this sale. Consignment details will be sent to those who request this information. The consignment deadline is December 31, 1998, but many categories fill up long before that date.

The Conditions of Sale

All lots sold in this auction are subject to the following conditions: please read carefully.

Terms of Sale. All lots will be sold, in the numerical sequence of this catalogue, to the highest bidder as determined by the auctioneer. In the case of disputed bids, the auctioneer shall have the sole discretion of determining the purchaser, and may elect to reoffer the lot for sale. We will accept cash, travelers checks, or personal checks with acceptable identification or if the buyer is known to us; we reserve the right in some cases to ship the lot to the purchaser after their check has cleared.

Sales Tax. All lots are subject to 6.75% Illinois state sales tax unless a valid tax exemption form has been filed with us; proof of sales tax exemption status may be required, i.e., a xerox copy of your sales tax registration form.

Absentee Bids. A form for absentee bids is available. We will be happy to execute your bid for you as if you were present at the auction. When you do this, it does not mean that the bidding will commence with your bid, it simply means that we will not bid for you above the amount you indicate. It is advantageous to place these absentee bids as early as possible. In the case of identical bids, the bid from the floor will take precedence; for identical absentee bids, the earlier-dated bid will take precedence. Please read shipping information below.

Bidding Increments. Bidding increments are totally at the discretion of the auctioneer. However, the following increments are typically used: under $50, increments of $5; $50-$300, increments of $10; $300-$500, increments of $25; $500-$1,000, increments of $50; $1,000-$3,000, increments of $100; $3,000-$5,000, increments of $250; $5,000-$10,000, increments of $500; above $10,000, increments of $1,000.

Shipping and Handling Fees. We offer the possibility of shipping your purchases anywhere. For the United States and Canada, the flat charge for this service is <u>**$15 per lot**</u> for lots whose sale price is less than $1000; the charges will be higher for the lots valued over $1000 due to insurance charges. Lots which consist of large items can be shipped, with actual shipping charges to be paid by the purchaser.

Shipping purchases to Europe is also possible. **<u>There is an initial charge of $75 for this service; additional lots will be included at the actual shipping cost, which may go above that amount if several lots are purchased.</u>** Absentee bidders will be sent an invoice for the shipping charges and balance due; we offer the convenience of accepting payment in all major European currencies. We normally use United Parcel Service or DHL to ship to Europe, and in most cases we cannot use the Postal Service. United Parcel Service is highly reliable and extremely rapid. However, please note that the minimum charge for a small parcel sent by UPS to Europe is $75. Parcels consisting of several lots may cost twice that amount. <u>Lots which are shipped outside the United States are subject to customs duties in the destination country, which is based upon the purchase price of the lot and we are required to state it. It is the responsibility of the purchaser to determine the amount of these duties and to pay them in full.</u>

Price Estimates and Reserves. Some lots, typically those with a value in excess of one thousand dollars, are offered for sale with a "reserve price." The reserve is a confidential minimum price below which the lot will not be sold. The reserve price for any lot in this sale is usually well below the low estimate and is never allowed to be higher than the estimates. The estimates are merely a range within which we believe the lot may find a buyer, but of course many lots may be sold at prices well below or well above these estimates, depending on the wishes of the bidders.

Buyer's Premium. A buyer's premium of 10% will be added to the hammer price of all lots, to be paid by the buyer as a part of the purchase price.

Condition of Lots. While we attempt to describe the condition of each lot as accurately as possible, as in all auctions, the lots here are sold "as is." We attempt to mention in the descriptions any negative aspect we think bidders need to know, for example: [label absent], [chip to stopper], etc. However, many factors relating to condition cannot be adequately described in the short captions of this catalogue, and this is especially true in the case of miniature or group lots. Very many perfume bottles have exceedingly tiny chips around the opening where the stopper enters the bottle. Sometimes these may also be found on the tongue of the stopper or on the base of the bottle. The boxes and labels of commercial bottles all show varying signs of usage and age, such as discoloration and fraying, and unless we note that the box is in pristine condition, such signs of age should be expected. All bottles, and especially commercial ones, may contain perfume residue and other internal stains. Not all stoppers fit into the bottle with perfect snugness and symmetry, especially those of Czechoslovakian manufacture. <u>Therefore, bidders should inspect each lot they wish to bid on prior to purchase.</u> We would also be happy to discuss the condition of any lot prior to the sale. Measurements given in this catalogue are in inches and centimeters, rounded in most cases to the nearest quarter inch or half-centimeter. Unless stated otherwise, the bottles are empty of perfume.

In cases where glass by a particular maker is described as unsigned, the catalogue can only provide a reasonable surmise, not a guarantee, as to the maker. Many of the early French glass makers produced glass of similar quality and design. In these cases, the buyer should consult the available reference works and thereafter make their own determination. The glass made by Lalique & Cie. is all grouped together; this includes bottles designed after René Lalique's death by Marc and Marie Claude Lalique. Following the convention used in Utt [1990], perfume bottles produced for sale by R. Lalique & Cie. are referred to as Maison Lalique or Cristal Lalique.

Reference numbers are provided for Lalique, Baccarat, and in many cases for Czech glass and commercial bottles, as described in Utt [1990], Compagnie des Cristalleries de Baccarat [1986], North [1990], Forsythe I & II [1982 & 1993], and Lefkowith [1994] and Leach [1997]. These reference numbers are also used in the article section of the catalogue.

Consignments. We will be accepting consignments for our ninth auction, to be held May 15, 1999, and we are particularly in search of fine perfume bottles. Our rates of consignment are very competitive with other auctions, and we can offer exposure of your bottles to a specialized buying audience. We guarantee confidentiality. We also purchase individual bottles or entire collections outright, if that avenue of sale is preferred. Contact us and we would be happy to discuss these terms with you. We are especially interested in perfume bottles of high quality, not broken or damaged pieces. Please bear in mind that consignments for the 1999 auction must be completed by <u>December 31, 1998</u> to allow sufficient time to prepare and publish the catalogue; many categories fill up well before that date.

Bibliography on the Collection of Perfume:

Atlas, M. and Monniot, A. *Guerlain - Les Flacons à Parfum Depuis 1828.* Toulouse, France: Editions Milan, 1997.

Atlas, M. and Monniot, A. *Un Siècle d'Echantillons Guerlain.* Toulouse, France: Editions Milan, 1995.

Ball, J. D. and Torem, D. H. *Commercial Fragrance Bottles.* Atglen, Pennsylvania: Schiffer Publishing Co., 1993.

Ball, J. D. and Torem, D. H. *Fragrance Bottle Masterpieces.* Atglen, Pennsylvania: Schiffer Publishing Co., 1996.

Barille, Elisabeth. *Coty.* Paris: Editions Assouline, 1995.

Berger, C. & D. *Tous les Parfums du Monde.* Toulouse: Editions Milan, 1995.

Bonduelle, J. P. et Lancry, J. M. *Flacons à Parfums Catalogues pour les Ventes aux Enchères Publiques*: March 31, 1990; March 24, 1991; June 16, 1991; October 24, 1991; June 21, 1992; May 16, 1993; November 21, 1993; March 27, 1994; November 20, 1994; June 18, 1995; December 3, 1995; June 16, 1996; December 1, 1996; June 15, 1997; expert: J.-M. Martin-Hattemberg.

Bonhams *Scent Bottle and Lalique auction catalogues*: November 29, 1989; October 18, 1990; November 21, 1990; April 24, 1991; October 24, 1991; October 28, 1991; April 28, 1992; October 29, 1992; April 7, 1993; June 28, 1993; October 20, 1993; expert: Juliette Bogaers; September 29, 1997; experts Isobel Muston, Eric Knowles, and Emma Thommeret.

Bowman, Glinda. *Miniature Perfume Bottles.* Atglen, Pennsylvania: Schiffer, 1994.

Byrd, Joan. *DeVilbiss Perfumizers & Perfume Lights: The Harvey K. Littleton Collection.* Cullowhee, North Carolina: Western Carolina University, 1985.

Cabré, Monique. *La Légende du Chevalier d'Orsay: Parfums de Dandy.* Toulouse: Editions Milan, 1997.

Charles-Roux, Edmonde. *Chanel and Her World.* New York: Vendome Press, 1981.

Christin, Jean. *Flacons à parfum du XXe siècle.* September 29, 1996, Hotel des Bergues, Geneva, Switzerland.

Chassaing, Rivet, Fournié. *Flacons à Parfums Catalogue pour la Vente aux Enchères Publiques*: June 27, 1994, Toulouse, France; expert: Geneviève Fontan.

Cohet et Feraud *Floréal Perfume Bottle Auction Catalogue,* Toulouse, France, April 15-16, 1995; November 4, 1995; expert: Flora Entajan.

Colard, Grégoire. *[Caron] The Secret Charm of a Perfumed House.* Paris: J. C. Lattès, 1984.

Compagnie des Cristalleries de Baccarat. *Baccarat Les Flacons à Parfum/The Perfume Bottles.* Paris: Henri Addor & Associés, 1986.

Courset, J-M. *5000 Miniatures de Parfum.* Toulouse: Editions Milan, 1995.

Coutau-Bégarie, O. *Flacons à Parfums Catalogues pour les Ventes aux Enchères Publiques*: December 6, 1993; October 24, 1994; June 12, 1995; November 27, 1995; June 3, 1996; December 1, 1997; expert: Régine de Robien.

Drouot-Richelieu, Neret-Minet, Coutau-Begarie. *Flacons à Parfums Catalogues pour les Ventes aux Enchères Publiques*: June 23, 1986; April 2, 1987; Nov. 4, 1987; April 13, 1988; Nov. 7, 1988; May 20, 1989; Nov. 13, 1989; May 21, 1990; Nov. 24, 1990; April 8, 1991; May 27, 1991; Nov. 15, 1991; December 14, 1992; expert: Régine de Robien.

Drouot-Richelieu, Neret-Minet. *Flacons à Parfums Catalogue pour la Vente aux Enchères Publiques*: December 14, 1992; expert: J.-M. Martin-Hattemberg.

Drouot-Richelieu, Millon & Robert. *Flacons à Parfums: Catalogue pour la Vente aux Enchères Publiques*: December 6, 1991; expert: Régine de Robien.

Duchesne, Clarence, ed. *La Mémoire des Parfums,* Numeros 1-11. Paris, 1988-1991.

Duval, René. *Parfums de Volnay.* Catalogue of the Company, 1928.

Fellous, Colette. *Guerlain.* Paris: Denoël, 1987.

Fleck, F. *Flacons à Parfum, Catalogue* for the Perfume Bottle Auction, March 12, 1994; expert: Anne Meter-Seguin.

Fontan, Geneviève. *Parfums d'Extase.* Toulouse: Arfon, 1996.

Fontan, Geneviève, and Barnouin, Nathalie. *Cote Générale des Echantillons de Parfum.* Toulouse: Editions Fontan & Barnouin, 1996.

Fontan, Geneviève, and Barnouin, Nathalie. *L'Argus des Echantillons de Parfum.* Toulouse: Editions Milan, 1992.

Fontan, Geneviève, and Barnouin, Nathalie. *La Cote Internationale des Echantillons de Parfum, 1995-1996. Les Echantillons Anciens.* Toulouse: 813 Edition, 1994.

Fontan, Geneviève, and Barnouin, Nathalie. *La Cote Internationale des Echantillons de Parfums Modernes.* Toulouse: 813 Edition, 1995.

Fontan, Geneviève, and Barnouin, Nathalie. *Les Intégrales: Rochas* and *Les Intégrales: Ricci.* Toulouse: Editions Fontan & Barnouin, 1996.

Forsythe, Ruth. *Made in Czechoslovakia.* Marietta, Ohio: Richardson Printing Co., 1982; *Made in Czechoslovakia, Book 2.* Marietta Ohio: Richardson Printing Co., 1993.

Frankl, Beatrice. *Parfum-Flacons.* Augsburg: Battenberg Verlag, 1994.

Gerson, Roselyn. *Vintage Ladies' Compacts.* Paducah, KY: Collector Books, 1996.

Gerson, Roselyn. *Vintage and Contemporary Purse Accessories.* Paducah, KY: Collector Books, 1997.

Ghozland, F. *Perfume Fantasies.* Toulouse: Editions Milan, 1987.

Guinn, Hugh D. *The Glass of René Lalique at Auction.* Tulsa, Oklahoma: Guindex Publications, 1994.

Hymne au Parfum: Catalogue de l'exposition, 1990-1991. Paris: Comité Français du Parfum, 1991.

Kaufman, William I. *Perfume.* New York: E. P. Dutton & Co., 1974.

Killian, E. H. *Perfume Bottles Remembered.* Traverse City, Michigan: E. Killian, 1989.

La Quinzaine du Parfum. *Perfume Bottle Auction Catalogue* for the sale of October 21, 1994; expert: Creezy Courtoy. Brussels, Belgium.

Latimer, Tirza True. *The Perfume Atomizer: An Object with Atmosphere.* West Chester, Pennsylvania: Schiffer Publishing, 1991.

Leach, Ken. *Perfume Presentation: 100 Years of Artistry.* Toronto: Kres Publishing, 1997.

Lefkowith, Christie Mayer. *The Art of Perfume.* New York: Thames and Hudson, 1994.

Le Louvre des Antiquaires. *Autour du Parfum du XVIe au XIXe Siècle.* Paris: Le Louvre des Antiquaires, 1985.

Marcilhac, Félix. *R. Lalique: Catalogue Raisonné de l'Oeuvre de Verre.* Paris: Editions de l'Amateur, 1989.

Martin, Hazel. *Figural Perfume and Scent Bottles.* Lancaster, CA: Hazel Martin, 1982.

Martin-Hattemberg, Jean-Marie. *Précieux Effluves / Scentsfully Precious.* Toulouse: Milan Editions, 1997.

Matthews, Leslie G. *The Antiques of Perfume.* London: G. Bell & Sons, 1973.

Mini Flacons. Wiesbaden, Germany: SU Verlag, 1993.

Mueller, Laura M. *Collector's Encyclopedia of Compacts: Volumes 1 and 2.* Paducah, KY: Collector Books, 1996.

Neret-Minet. *Flacons à Parfums Catalogue pour les Ventes aux Enchères Publiques,* November 14, 1991; expert: Elisabeth Danenberg.

North, Jacquelyne. *Commercial Perfume Bottles.* West Chester, Pennsylvania: Schiffer Publishing Co, 1987.

North, Jacquelyne. *Czechoslovakian Perfume Bottles and Boudoir Accessories.* Marietta, Ohio: Antique Publications, 1990.

North, Jacquelyne. *Perfume, Cologne, and Scent Bottles.* West Chester, Pennsylvania: Schiffer Publishing Co, 1986.

Parfum, Art, et Valeur. Catalogue de Vente, November 15, 1995. Expert: Geneviève Fontan.

Paulson, Paul L. *Guide to Russian Silver Hallmarks.* Paulson: Washington DC, 1976.

Pavia, Fabienne. *The World of Perfume.* New York: Knickerbocker Press, 1995.

Phillips Auctions. *Perfume Presentations.* October 6, 1996, October 26, 1997. Geneva, Switzerland. Expert: Christie Mayer Lefkowith.

René Lalique and Cristal Lalique Perfume Bottles (The Weinstein Collection). New York: Christie's/Lalique Society of America, 1993.

René Lalique et Cie. *Lalique Glass: The Complete Illustrated Catalogue for 1932.* Reprinted by The Corning Museum of Glass, Corning, New York. New York: Dover Publications, 1981.

Restrepo, Federico. *Le Livre d'Heures des Flacons et des Rêves.* Toulouse: Editions Milan, 1995.

Scent Bottles Through the Centuries: the Collection of Joan Hermanowski. St. Petersburg, Florida: Museum of Fine Art, 1997.

Sloan, Jean. *Perfume and Scent Bottle Collecting.* Lombard, Illinois: Wallace-Homestead Co., 1986.

Truitt, R. and D. Czech Glass 1918-1939. *Glass Collector's Digest,* Vol. 10, #6, May 1997. pp. 39-46.

Utt, Mary Lou and Glenn. *Lalique Perfume Bottles.* New York: Crown Publishers, 1990.

Watine-Arnault, D.. *Flacons à Parfums Christian Dior: Catalogue pour la Vente aux Enchères Publiques*: April 12, 1992; expert: Régine de Robien.

Whitmyer, M. & K. *Bedroom and Bathroom Glassware of the Depression Years.* Paducah, Kentucky: Collector Books, 1990.

Books Available from Monsen and Baer:

Baccarat Les Flacons à Parfum/The Perfume Bottles [Cie. des Cristalleries de Baccarat] @ $85 + $7 shipping. Hardcover§

Commercial Fragrance Bottles [J. Ball and D. Torem] @ $79.95 + $7 shipping. Hardcover§

Commercial Perfume Bottles [J. Jones-North] @ $69.95 + $7 shipping. Hardcover§

Fragrance Bottle Masterpieces [J. Ball and D. Torem] @ $69.95 + $7 shipping. Hardcover§

Guerlain: A Century of Minis: 1895-1995 [M. Atlas and A. Monniot] *Milan Editions 160 pp, text in English and French.* Hardcover @ $60 + $7 shipping.

Guerlain: The Perfume Bottles since 1826 [M. Atlas and A. Monniot] @ $69.95 + $9 shipping. Hardcover§

Lalique Perfume Bottles [M. L. and G. Utt and P. Bayer] @ $35 + $7 shipping. Hardcover§

The Legende of the Chevalier d'Orsay: Parfums de Dandy [M. Cabré] @ $48 + $7 shipping. Text in French and in English, Hardcover§

Made in Czechoslovakia, Book 2 [R. Forsythe] @ $29.95 + $5 shipping. Softcover¶

Perfume, Cologne, and Scent Bottles [J. Jones-North] @ $69.95 + $7 shipping. Hardcover§

The Perfume Atomizer [T. T. Latimer] @ $69.95 + $7 shipping. Hardcover§

Scentsfully Precious [J.-M. Martin-Hattemberg & F. Ghozland] @ $48 + $7 shipping. Hardcover§

We can ship the above books to Europe, but the airmail cost is as follows: §These books can be shipped to Europe for an additional $27 each. ¶These books can be shipped to Europe for an additional $16 each.

Important New Books Available through Monsen and Baer:

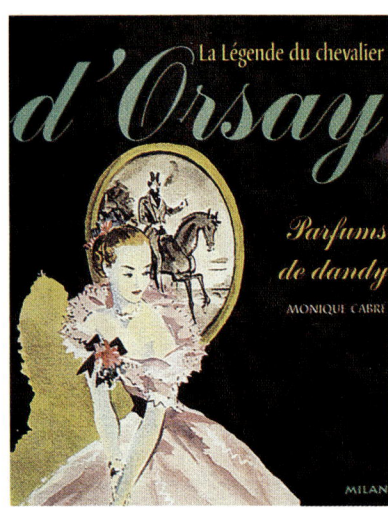

The Legende of the Chevalier d'Orsay: Parfums de Dandy, by Monique Cabré. Toulouse, France: Editions Milan, 1997. A history of d'Orsay, beautifully illustrated, with text in English and French, Hardcover, 126 pp.
Price: $48, plus $7 shipping.

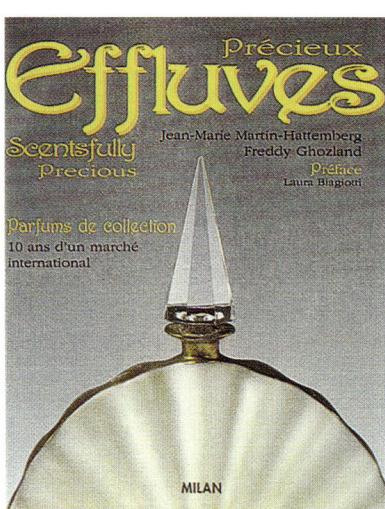

Scentsfully Precious/Précieux Effluves by J.-M. Martin-Hattemberg and Freddy Ghozland. Toulouse, France: Editions Milan, 1996. Beautifully illustrated, with text in French and English, Hardcover, 126 pp.
Price: $48, plus $7 shipping.

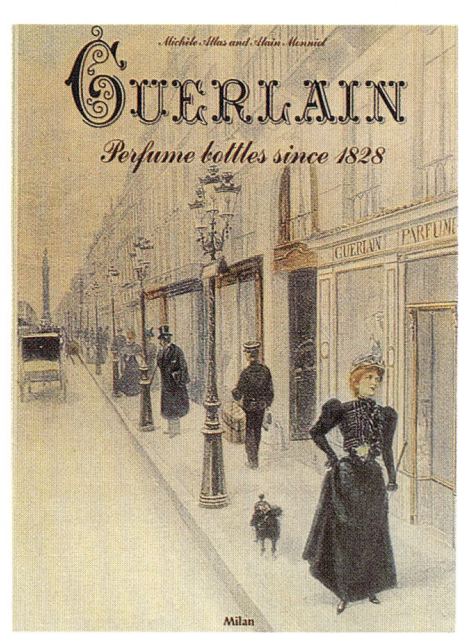

Guerlain: The Perfume Bottles since 1826, by Michèle Atlas and Alain Monniot. Toulouse, France: Editions Milan, 1997. This is a definitive history of Guerlain, beautifully illustrated, with the text in English, Hardcover, 320 pp.
Price: $69.95, plus $9 shipping.

The following auction catalogues are also available, all **postpaid** and with Prices Realized:

SOFTCOVER

Monsen and Baer Perfume Bottle Auction I,
Chicago, April 6, 1991 @ $18.00. ($25 for International shipment).
Monsen and Baer Perfume Bottle Auction II,
Atlanta, May 16, 1992 @ $25.00. ($30 for International shipment).
Monsen and Baer Perfume Bottle Auction III,
Dallas, May 1, 1993 @ $28.00. ($35 for International shipment).
Monsen and Baer Perfume Bottle Auction IV,
Washington, D. C., May 14, 1994 @ $29.00. ($35 for International shipment).
Monsen and Baer Perfume Bottle Auction V,
Chicago, Illinois, May 6, 1995 @ $35.00. ($40 for International shipment).

HARD COVER

The Beauty of Perfume, Monsen and Baer Perfume Bottle Auction VI,
San Francisco, California, May 11, 1996. @ $35.00. ($45 for International)
The Legacies of Perfume, Monsen and Baer Perfume Bottle Auction VII,
Washington D. C., May 3, 1997. @ $45.00 ($50 for International shipment.)
Memories of Perfume, Monsen and Baer Perfume Bottle Auction VIII,
Chicago, Illinois., May 16, 1998. @ $45.00 ($50 for International shipment.)

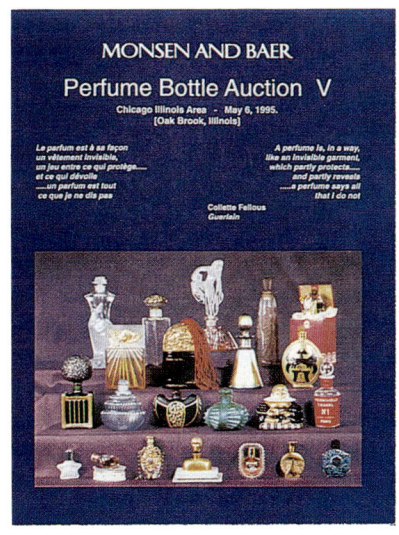
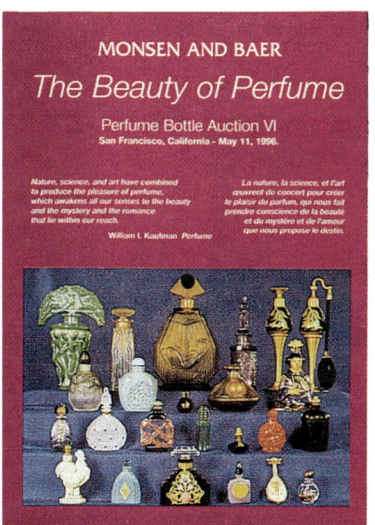
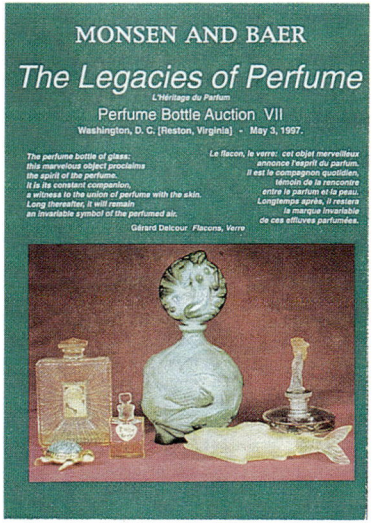

Monsen and Baer publish these books on American Art Pottery: *The Collectors' Compendium of Roseville Pottery, Volumes I and II.*

These books include new historical research and color photos of all the pieces in the pottery lines covered. Price guide information is included in Volume I and a separate price guide accompanies Volume II. Both books are 128 pp each, hardcover, and prices are postpaid.

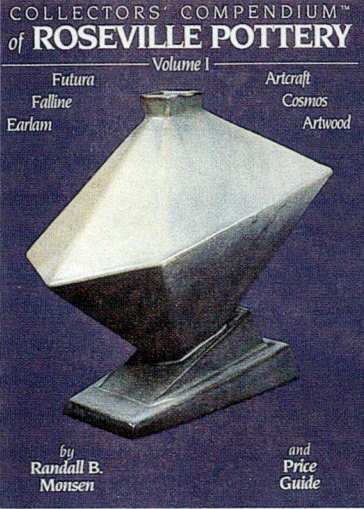
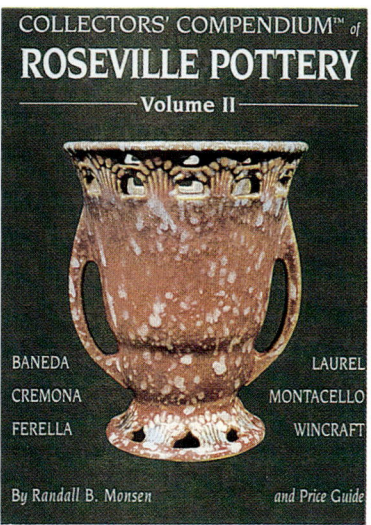

Volume I - $35   Volume II - $45

Les Parfums Lucien Lelong
Randall B. Monsen

Lucien Lelong was one of the great fashion designers of the twentieth century, and one of the century's greatest masters of the art of perfume. He was also a great French patriot. His perfume creations are among the most treasured objects in many collections of historically important perfumes. Every collector has at least one favorite to treasure as the centerpiece of their collection. Not only were Lelong perfumes commercially successful in their time, but they were artistically so beautiful that they will surely be treasured by each successive generation of collectors who falls under their spell; long after the perfume has vanished, lovers of perfume covet and protect the perfumes' beautiful boxes and glass bottles. This article is motivated by a desire to share with other collectors our admiration for this wonderful company, and by the occasion of the re-introduction of one of Lelong's greatest fragrances, *Indiscret,* in October of 1997.

Lucien Lelong was born in Paris on October 11, 1889, to Arthur and Valentine [Lambelet] Lelong. His father was in the textile business, and since Lucien was expected to carry on his father's business, he prepared for a commercial career by attaining his diploma in Hautes Etudes Commerciales in 1913. His father had trained him in the suitability of different fabrics for different fashions, and Lucien Lelong decided, possibly as a means of promoting sales of textiles, to become a couturier. At the young age of 24, he prepared a collection of gowns to be presented to the fashion world, but two days before the scheduled opening of his collection, he was drafted for combat. Lelong fought for France throughout World War I, and just before the end of the hostilities, he was hit by a shell and hospitalized during an entire year. When the war ended, he found himself without financial resources, but he managed somehow to borrow $2,500 from a friend, and with this money [the sum must have been very substantial at the time] he opened a *maison de couture* on the Place de la Madeleine. His first collection was a great success, and he soon became a leader of the French fashion industry along with Worth, Patou, Lanvin and Chanel. Lelong was awarded the *Croix de Guerre* after the war and

Lucien Lelong était un des grands couturiers du XXème siècle et un des plus grands maîtres de l'art du parfum. C'était aussi un grand patriote. Ses créations figurent parmi les joyaux les plus prisés dans de nombreuses collections de parfums historiquement reconnues. Chaque collectionneur a au moins une préférence parmi les pièces de choix de sa collection. Non seulement les parfums Lelong étaient un succès commercial, mais ils étaient si beaux d'un point de vue artistique qu'ils seront certainement recherchés par des générations successives de collectionneurs captivés par leur charme; bien après la disparition du parfum lui-même, les amateurs de parfums recherchent et protègent leurs beaux flacons et coffrets. Ces lignes sont nées du désir de partager avec d'autres collectionneurs le bonheur d'être entouré d'objets chers à notre coeur à l'occasion du relancement en octobre 1998 d'un de ses plus grands parfums, *Indiscret.*

Lucien Lelong est né à Paris le 11 octobre 1889, fils d'Arthur et de Valentine [Lambelet] Lelong. Son père avait une affaire de textiles, et comme Lucien devait reprendre l'affaire de son père, il se prépara à une carrière commerciale en obtenant un diplôme de l'École des Hautes Études Commerciales. Son père l'avait formé dans la connaissance de différents textiles pour différents articles, et Lucien Lelong décida, peut-être pour promouvoir la vente de textiles, de devenir couturier. À l'âge précoce de 24 ans, il avait préparé une collection de robes de mode, mais deux jours avant le défilé, il fut mobilisé. Lelong fit toute la Guerre de 14, et juste avant la fin des hostilités il fut blessé par un obus et hospitalisé pendant une année entière. Sans ressources financières à la fin de la guerre, il réussit à emprunter 12.500 francs à un ami; une somme considérable à l'époque, et il ouvrit sa maison de couture Place de la Madeleine. Sa première collection fut une grande réussite, et il devint vite, avec Worth, Patou, Lanvin, et Chanel, un géant de l'industrie de la mode. Lelong fut décoré de la Croix de Guerre et en 1926 il fut nommé chevalier de Légion d'Honneur.

En 1924 Lelong fonda la Société des Parfums Lucien Lelong. Il estimait que le parfum était un élément

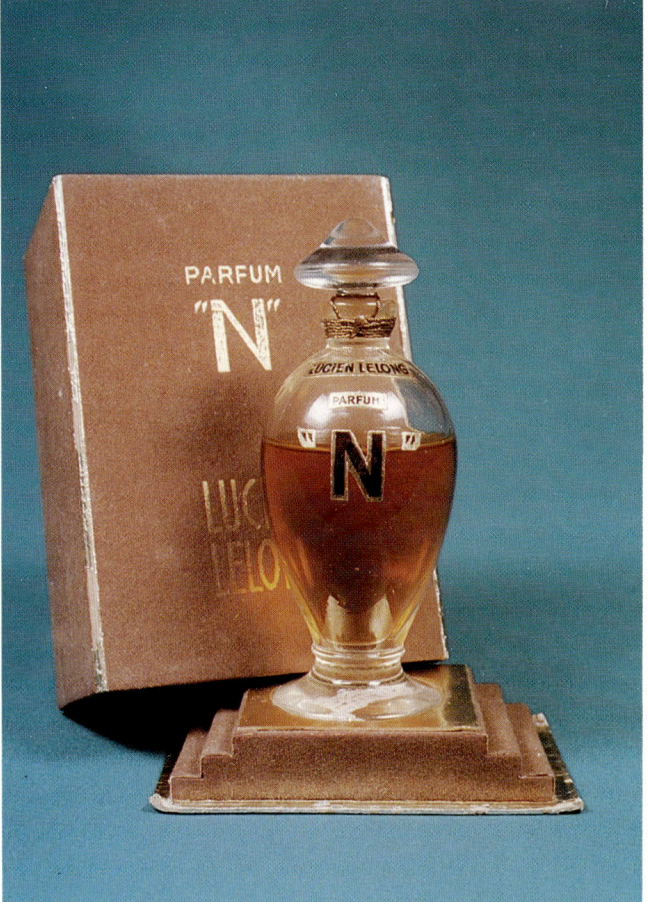

Figure 1. The perfume *N*, in a baluster-shaped bottle and in a presentation not seen in other published sources. Collection of Randall B. Monsen and Rodney L. Baer.

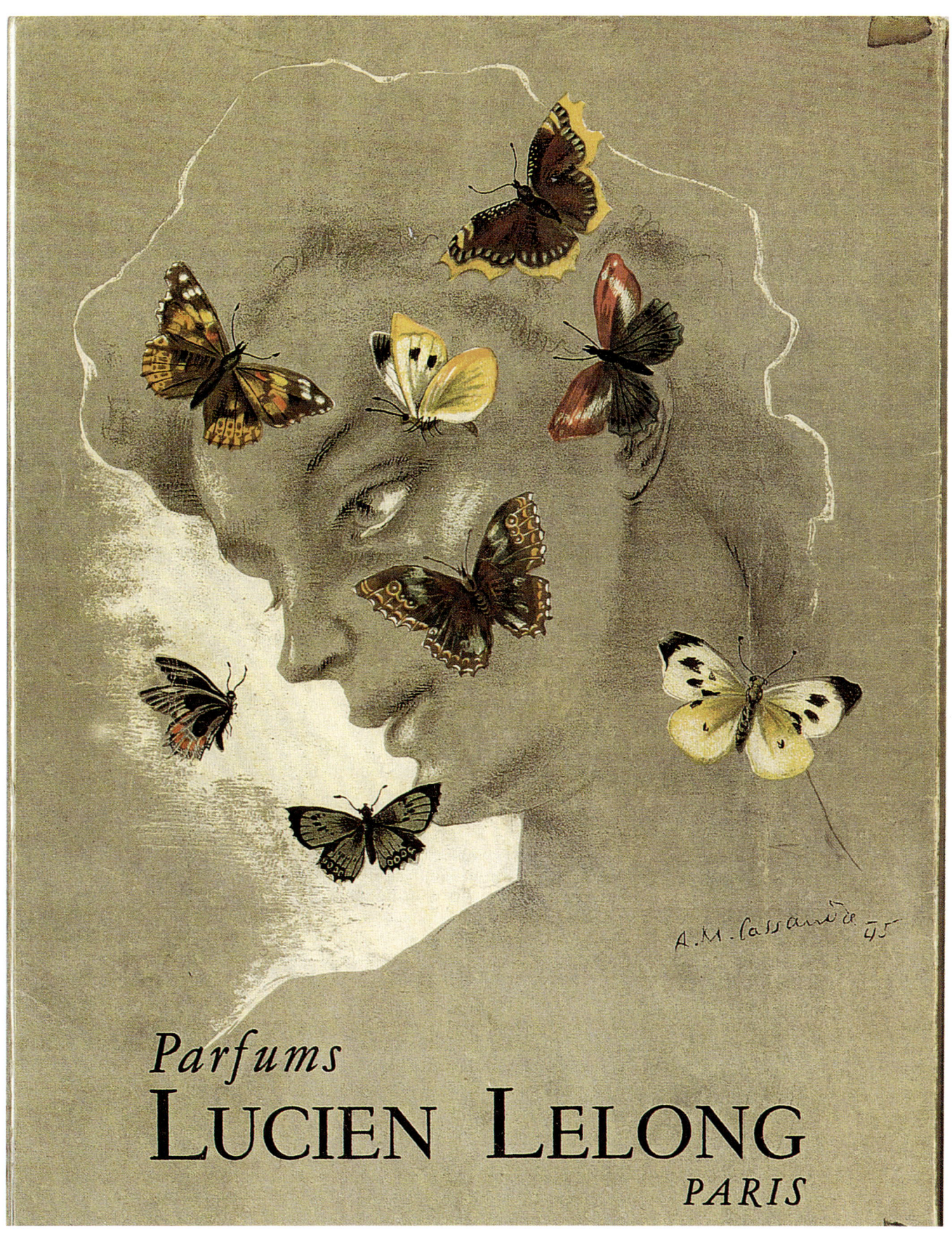

Figure 2. Lucien Lelong used beautiful artwork in their publicity. This advertisement dates from February, 1945. Collection of Randall B. Monsen and Rodney L. Baer.

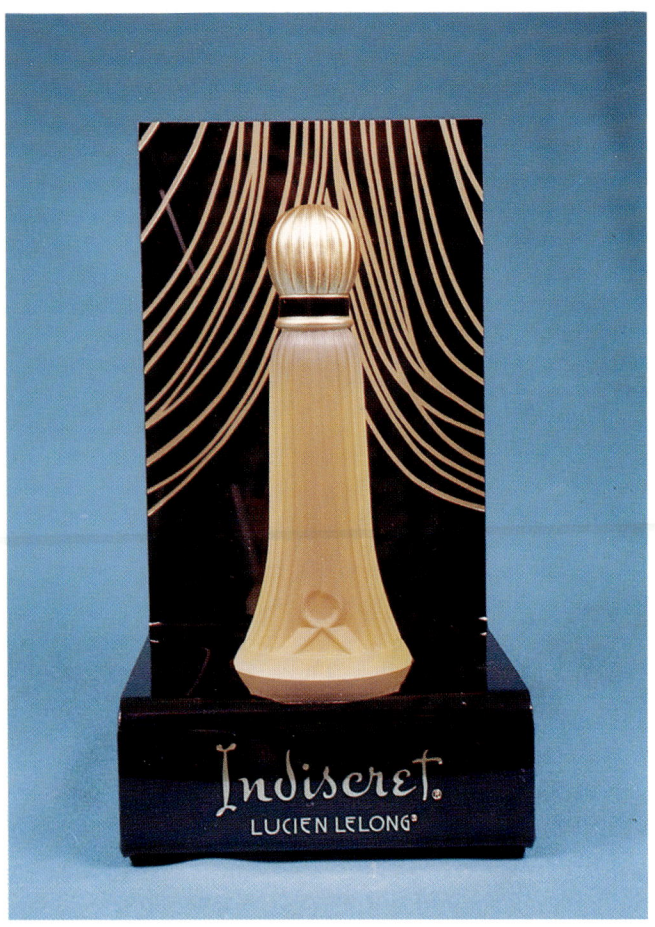

Figure 3. The *Indiscret* Eau de Parfum, on its elegant black and gold display stand. Courtesy of *Parfums Lucien Lelong*.

in 1926 was made a *Chevalier de la Legion d'Honneur*.

In 1924 Lelong established the *Societé des Parfums Lucien Lelong*. Lelong's view of perfume was that it formed an essential part of the woman's dress, her fashion, and her style. He also believed that a woman should try different perfumes until she found her own true perfume, and that she should then wear it exclusively so that her very identity was partially defined by it. *Current Biography* of 1955 quotes a 1946 newspaper story to the effect that Lelong felt "the only time a woman should change her perfume is when she is using some other perfumer's product and she changes to one of mine." Lelong's first perfume is said to be *N,* named in honor of his second wife the Princess Nathalie Paley. Actually, Lelong used initials often as perfume names, thus associating the perfume with the romance of the mysterious persona for whom the perfume might be named. Thus, the perfume presentation becomes a *parfum à clef*. This is an interesting counterpoint to Chanel's use [...and Molyneux's use] of numbers for perfume names, which accomplished the same thing, as if each perfume were a specially commissioned creation for a great lady, whose identity must not be known.

Lelong eventually became a forceful leader of the fashion industry in Paris. In 1937 he was elected President of the *Chambre Syndicale de la Couture Française*, that is, the Trade Association for French Fashion. But by the late 1930's, Europe was descending into the darkness of fascism. Lucien Lelong is widely credited with having successfully shepherded his profession through

fondamental de l'habillement, de la mode, du style d'une femme. Il croyait aussi qu'une femme devait expérimenter différents parfums avant de trouver son vrai parfum, et qu'ensuite elle devait le porter exclusivement de manière à en faire une partie de son identité personnelle. *Current Biography* de 1995 cite un article de journal de 1946 faisant état de l'opinion de Lelong "qu'une femme ne devrait changer de parfum que pour passer du produit d'un autre à un des miens". Le premier parfum de Lelong aurait été *N*, en l'honneur de sa seconde femme la Princesse Nathalie Paley. En fait, Lelong a souvent utilisé des monogrammes pour des noms de parfum, associant ainsi au parfum l'aura romantique de la personne mystérieuse en mémoire de laquelle le parfum aurait été créé. La présentation d'un parfum devient donc un parfum à clef. Elle fait un contrepoint intéressant à l'habitude de Chanel [et Molyneux] d'utiliser des nombres comme noms de parfums, ce qui avait le même effet, comme si chaque parfum était une création spéciale pour une grande dame, dont l'identité doit rester secrète.

Lelong devint un chef important de l'industrie de la mode à Paris. En 1937 il fut élu président de la Chambre Syndicale de la Couture Française. Mais vers la fin des années 30, l'Europe glissait vers l'obscurité du fascisme. Lucien Lelong est reconnu pour avoir guidé sa corporation avec succès dans ces années sombres et difficiles. Pendant l'occupation, Lelong était responsable des restrictions de production et des matériaux pour l'industrie de la mode. Son but semble avoir été de maintenir l'industrie de la mode pendant la guerre afin qu'elle puisse reprendre une fois la paix revenue. Il ne tolérait aucun carcan à la liberté créative individuelle, qu'il pensait la raison d'être de la couture, et il encourageait les couturiers à continuer leur travail quelles que soient leurs difficultés ou frustrations. Quelques couturiers favorisaient le bleu, le blanc, et le rouge en

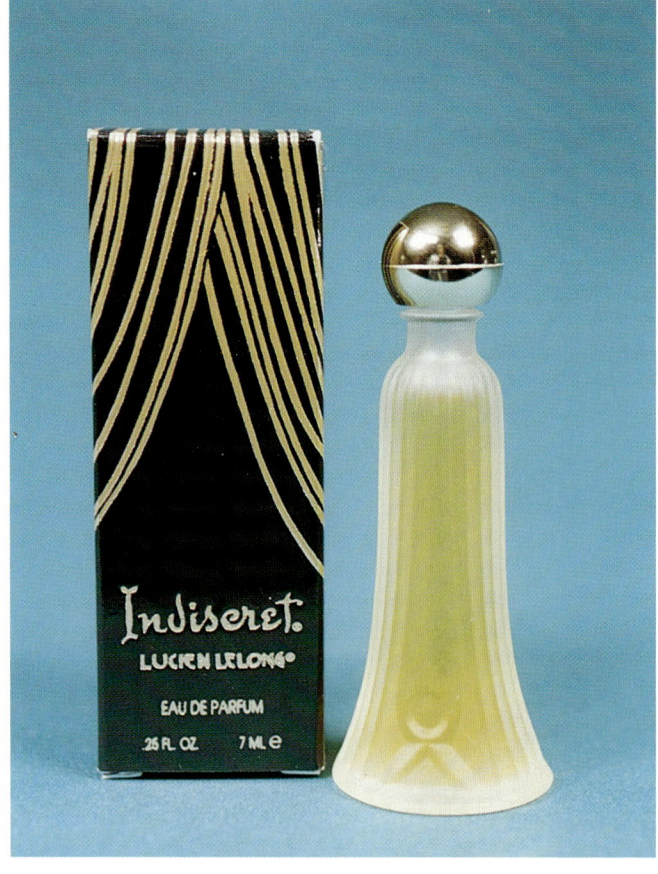

Figure 4. The *Indiscret* deluxe replica miniature, in its box. Courtesy of *Parfums Lucien Lelong*.

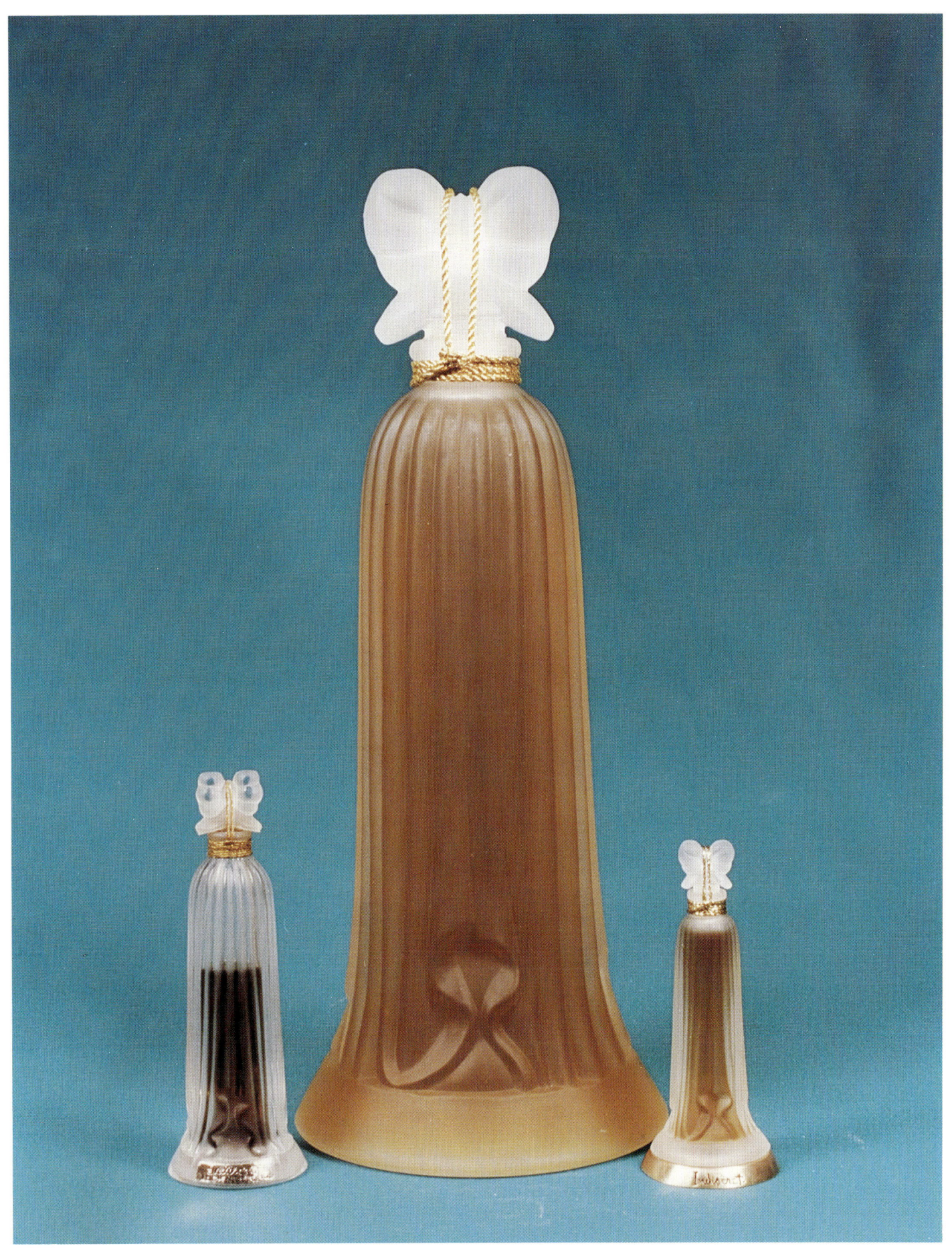

Figure 5. Lucien Lelong *Indiscret*, the old and the new. At the far left, the *Indiscret* bottle circa late 1930's [Collection of Randall B. Monsen and Rodney L Baer]; in the middle, the giant factice for the re-introduction of *Indiscret,* and to the right the *Limited Edition Parfum,* both courtesy of *Parfums Lucien Lelong*. Note the different shape of the drapery near the base of the bottles.

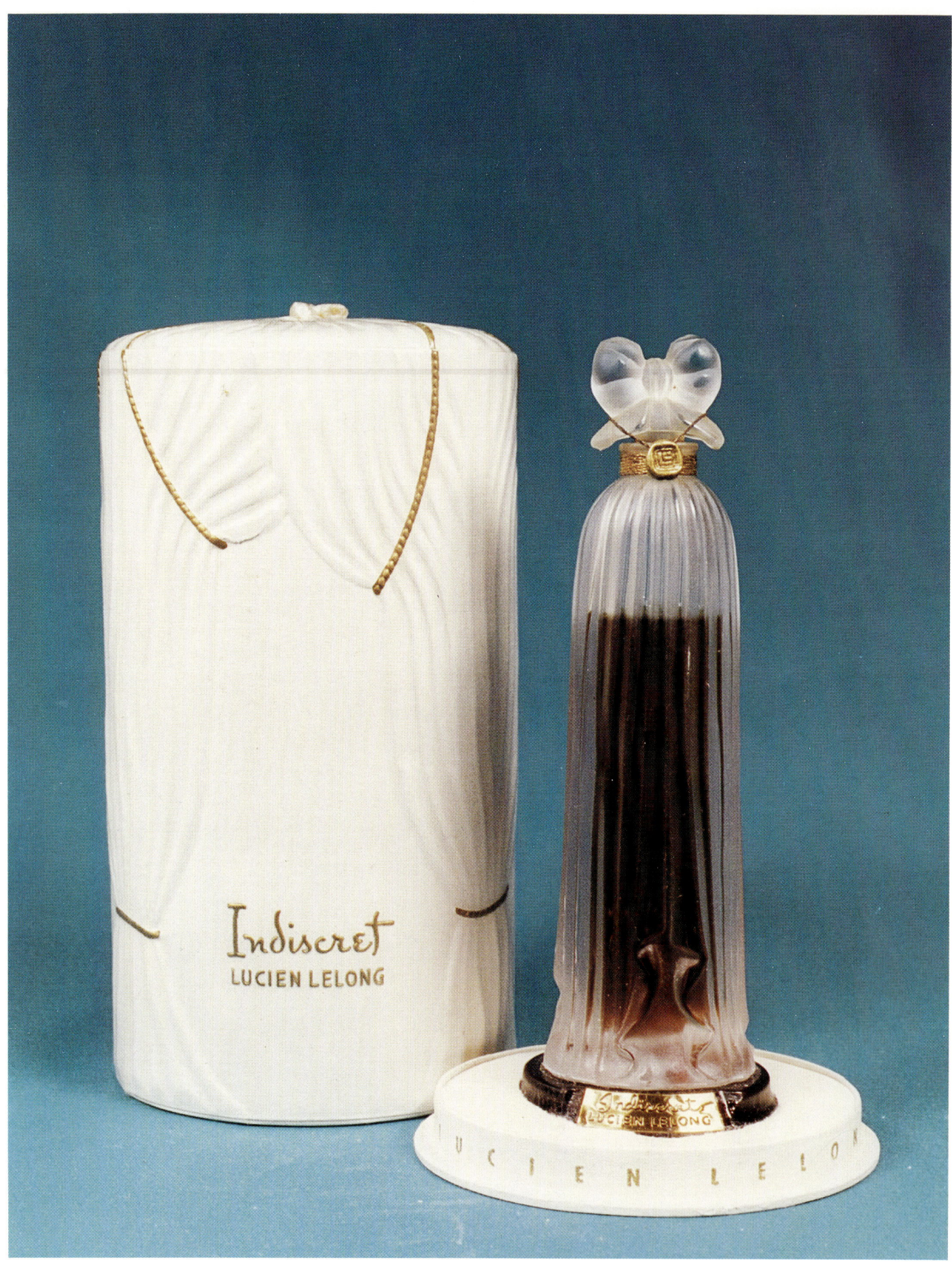

Figure 6. Lucien Lelong *Indiscret*, the original presentation. The box, in its light cream color, continues the theme of the design. Note that this particular bottle differs from both the old *and* the re-introduced *Indiscret* shown in Figs. 5 and 7 in that the base of the bottle is made of wood, rather than totally of glass. Collection of Randall B. Monsen and Rodney L. Baer.

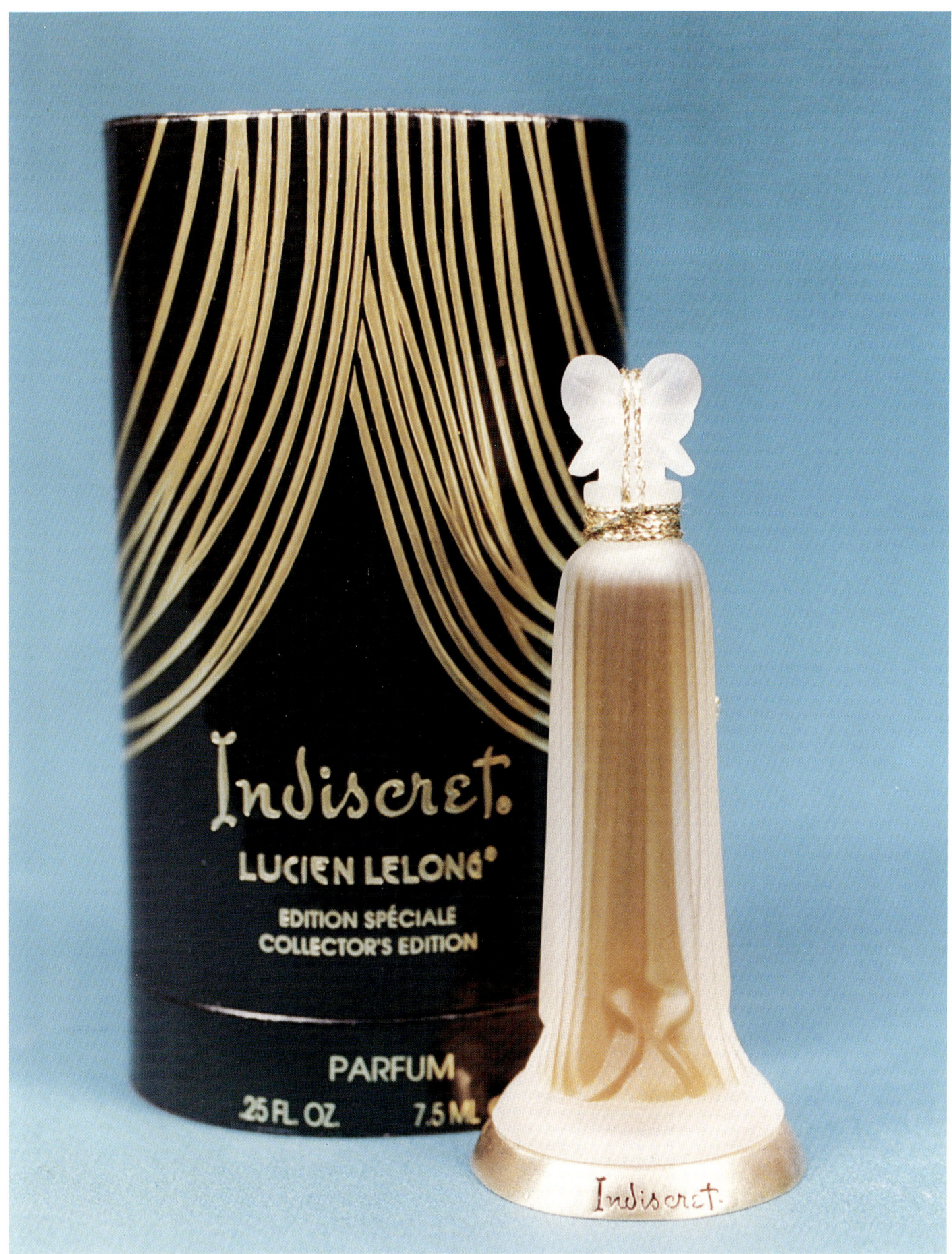

Figure 7. Lucien Lelong *Indiscret*, re-introduced in an elegant collectors' *Limited Edition*. Courtesy of *Parfums Lucien Lelong*.

this darkest and most difficult of times. When France became an occupied country in World War II, Lelong was put in charge of restrictions in production and materials for the fashion industry. His goal seems to have been to keep the fashion industry alive during the war so that it would be able to flourish after the war. He would not tolerate any interference with individual creative liberty, which he felt was the *raison d'être* of couture, and he encouraged designers to continue their work no matter what difficulties and frustrations they encountered. Some designers tended to favor the colors red, white, and blue in abundance in their fashion collections, colors which of course represented the French flag. In fact, the fashion establishment of Mme. Grès was ordered closed by General Joseph Goebbels precisely because of the too prominent use of these three colors in one of her collections. In order to keep as many people working as possible, Lelong urged the fashion establishments to continue to show collections during the war years, even though, of course, money could only be lost, not made, by doing so. In 1943, Joseph Goebbels wanted to move the fashion industry to Berlin, and Lelong derailed this plan by every means possible, including both subterfuge and outright refusal, and the historical record shows that Goebbels' plan did not in fact take place. When the war was finally over, Lelong was given many tributes for his work in preserving the fashion industry. And the French fashion industry did blossom after the war, with unprecedented growth and productivity.

In fact, the seeds of post-war success in fashion were planted and nourished during the bleakest war years, and more than anywhere else, this happened at the house of Lucien Lelong. Pierre Balmain and Christian Dior joined the staff of Lelong in 1941; Hubert de Givenchy also worked there. In *The Glass of Fashion* by Cecil Beaton, Christian Dior testified that he learned much from Lelong's intuitive understanding of fabrics and their integral importance in the creation of a dress, to the extent that a given design could be a great success if made in one fabric, and a dismal failure if made in another. In other words, fabric and design must be understood together and in the same context. This knowledge was passed from Lelong to Dior, Balmain, and de Givenchy and from them in turn to other designers who started their careers with them. As is well known, Balmain, Dior, and de Givenchy each established their own houses of fashion in the mid 1940's and each became a great success.

By late 1945, Lelong had already served as President of the *Chambre Syndicale de la Couture* for eight years, and the members wanted to re-elect him once again to this position. However, he requested to be released from these very time-consuming duties, and was given the title of honorary President, which title he continued to hold throughout the 1950's. Then, in 1948, Lelong became seriously ill, and acting on his doctor's orders, he stopped working and simply closed his maison de couture. He could easily have sold it instead, but he decided that if he himself could not direct it he would rather see it closed. Nonetheless, he did continue to direct his perfume business, which was very successful and which continued uninterrupted, producing at least ten different perfumes at any one time. He personally selected the designs for the glass bottles and the boxes. These perfumes matched the luxuriousness and brilliant design of his dresses.

Lelong himself was a rather short man, with a very direct manner and a sharp business acumen. For sport, he

abondance dans leurs collections, des couleurs qui n'étaient pas en vogue officielle en tout cas. D'ailleurs la maison de Mme. Grès dut fermer sur ordre de Goebbels précisément à cause d'un usage abusif de ces trois couleurs dans une de ses collections. Afin de maintenir autant d'emplois que possible, Lelong encouragea les maisons de couture à montrer des collections pendant la guerre, même si, de toute évidence, ils ne pouvaient que perdre de l'argent en le faisant. En 1943 Goebbels voulut déplacer l'industrie de la mode à Berlin, et Lelong réussit à faire échouer ce plan par tous les moyens, y compris le subterfuge et le refus catégorique. L'histoire montre que les idées de Goebbels furent abandonnées. La guerre enfin finie, Lelong reçut de nombreuses accolades pour ses efforts en faveur du maintien de l'industrie de la mode. Et en fait, l'industrie de la mode française a prospéré après la guerre, avec une croissance et une productivité sans précédant.

En fait, les graines du succès d'après-guerre dans la mode furent plantées et protégées pendant les années les plus sombres de la guerre, et nulle part autant que dans la maison de Lucien Lelong. Pierre Balmain et Christian Dior en firent partie dès 1941; Hubert de Givenchy y travailla aussi. Dans *The Glass of Fashion* de Cecil Beaton, Christian Dior déclara qu'il apprit beaucoup de la connaissance intuitive des tissus et de leur importance de base dans la création d'une robe, au point qu'une conception donnée peut être une grande réussite faite dans un tissu et un lamentable échec dans un autre. Autrement dit, le tissu et la conception ne font qu'un. Cette vérité fut transmise de Lelong à Dior, Balmain et de Givenchy et par eux ensuite avec les dessinateurs qui ont démarré chez eux.

À la fin de 1945, Lelong avait déjà été président de la

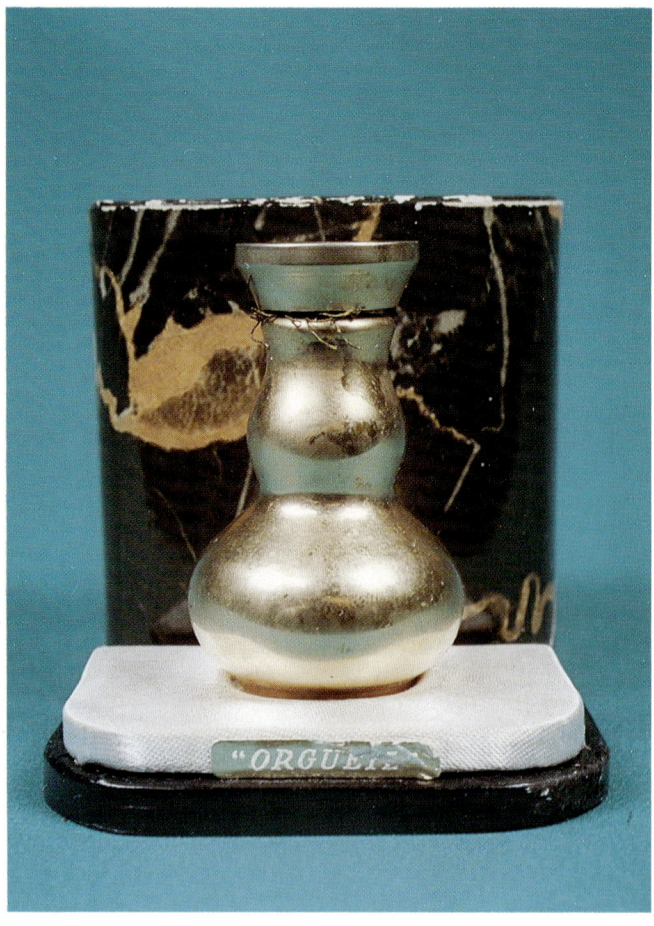

Figure 8. Lucien Lelong *Orgueil* ['Pride'], in a very tiny first size. Collection of Randall B. Monsen and Rodney L. Baer.

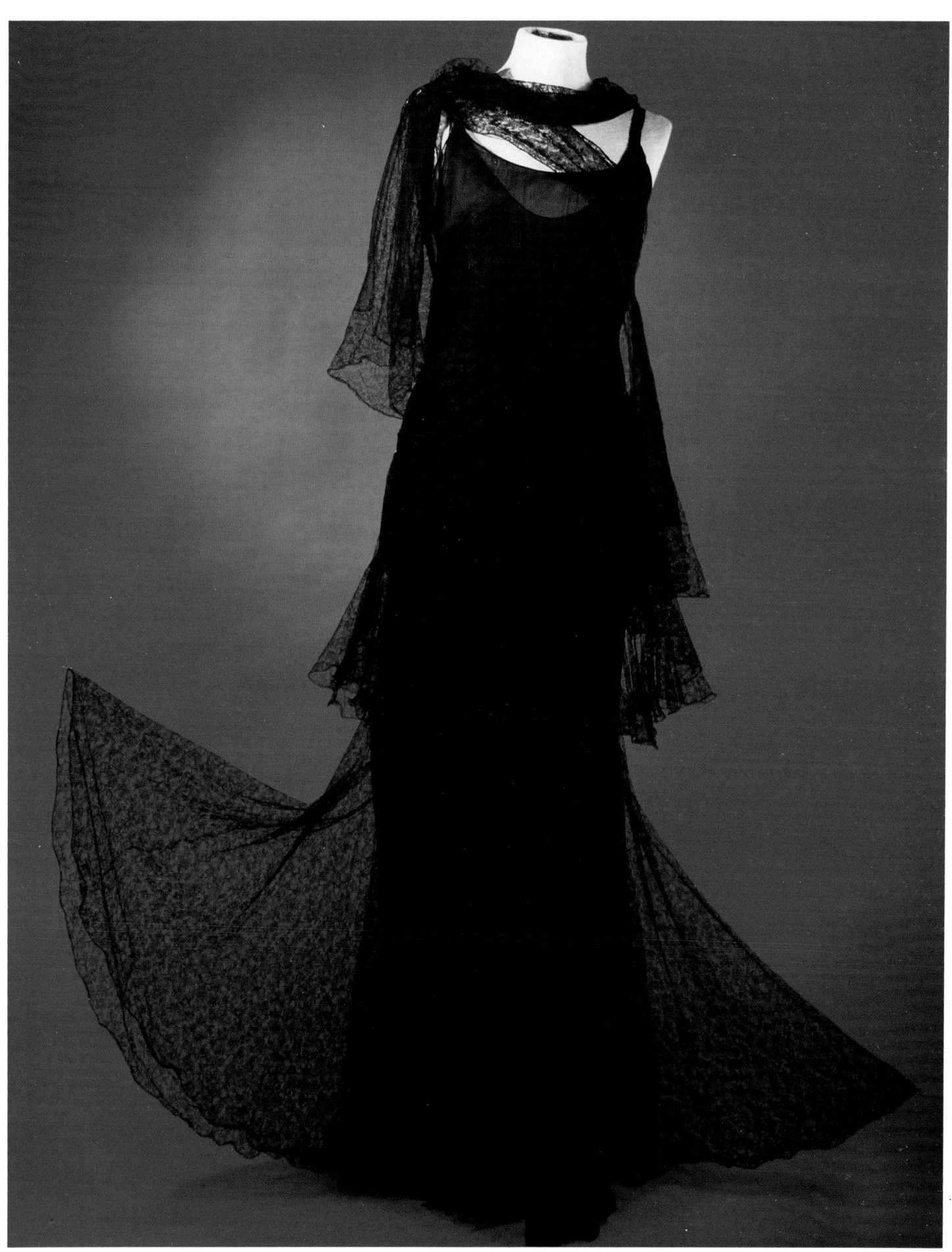

Figure 9. An evening dress in black silk chiffon and black Chantilly lace by Lucien Lelong, circa 1932. Collection of Arnold and Lucy Neis, *Parfums Lucien Lelong*.

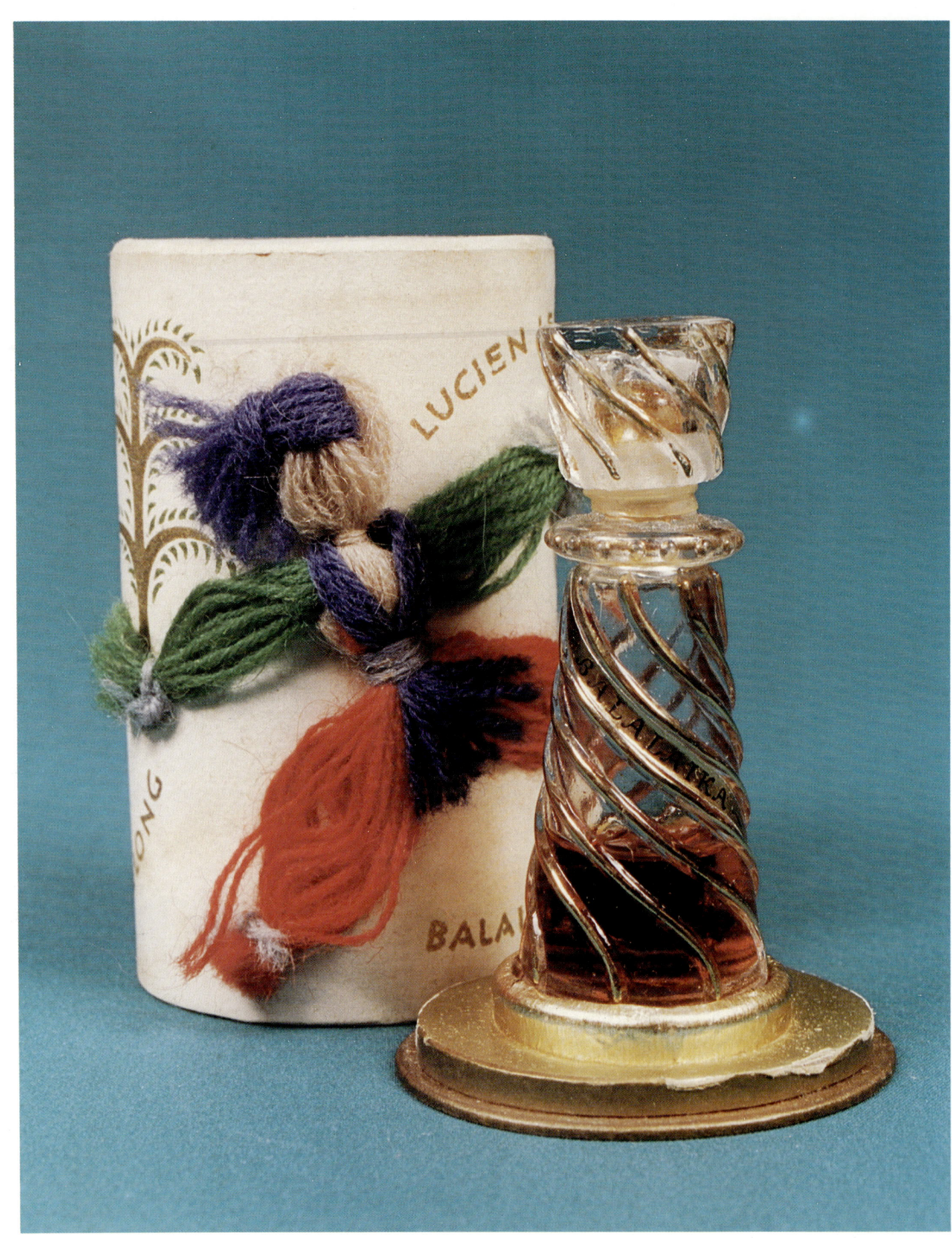

Figure 10. Lucien Lelong *Balalaika*, in its box decorated with a tiny doll of yarn. Collection of Randall B. Monsen and Rodney L. Baer.

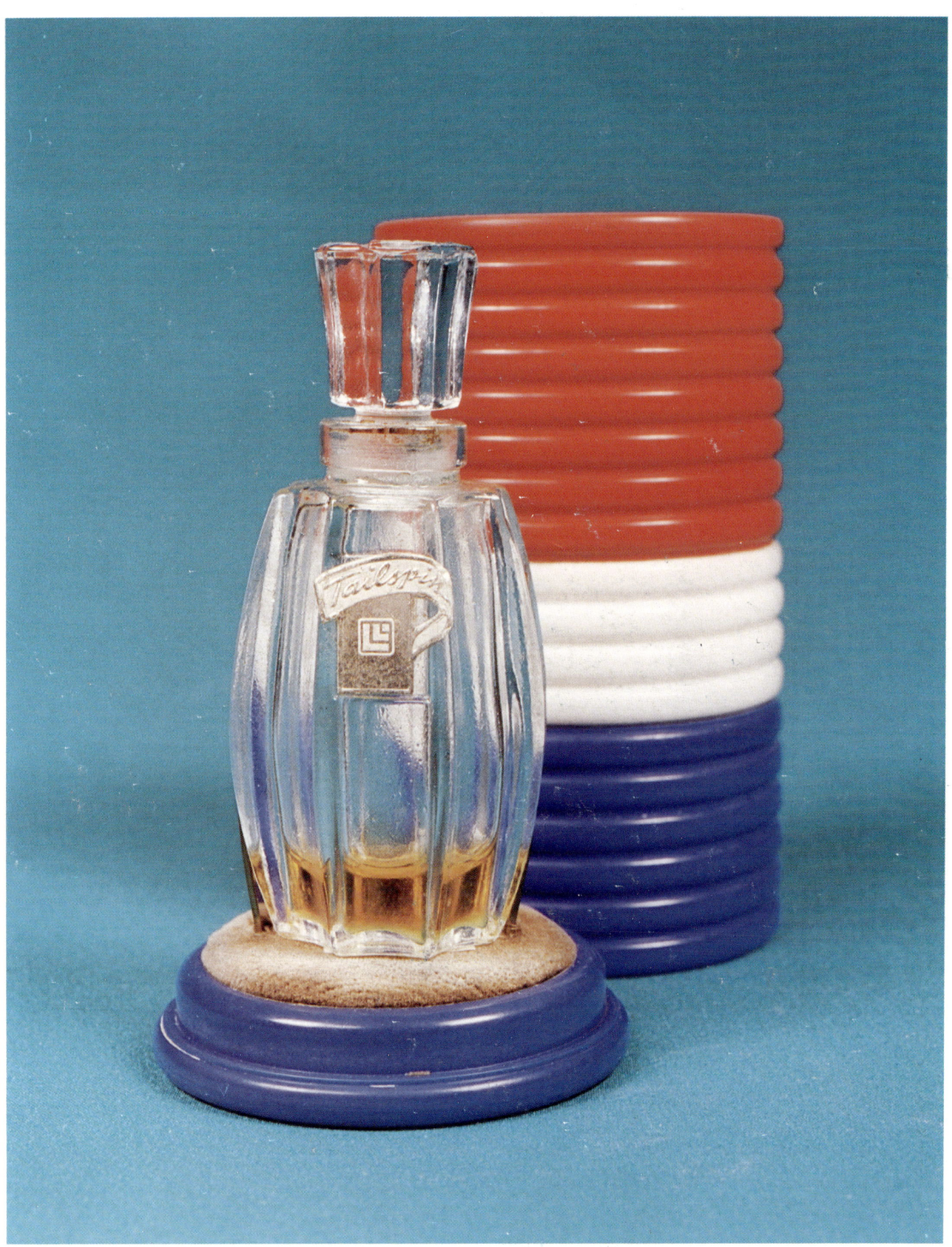

Figure 11. Lucien Lelong *Tailspin*, in its box molded as a stack of poker chips, where the order of the colors is identical to that of the French flag. Collection of Randall B. Monsen and Rodney L. Baer.

is said to have enjoyed both horses and golf. He also had a studio in Montparnasse, where he not only created dress designs, but also displayed his talents as a sculptor. He was also a great collector, with a passion for Chinese porcelain of the fifteenth to the eighteenth centuries, and for Russian glass produced from the era of Elizabeth I to Catherine the Great [that is, from the seventeenth to the eighteenth centuries]. These facts are not without importance in understanding his use of glass for perfume bottles. He is said to have purchased, in 1928, the Imperial collection of Russian glassware owned by Nicholas II. Lelong had a daughter, Nicole, from his first marriage in 1919 to Nelle Audey. His second marriage, to Nathalie Paley, ended in divorce in 1935. In 1954 he married Mme. Dancovici, and together they spent much of their time in Biarritz. Lucien Lelong died on May 10, 1958.

In the 1920's, Lelong created at least five perfumes whose names are merely letters: *A, B, C, J, N*. The perfume *L* has come to light this year due to the fact a tester for this fragrance is to be found in the 1998 Monsen and Baer auction. Of these 'letter' perfumes, the best known are *J* and *N*. Around 1928 or 1929 René Lalique created a beautiful bottle and a stunning modern box used at least for the perfumes *J* and *N,* as well as possibly others. This bottle resembles a modern skyscraper in its overall outline, but it is decorated in black enamel garlands in such a way that it has a very soft and subtle appeal. The box for this perfume, also thought to have been designed by René Lalique, is no less spectacular than the bottle. It duplicates exactly the overall shape of the bottle in chrome metal decorated with enamel of various hues, and with a velvet lining. This box may be found in several different colors, including green, red, and cream, in addition to black. The different colors of the boxes probably corresponded to different fragrances.

A different bottle designed by René Lalique for Lucien Lelong is referred to by Utt [1985] as *Etoile de Mer*, or 'Starfish.' It is an unusual design which uses an eight-pointed star in the form of a column; the stopper conforms perfectly, but on a smaller scale. The points of the star are created with small steps, and frosted so as to give the design greater depth; there is definitely an important architectural feeling to the design of this bottle as well. A silver label goes around the neck of the bottle. This bottle may well have been used for the well known letter-named perfumes, as well as for floral scents, such as *Gardenia*. This very same Lalique design was then also produced by a different glassmaker in glass of a different quality. A boxed example shown here is that of the fragrance *Gardenia*. The black and gold *faux marbre* paper that is used for this box must have been a personal favorite of the designer, as it was also used in many other presentations. A totally different presentation of the perfume *N* was done in an urn shape bottle with the letter name placed very prominently on the side of the bottle.

The perfumes *Indiscret* and *Mon Image* were possibly the two most successful perfumes of Lucien Lelong. *Indiscret,* which is the French word for the English indiscreet, was presented in a beautiful frosted glass bottle which is thought to have been inspired by the act of a lady dropping her handkerchief. The *Indiscret* bottle makes reference to Lelong's talent as a great couturier and it evokes at the same time the sensation of something being revealed, something beautiful hidden below the folds and folds of soft material. The graphics for the box beautifully reinforce these themes.

chambre syndicale pendant 8 ans, et les membres voulaient reconduire son mandat. Mais il demanda d'être relevé de ces charges très lourdes et il devint président honoraire, un titre qu'il continua à porter dans les années 50. Puis en 1948 Lelong devint dangereusement malade, et sur ordre de son médecin, il cessa de travailler et ferma tout simplement sa maison de couture. Il aurait pu la vendre facilement, mais il décida que s'il ne pouvait pas la diriger lui-même, il préférerait la fermer. Il continua néanmoins son activité parfumière qui resta prospère et se poursuivit sans interruption produisant au moins dix parfums à la fois pendant cette période. C'est lui qui choisissait personnellement les dessins des flacons et des boîtes. Ses parfums étaient aussi luxueux et brillants que l'étaient ses robes.

Lelong était un homme assez petit, avec une manière très directe, et un sens aigu des affaires. Pour le sport, il préférait les chevaux et le golf. Il avait aussi un studio à Montparnasse, où il créait non seulement des robes mais où il s'adonnait aussi à la sculpture. Il était aussi grand collectionneur, avec une passion pour la porcelaine chinoise du XVème au XVIIIème siècles, et pour le verre russe produit de l'époque d'Élizabeth Ière à Catherine la Grande. Ces faits ne sont pas sans importance pour la compréhension de son usage du verre pour ses flacons de parfum. On dit qu'en 1928 il acheta la collection de verre russe ayant appartenue à Nicolas II. Lelong eut une fille, Nicole, de son premier mariage avec Nelle Audey en 1919. Son second mariage, à Nathalie Paley, fut dissout en 1935. En 1954 il épousa Mme. Dancovici, et ils passèrent beaucoup de leur temps à Biarritz. Lucien Lelong mourut le 10 mai 1958. Au cours des années, les Parfums Lelong devinrent une division de Coty International et c'est maintenant une société indépendante appartenant à Arnold et Lucy Neis.

Pendant les années 20, Lelong créa au moins 5 (peut-être plus) parfums dont les noms ne sont que des lettres: *A, B, C, J, N*. Les plus connus sont *J* et *N*. En 1928 ou 1929 René Lalique créa un beau flacon et une boîte moderne très originale utilisée pour les parfums *J* et *N*, et peut-être d'autres. Ce flacon ressemble à un gratte-ciel moderne dans ses lignes générales, mais est décoré avec des guirlandes en émail noir de manière à lui donner un attrait très doux et subtil. La boîte de ce parfum, attribuée aussi à René Lalique, n'est pas moins spectaculaire que le flacon. Il reproduit exactement les lignes générales du flacon en métal chromé décoré d'émaux de différentes couleurs, y compris le vert, le rouge, et le crème, en plus du noir. Les différentes couleurs des boîtes correspondent probablement aux différents parfums.

Un flacon différent conçu aussi par Lalique pour Lucien Lelong est appelée par Utt [1985] *Étoile de mer*. C'est une conception inhabituelle utilisant une étoile à huit pointes en forme de colonne; le bouchon est parfaitement conforme mais plus petit. Les pointes de l'étoile sont constituées de petites indentations, et glacées afin de donner une impression de profondeur; ce flacon a aussi manifestement une dimension architecturale. Une étiquette en argent fait le tour du goulot. Ce flacon a très bien pu être utilisé pour les parfums à lettre, ainsi que les parfums floraux, tels que *Gardenia*. Ce même dessin de Lalique a ensuite été produit par un autre fournisseur dans un verre d'une autre qualité. Un exemple avec boîte illustré ici est celui de *Gardenia*. Le papier faux marbre noir et or utilisé pour cette boîte devait plaire au concepteur, car il fait partie de nombreuses autres présentations. Une présentation entièrement différente du parfum *N* utilise un flacon en forme d'urne avec une lettre en

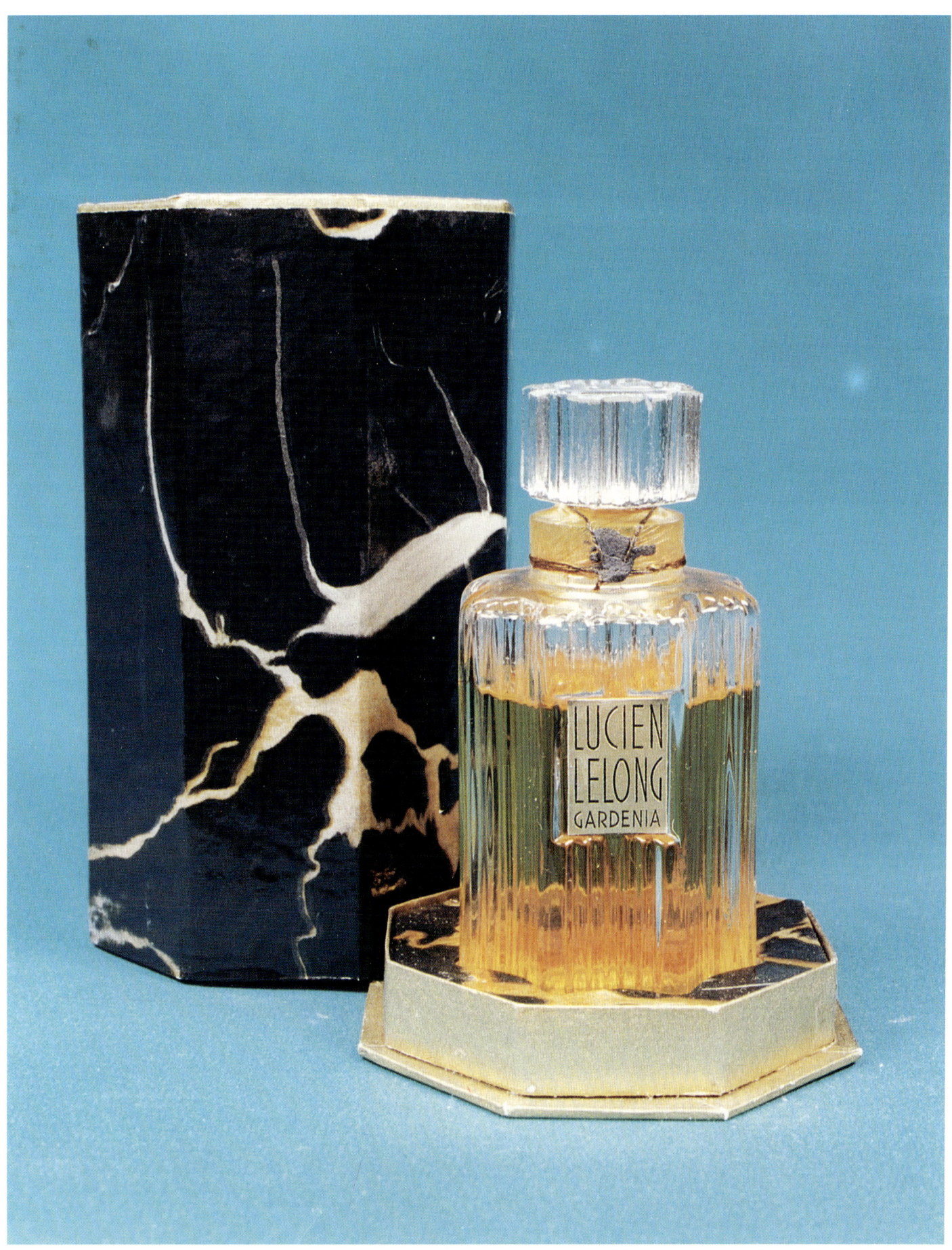

Figure 12. Lucien Lelong *Gardenia*, in a production bottle similar to the design by René Lalique. Note the use of *faux marbre* paper which imparts an architectural appearance to the presentation. Collection of Randall B. Monsen and Rodney L. Baer.

The perfume *Jabot* also makes reference to couture. The bottle for *Jabot,* a woman's silk bow, is quite literally a jabot cast in glass, and it is presented in an elegant hatbox.

The perfume *Mon Image* ['My Image'] evokes the image of the youth Narcissus, and the perfume itself is an intoxicating replication of the flower of the same name. Because of Narcissus' fascination with his reflected image in a pool of water, this perfume is presented in a unique box of mirrors. The bottle itself is a geometric structure with the Lelong logo impressed into the top, and the bottle has a distinct architectural aspect to it.

The perfume *Orgueil* ['Pride'] is somewhat unique among Lelong creations in that it is a glass bottle encased in gold. It was produced at the end of World War II as a celebration of the Liberation of France, and the significance of the name is more in the sense of patriotism than of personal vanity. It is a bottle that says "We prevailed," and it is presented on a stage of white satin in a box of faux black and gold marble. During World War II, many perfume companies in Allied countries produced perfumes and other cosmetic products with names such as *Courage* [Bourjois] and *Winged Victory* [Elizabeth Arden]. Immediately after the war, many of the great French perfumers commemorated the Liberation with perfumes, although the political significance of the names has by now been forgotten: Patou *L'Heure Attendue* ['The Awaited Hour'], Guerlain *Fleur de Feu* ['Flower of Fire'], Chanel *No. 46*, Schiaparelli *Le Roy Soleil,* and Molyneux *Magnificence.*

Eventually, Parfums Lucien Lelong became a division of Coty International, and it is now an independent company owned by Arnold and Lucy Neis, who are themselves collectors of perfume and couture. *Indiscret* was re-introduced in the fall of 1997. The bottles for the 1997 presentation are faithful to the original Lelong design, and they represent a superb model for how a historically important perfume should be re-introduced to the market of today. There are two sizes of eau de parfum [1.7 and 3.4 oz], both with atomizers and a gold and black round cap, an adorable deluxe miniature with a round gold cap, and a perfume which brings to life the original design with great beauty and vitality. Differences that collectors will notice between the old and new bottles are that the folds of drapery are slightly different near the bottom of the bottle, the stopper has a plastic tip, and the bottle is attached to a gold metal base; the presentation box is also different in quite unmistakeable ways. *The beauty and faithfulness of this presentation does honor to the original design, yet it could never be confused with it.* The boxes for the 1997 presentation are all in black and gold and are lined in bright pink satin. Marc Rosen acted as the consultant on the packaging of the re-introduction of *Indiscret*. The scent of the 1997 *Indiscret* is a complex green fruity floral scent "designed to blend sparkling, bright freshness with the warm and sensual." It has top notes of Mandarin, Tiger Orchid, Orange Blossom, Italian Bergamot, White Peach Blossom, Galbanum and Moroccan Neroli. The middle bouquet of the fragrance includes Iris, Rose Geranium, French Tuberose, Algerian Jasmine, Ylang Ylang, Indonesian Clove, Basil, Violet Leaves and Cypress. A wealth of warm, exotic naturals and wood notes comprise the fragrance base—Scarlet Oak Moss, Vetiver Haiti, and Guaiacwood are surrounded by the sensuality of Patchouli Madagascar, Sandalwood, White Musk, and Egyptian Amber.

Two themes dominate in the beautiful perfume presentations of Lucien Lelong. One theme is the couture motif

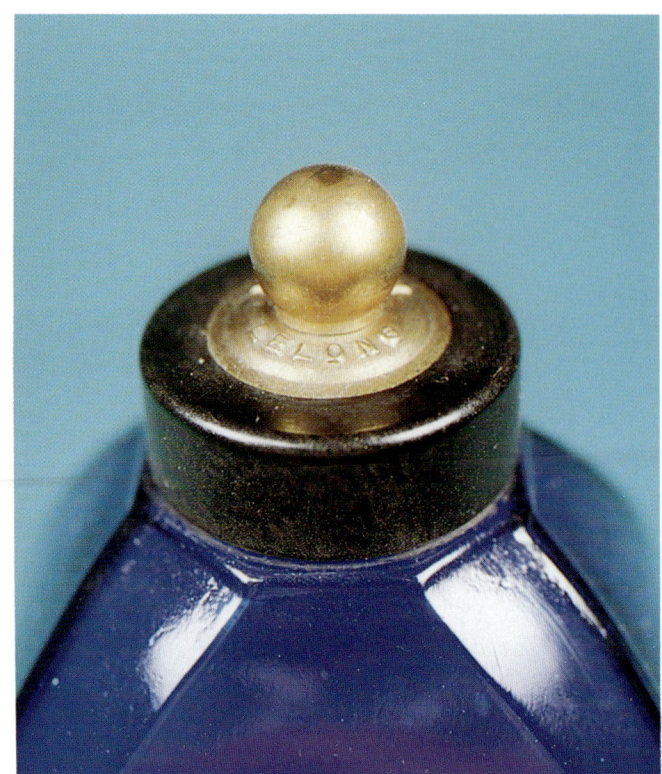

Figure 13. A close-up of the bottle shown on the opposite page. The gold stopper is marked *Lucien Lelong*.

évidence sur un côté du flacon.

Les parfums *Indiscret* et *Mon Image* étaient probablement les plus grandes réussites de Lucien Lelong. *Indiscret* était présenté dans un magnifique flacon en verre glacé qui serait inspiré par le geste d'une femme laissant tomber son mouchoir. Le flacon d'*Indiscret* fait allusion au talent de Lelong comme grand couturier et il évoque aussi la sensation de quelque chose qui se dévoile, quelque chose de beau caché sous des plis et des plis de tissus. Le graphisme de cette boîte renforce ces thèmes. Le parfum *Jabot* fait aussi allusion à la couture. Le flacon pour *Jabot*, un nœud en soie pour femme, est littéralement un jabot coulé en verre présenté dans une élégante boîte à chapeau.

Le parfum *Mon Image* évoque l'image du jeune Narcisse, et le parfum lui-même est une réplique de la fleur du même nom. Ce parfum est présenté dans une boîte faite de miroirs, en évocation de Narcisse qui était fasciné par sa réflexion dans l'eau. Le flacon lui-même est de forme géométrique très architectural avec la griffe Lelong sur le bouchon.

Le parfum *Orgueil* est assez particulier parmi les créations Lelong dans la mesure où c'est un flacon de verre chassé en or. Produit à la fin de la Deuxième Guerre Mondiale en célébration de la Libération, son nom est plus une affirmation patriotique qu'une vanité personnelle. C'est un flacon qui proclame "nous avons vaincu", présenté sur un plateau en satin blanc dans une boîte en faux marbre noir et or. Nombreux furent les parfumeurs français qui célébraient la fin de la guerre par des créations nouvelles, même si la signification politique de ces noms a été largement oubliée: Patou *L'Heure Attendue*, Guerlain *Fleur de Feu*, Chanel *#46*, Schiaparelli *Le Roy Soleil*, et Molyneux *Magnificence.*

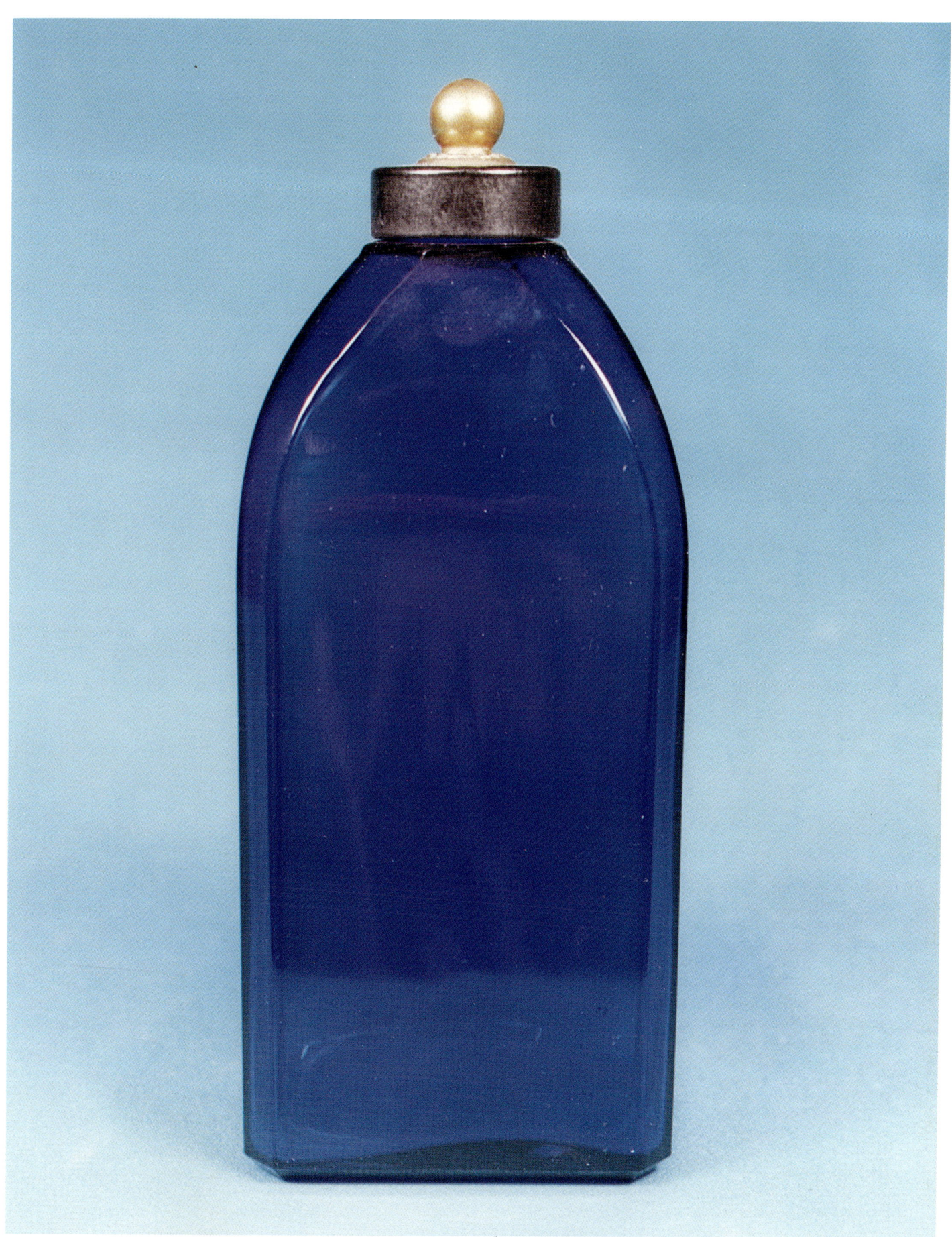

Figure 14. Lucien Lelong rare store dispenser bottle, of very large size. Collection of Randall B. Monsen and Rodney L. Baer.

which provides a direct visual link between fashion and perfume. The couture motif is the replication of fabrics, garlands, and feathers in the medium of glass. Some of the perfumes which use this motif are *Indiscret, Jabot, Les Plumes,* and *Cachet*. The other frequent motif is that of modern architecture. Many Lelong creations resemble buildings or use architectural motifs: *N, Mon Image, Balalaika, Murmure, Castel, Impromptu, Opening Night,* and *Penthouse,* a presentation of four miniatures. The Lelong logo itself is a geometric design based upon an L inside an L. It is a brilliant logo because of its identifiability on the one hand and beautiful geometric symmetry on the other hand, and it lends itself perfectly to architectural themes. It is found impressed on a great many Lelong bottles, and on almost all the graphics of the boxes for the perfumes. Perfume collectors of today and of tomorrow will always admire the ability of Lelong to use the softness of the couture motif with the strength of the architecture motif in perfect harmony with each other. Just as Lelong's success in fashion was based upon his knowledge of the importance of fabric to the dress design, his success in the artistry of perfume was based no less on his knowledge of the importance of the design of the glass bottle, the perfume name, and the entire presentation to the very identity of the fragrance and thus to its eventual success.

Deux thèmes dominent les magnifiques présentations de parfum de Lucien Lelong. L'un est celui de la couture, lien palpable entre la mode et le parfum. Il transparaît dans la reproduction de tissus, de guirlandes, et de plumes, tous de verre. Certains parfums utilisant ce motif sont *Indiscret, Jabot, Les Plumes,* et *Cachet*. L'autre motif fréquent est l'architecture: *N, Mon Image, Balalaïka, Murmure, Castel, Impromptu, Opening Night,* et *Penthouse,* un quatuor en miniature. La griffe Lelong est un dessin géométrique fait d'un L encastré dans un autre L. La griffe est brillante, car elle est immédiatement identifiable d'une part, avec une belle symétrie géométrique d'autre part, et elle se prête admirablement aux thèmes architecturaux. On la retrouve gaufrée sur beaucoup de flacons Lelong, et sur presque toutes les boîtes de parfum. Les collectionneurs de parfums d'aujourd'hui et de demain admireront toujours la capacité de Lelong à marier la douceur du motif couture avec la force du motif architectural dans une harmonie parfaite. Tout comme le succès en couture de Lelong procédait de la reconnaissance de l'importance du tissu dans la conception d'une robe, son succès dans l'art du parfum partait de l'appréciation de l'art du flacon, du nom du parfum, de l'art de présentation du parfum, jusqu'à l'identité elle-même du parfum.

Bibliography

Ball, J. D. and Torem, D. H. *Commercial Fragrance Bottles*. Atglen, Pennsylvania: Schiffer Publishing Co., 1993.

Berger, C. & D. *Tous les Parfums du Monde*. Toulouse: Editions Milan, 1995.

Calasibetta, C. *Fairchild's Dictionary of Fashion*. New York: Fairchild, 19

Compagnie des Cristalleries de Baccarat. *Baccarat Les Flacons à Parfum/The Perfume Bottles*. Paris: Henri Addor & Associés, 1986.

Courset, J-M. *5000 Miniatures de Parfum*. Toulouse: Editions Milan, 1995.

Current Biography 1955. New York: H. W. Wilson, 1955.

Dior, C. *Christian Dior and I*. New York: E. P. Dutton, 1957.

Fontan, Geneviève, and Barnouin, Nathalie. *La Cote Internationale des Echantillons de Parfum, 1995-1996.* ΙȜ Echantillons Anciens. Toulouse: 813 Edition, 1994.

Hart, A. Lucien Lelong. *Mini-Scents*, Vol 4, #2, Spring 1996.

Leach, Ken. *Perfume Presentation: 100 Years of Artistry*. Toronto: Kres Publishing, 1997.

Lefkowith, Christie Mayer. *The Art of Perfume*. New York: Thames and Hudson, 1994.

Lucien Lelong: *A Retrospective Catalogue of the Exhibition of vintage couture and antique fragrance packaging of Lucien Lelong*. September 9-24, 1997. New York: French Institute and the Aliance Française.

North, Jacquelyne. *Commercial Perfume Bottles*. West Chester, Pennsylvania: Schiffer Publishing Co, 1987.

Nystrom, P. *Economics of Fashion*. New York: Ronald Press, 1928.

Utt, Mary Lou and Glenn. *Lalique Perfume Bottles*. New York: Crown Publishers, 1990.

The Lucien Lelong Catalogue: A Work-in-Progress

There is unfortunate confusion in published sources among fragrances [i.e., *Mon Image*] and presentation names [i.e, *Penthouse*], and even names of lines of lipstick and make-up [i.e., *Duveytn, Nicole*]; in addition, confusion exists between names which represent different perfumes and those which are merely translations from French to English of the very same name [i.e, between *Murmure* and *Whisper*, the name used in the English-speaking market]. Furthermore, there are irreconcilable discrepancies, not to say errors, in some published sources, and these have been replicated from book to book. An additional complication is that the Lelong company sometimes relaunched its fragrances under new names, cf. *N* and *Taglio; Orage* was later re-launched under the name *Opening Night*, not in the usual pyramid bottle, but a hemispherical one. In compiling this catalogue of fragrances, we rely on a variety of sources, including advertisements, our personal collection, data from our auctions and those of others, and, especially where trademark dates are concerned, North [1987], Berger [1995], and Leach [1997]. We gratefully acknowledge the advice of Helen Farnsworth, Lenore Hiers, and Arnold and Lucy Neis and Eileen Paley of *Parfums Lucien Lelong* in compiling this list. <u>Note that those names we have listed as fragrance names we have verified either by seeing the actual bottle, a picture of it, or an advertisement in which it is pictured.</u>

According to Baccarat [1986], Lelong used a Baccarat flacon in 1933 for one of its fragrances, although it is not clear which fragrance that might have been. It was Baccarat bottle #26, originally from 1908 production.

The following are names which were trademarked by Lelong, but for which we have no other existing reference, and which we are not able to affirm that they were ever put into production or that they are indeed fragrance names: *Abra Ca Dabra* [possibly a lipstick/compact], *Balaiza, Big Moment, Cabochon* [possibly a lipstick/compact], *Carousel, Cologne of the Hour, Cool Mist, Double Life, Falbalas, Fan Fare, Flippant, Grand Bouquet, Hearsay, High Time, Ingénue, Papotage, Philtre d'Amour, Round Trip, Sahara, Sextet, Take Two, Turbulent*. Some of these may well exist as perfumes, and if they do exist we will add them to this catalogue-in-progress as they come to light. However, we believe that most of these either were never put into production, or they are possibly names of compacts, make-up, or of presentation names of standard Lelong perfumes.

Lucien Lelong Fragrance Names

Fragrance [English Market Name/'translation']	™Date	Probable Introduction	Fragrance [English Market Name/'translation']	™Date	Probable Introduction
A, B, C, J, L, N		1924-1928	**Opening Night** 'La Première'	1934	late 1930's
6, 7		1951	**Orage**	1942	1940's
Balalaika	1939	1940's	**Tempest**, later **Opening Night**		
Cachet		1950's	**Orgueil** 'Pride'	1946	1946
Carefree	1939	1940's	**Passionément** 'Passionately'	1940	1940's
Concentration 44		1930's	**Tailspin**		
Edition Limitée [Limited Edition of 200]	1951	1951	**Sirôcco**	1934	late 1930's, 1940's
Elle. Elle.... 'Her. She....' Also a pun referring to LL.	1937	1940's	**Spring and Summer Cologne**		1950
Gardenia		1930's	**Taglio** [= reprise of the original **N**]	1945	1945-1950
Impromptu	1937	late 1930's, 1940's	Florals:		
Indiscret	1935	late 1930's; re-introduced 1997	**Chevrefeuille** 'Honeysuckle'		late 1930's, 1940's
Jabot	1939	1940's	**Extra Sec**		1940's
			Gardenia		1930's, 1940's
Joli Bouquet 'Pretty Bouquet'	1953		**Lavande** 'French Lavender'		late 1930's, 1940's
Mon Image 'My Image'	1933	mid 1930's	**Lilac**		late 1930's, 1940's
			Magnolia		late 1930's, 1940's
			Mignonette		1940's
			Mimosa		1940's
			Petunia		1940's
Murmure Whisper	1932	mid 1930's	**Pois de Senteur** 'Sweet Pea'		late 1930's, 1940's
			Violette		late 1930's, 1940's

Lucien Lelong Presentation Names

Presentation Name - ™Date; or Prob. Introduction Translation/Fragrances contained

Armoire Louis XIV - 1940's - *Sirôcco*, prob. others
Bath Condiments - 1938 - talc/bath oil, designed as sugar shakers
Botticelli Bottle - 1954 - *Tailspin, Sirôcco Cologne*
Castle/Le Castel - **1940**; 1940's - *Indiscret, Impromptu, Tailspin, Carefree*, prob. others
Christmas Carolers - 1938 - various
Christmas Wreath - 1938 - *Indiscret, Impromptu, Opening Night*
Christmas Tree[1] - various miniatures [standing tree]
Christmas Tree[2] - *Tailspin*, poss. others
Cologne Fantasy - 1954 - Cologne minis of *Indiscret, Tailspin, Sirôcco, Balalaika*
Dress Clips - 1940's - *Indiscret, Jabot*, poss. others
Ensemble - 1930's - Compact and Cigarette case
Les Fleurs de Lucien Lelong - 1938 - *Mimosa, Gardenia*, etc. 'The Flowers of L. L.'
Flower Caddy - 1940's - *Petunia, Mignonette, Honeysuckle*
Flower Pot - 1940's [?] - all then current perfumes
Fragrance Delight - 1954 - Perfume & Cologne minis of *Indiscret & Sirôcco*
Gyroscope - 1940's [?] - various
Jeweled Perfumes - 1954 - minis of *Indiscret, Tailspin, Sirôcco, Orgueil*
Joli Bouquet - 1930's - 'Pretty Bouquet'
Joli Petits Parfums - 1930 - various cologne minis - 'Pretty Little Perfumes'
Little Cherub - 1938 - various
Party-Party - three triangular minis, similar to *Tout Lelong*
Perfume Album - various
Penthouse - 1934 - late 1930's - various
Le Petit Chapeau - various fragrances; 'The Little Hat'
Petits Fours - 1949 - 1950's - various

Les Plumes - late 1930's - various; 'The Feathers'
Place Vendôme - 1950's - various
Poker Chips - 1940's - *Tailspin*
Purser in Slipper - 1954 - *Indiscret, Tailspin, Sirôcco* purse size in a shoe
Remembrances de Versailles - 1950's - *Indiscret*, prob. others
The Royal Box - *Indiscret, Orgueil, Sirôcco, Tailspin*
Santa Claus - 1940's - *Whisper/Murmure*, poss. others
Shadow Box - 1954 - *Indiscret, Tailspin, Sirôcco*
Ting-A-Ling - 1949 - 1950's - *Taglio, Indiscret*, poss. others; *Ting-A-Ling* compact was also made
Tout Lelong - 1925 - 1930's - various; 'All Lelong/Lelong Elite'
Two for Travel - 1954 - *Balalaika + Indiscret* or *Sirôcco + Tailspin*
Valentine Heart - 1940's [?] - *Sweet Pea, Magnolia, Lilac, Honeysuckle*
Weekend - 1940's - various, prob. all

Make-up Lines and Compacts

Baguette, also **Petite Baguette** - 'Chopstick' but in English it would appear to be intended as a diminutive of 'bag.'
Duvetyn - 1938 - Lipstick line: *Nicole Pink, Chardon, Blood Red*; also a line of powders: *Indiscret, Rose Rachel, Sirôcco*, and others.
Flower Shades - 1939 - Lipstick presentation: *Camellia, Pink Rose, Dianthus*
Havoc - A line of lipsticks
Nicole Pink - 1938; 1940's - A line of make-up
Paint Box - Make-up kit
Quick Change - mid 1940's - Lipstick presentation: *Robin Hood, Indiscrete, Nicole Pink*
Sealed Lips - Lipstick, color called *Big Top*
Tambourine - Compact
Tic Tac Toe - mid 1940's - Lipstick presentation

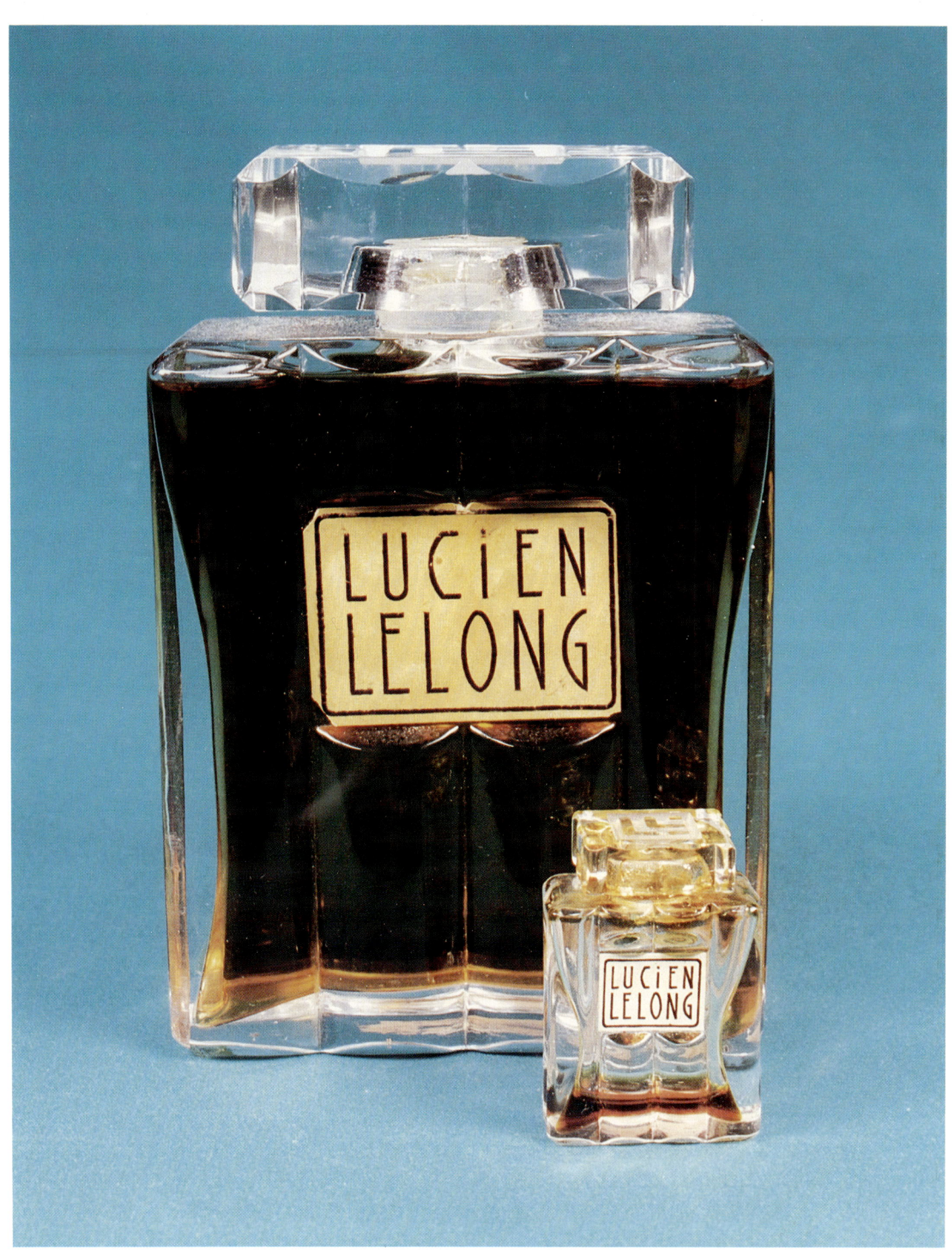

Figure 15. Lucien Lelong *Murmure* [*Whisper* in the English market], in a very rare factice size and a very small first size. Collection of Randall B. Monsen and Rodney L. Baer.

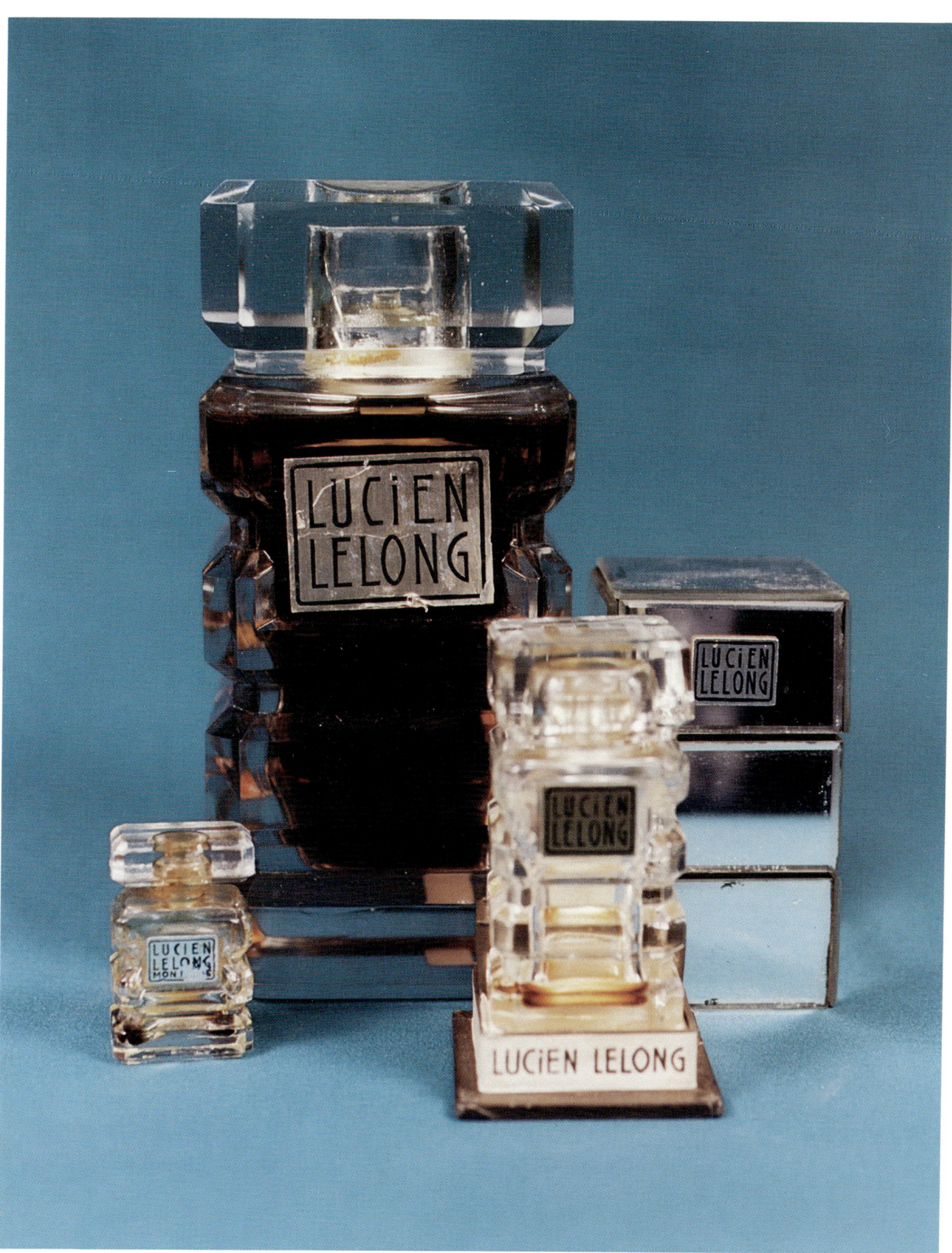

Figure 16. Lucien Lelong *Mon Image*, in a very large factice size, standard size, and miniature. All have a distinct architectural presence. Collection of Randall B. Monsen and Rodney L. Baer.

Die Parfüme Lucien Lelong

Lucien Lelong war einer der grossen Modeschöpfer des 20. Jahrhunderts sowie einer des Jahrhunderts grösster Meister der Parfümkunst. Er war auch ein grosser französischer Patriot. Seine Parfümkreationen befinden sich unter den meistgeschätzten Objekten vieler Kollektionen von historisch bedeutsamen Parfümen. Jeder Sammler hat mindestens einen hochgeschätzten Favoriten als Mittelpunkt seiner Kollektion. Lelong Parfüme waren zu ihrer Zeit nicht nur kommerziell erfolgreich sondern auch künstlerisch so herrlich, dass sie sicherlich von jeder nachfolgenden Generation von Sammlern, die ihrem Zauber erliegen, sehr geschätzt sein werden; lange nachdem das Parfüm verflogen ist, begehren und beschützen Parfüm-Liebhaber des Parfüm's schöne Schachteln und Glasflakons. Dieser Artikel ist motiviert durch das Verlangen, unsere Liebe zu dieser wundervollen Firma mit anderen Sammlern zu teilen und aufgrund der Begebenheit, dass einer der grössten Düfte Lelong's *Indiscret* im Oktober 1997 wieder herausgebracht wurde.

Lucien Lelong wurde am 11. Oktober 1889 in Paris als Sohn von Arthur und Valentine (Lambelet) Lelong geboren. Sein Vater war in der Textilbranche tätig, und da man annahm, dass Lucien seines Vater's Geschäft weiterführen würde, bereitete er sich auf eine kaufmännische Karriere vor und erwarb 1913 sein Diplom in *Hautes Etudes Commerciales*. Sein Vater hatte ihm die Sachkenntnis von verschiedenen Stoffen für verschiedene Moden beigebracht und Lucien Lelong entschloss sich, möglicherweise aus verkaufsfördernden Gründen bezüglich Textilien, Couturier zu werden. Im jungen Alter von 24 Jahren erstellte er eine Kollektion von Damenkleidern, die der Modewelt vorgestellt werden sollte, wurde jedoch zwei Tage vor der geplanten Eröffnung seiner Kollektion zum Wehrdienst eingezogen. Lelong kämpfte während des ganzen ersten Weltkrieges für Frankreich, wurde kurz vor dem Ende der Kriegshandlungen von einem Geschoss getroffen und für ein ganzes Jahr hospitalisiert. Nach Kriegsende war er ohne jegliche finanzielle Mittel, aber es gelang ihm irgendwie, von einem Freund 2.500,- Dollar zu leihen. Mit diesem Geld (die Summe muss zu dieser Zeit von sehr hohem Wert gewesen sein) eröffnete er ein *Maison de Couture* auf dem Place de la Madeleine. Seine erste Kollektion war ein grosser Erfolg und bald wurde er Leiter der französischen Modeindustrie, zusammen mit Worth, Patou, Lanvin und Chanel. Lelong wurde nach dem Krieg mit dem *Croix de Guerre* ausgezeichnet und in 1926 zum *Chevalier de la Legion d'Honneur* geschlagen.

In 1924 gründete Lelong die *Societé des Parfums Lucien Lelong*. Nach Lelong's Ansicht handelt es sich bei Parfüm um einen bedeutsamen Teil des Kleides einer Dame, ihrer Mode und ihres Stils. Er glaubte auch, dass eine Dame verschiedene Parfüme probieren sollte, bis sie ihr eigenes, wirkliches Parfüm gefunden hatte, um dieses dann einzig und allein zu benutzen, so dass ihre ureigene persönliche Identität teilweise dadurch gekennzeichnet sei. <u>Current Biography</u> aus 1995 zitiert einen Zeitungsbericht von 1946 bezüglich Lelong's Auffassung, dass "die einzige Zeit zu der eine Dame ihr Parfüm ändern sollte die sei, zu der sie eines anderen Parfümeur's Produkt benutzt und dann zu einem von meinen wechseln". Es wird gesagt, dass Lelong's erstes Parfüm *N* war, zu Ehren seiner zweiten Frau, der Prinzessin Nathalie Paley, genannt. Tatsächlich benutzte Lelong oft Initialen als Parfüm-Namen, womit er das Parfüm mit der Romanze der mysteriösen Person verknüpfte, nach der das Parfüm genannt sein mag. Und somit wird die Parfüm-Präsentation ein *parfum à clef*. Dies ist ein interessanter Kontrapunkt zu Chanel's (und Molyneux's) Gebrauch von Nummern zu Parfüm-Namen, was denselben Sinn erfüllte, nämlich als wäre jedes Parfüm eine eigens ausgeführte Kreation für eine grosse Dame, deren Identität man nicht kennen sollte.

Letztendlich wurde Lelong ein eindrucksvoller Leiter der Pariser Modeindustrie. In 1937 wurde er zum Präsidenten des *Chambre Syndicale de la Couture Francaise* gewählt, der Handelsassoziation der französischen Mode. Jedoch fiel Europa in den späten 1930'er Jahren der Finsternis des Faschismus anheim. Lucien Lelong wird allgemein dafür geehrt, dass er sein Geschäft erfolgreich durch diese dunkelste und schwierigste aller Zeiten behütet hat. Als Frankreich im zweiten Weltkrieg zu einem besetzten Land wurde, wurde Lelong mit der Einschränkung in der Produktion und bezüglich der Materialien für die Modeindustrie beauftragt. Es schien sein Ziel gewesen zu sein, die Modeindustrie während des Krieges am Leben zu erhalten, so dass sie danach wieder florieren konnte. Er tolerierte keine Einmischung in der individuellen kreativen Freiheit, die er als *raison d'être* der Couture empfand und ermutigte die Designer, ihre Arbeit fortzusetzen, egal welchen Schwierigkeiten und Frustrationen sie begegnen würden. Einige Modeschöpfer neigten dazu, die Farben blau, weiss und rot im Überfluss in ihren Modekollektionen zu bevorzugen; Farben, die zumindest offiziell nicht en vogue waren. Tatsächlich wurde das Modeunternehmen von Mme. Grès auf Befehl von General Joseph Goebbels geschlossen, exakt wegen des zu hervorstechenden Gebrauchs dieser drei Farben in einer ihrer Kollektionen. Damit so viel wie möglich Menschen ihre Arbeit behalten konnten, drängte Lelong die Modeunternehmen während der Kriegsjahre Modeschauen ihrer Kollektionen weiter durchzuführen, wenn auch natürlicherweise kein Gewinn damit erzielt werden konnte sondern lediglich Verluste. Joseph Goebbels wollte die Modeindustrie in 1943 nach Berlin verlagern und Lelong setzte sich diesem Plan mit allen nur möglichen Mitteln, einschliesslich von Ausreden und rundweger Ablehnung, entgegen. Die historische Aufzeichnung zeigt, dass Goebbel's Plan tatsächlich nicht stattfand. Nachdem der Krieg endlich vorüber war, erhielt Lelong viele Huldigungen für sein Werk in der Bewahrung der Modeindustrie, und die französische Modeindustrie erblühte nach dem Krieg in der Tat in beispiellosem Wachstum und noch nie dagewesener Produktivität.

Die Saat des Nachkriegserfolgs der Mode wurde tatsächlich in den freudlosesten Kriegsjahres gelegt und gepflegt, und mehr als irgendwo anders im Hause von Lucien Lelong. Pierre Balmain und Christian Dior schlossen sich in 1941 der Belegschaft von Lelong an; Hubert de Givenchy arbeitete ebenfalls dort. Christian Dior bezeugt in <u>The Glass of Fashion</u> (von Cecil Beaton), dass er sehr viel von Lelong's intuitivem Verständnis von Stoffen und deren wesentlicher Wichtigkeit bei der Kreation eines Kleides gelernt hat, soweit gehend, dass ein festgelegter Entwurf, wenn aus einem bestimmten Stoff gemacht, ein grosser Erfolg sein könnte; und ein grosser Misserfolg, wenn aus einem anderen. In anderen Worten: Stoff und Entwurf müssen miteinander in Gleichklang gebracht werden. Dieses Wissen wurde von Lelong an Dior, Balmain und de Givenchy weitergegeben und von diesen wiederum weiter an andere Designer, die ihre Karriere mit ihnen begannen. Wie sehr gut bekannt ist, gründeten alle ihre eigenen Modehäuser in der Mitte der 1940'er Jahre, und jeder einzelne von ihnen erzielte einen grossen Erfolg.

Zum Ende von 1945 hatte Lelong schon acht Jahre als Präsident des *Chambre Syndicale de la Couture* gedient und die Mitglieder wollten ihn noch einmal in dieser Position wählen. Er bat jedoch darum, von diesen sehr zeitaufwendigen Pflichten befreit zu werden und so erhielt er den Titel eines Ehren-Präsidenten, den er bis 1950 behielt. In 1948 wurde Lelong dann ernsthaft krank und hörte aufgrund der Anweisungen seiner Ärzte auf zu arbeiten und schloss sein *Maison de Couture*. Er hätte es stattdessen spielend verkaufen können, entschied jedoch, da er es selbst nicht leiten konnte, es lieber geschlossen zu sehen. Sein Parfüm-Unternehmen führte er nichtsdestoweniger weiter. Dieses war sehr erfolgreich, lief ohne Unterbrechung weiter und produzierte mindestens zehn verschiedene Parfüme zu jeglicher Zeit. Er selbst suchte die Entwürfe für die Glasflaschen und die Schachteln aus. Diese Parfüme waren dem Luxus und dem brillanten Design seiner Kleider ebenbürtig.

Lelong selbst war ein verhältnismässig kleiner Mann, von sehr direkter Art und Weise und einem starken Geschäftssinn. Im Sport, wird gesagt, fand er sowohl an Pferden wie auch an Golf Gefallen. Er hatte auch ein Studio am Montparnasse, wo er nicht nur Kleiderentwürfe schuf sondern auch sein Talent als Bildhauer zur Schau stellte. Auch war er ein grosser Sammler mit einer Leidenschaft für chinesisches Porzellan vom 15. bis 18. Jahrhundert und für russisches Glas, das von der Zeit von Elisabeth I bis zu der von Katharina der Grossen (also vom 17. bis zum 18. Jahrhundert) produziert wurde. Diese Fakten sind nicht ohne Wichtigkeit, um seinen Gebrauch von Glas für Parfüm-Flaschen zu verstehen. Es wird gesagt, dass er in 1928 die kaiserliche Kollektion russischen Glases kaufte, die Nikolaus II gehörte. Lelong hatte eine Tochter, Nicole, aus seiner ersten Ehe in 1919 mit Nelle Audey. Seine zweite Ehe mit Nathalie Paley wurde in 1935 geschieden. 1954 heiratete er Mme. Dancovici und verbrachte mit ihr die meiste Zeit in Biarritz. Lucien Lelong starb am 10. Mai 1958. Am Ende wurde aus den Parfums Lelong ein Teil von Coty International und sind jetzt ein unabhängiges Unternehmen im Besitz von Arnold und Lucy Neis.

In den 1920'er Jahren kreierte Lelong mindestens fünf (und möglicherweise mehr) Parfüme, deren Namen nur Buchstaben sind: *A*, *B*, *C*, *J*, *N*. Von diesen sind *J* und *N* die am besten bekannten. Um 1928 oder 1929 schuf René Lalique eine herrliche Flasche und eine überwältigend moderne Schachtel, die zumindest für die Parfüme *J* und *N* benutzt wurden. Möglicherweise auch für andere. Diese Flasche ähnelt in ihrem gesamten Aussehen einem modernen Wolkenkratzer, ist aber mit schwarzen Emaille-Girlanden in einer solchen Art und Weise dekoriert, dass sie einen sehr zarten und subtilen Anklang findet. Die Schachtel für dieses Parfüm, von der angenommen wird, dass sie auch von René Lalique geschaffen wurde, ist nicht weniger spektakulär als die Flasche. Sie dupliziert genau das Erscheinungsbild der Flasche und zwar in Chromstahl, dekoriert mit Emaille in verschiedenen Farbtönen und einem Futter aus Samt. Diese Schachtel kann man in mehreren unterschiedlichen Farben finden, einschliesslich grün, rot und cremefarben, im Zusatz zu schwarz. Die unterschiedlichen Farben der Schachteln entsprechen wahrscheinlich den unterschiedlichen Düften.

Auf eine andere Flasche, auch von René Lalique entworfen, wurde von Utt (1985) als *Etoile de Mer* (Seestern) Bezug genommen. Es handelt sich hier um einen ausserordentlichen Entwurf, der einen achteckigen Stern in Form einer Säule darstellt. Der Stöpsel stimmt in kleinerem Umfang genau damit überein. Die Spitzen des Sterns sind in kleinen Stufen geschaffen und mattiert, als ob dem Entwurf grössere Tiefe gegeben werden soll; ohne Zweifel liegt hier auch ein wichtiges architektonisches Gefühl im Entwurf dieser Flasche vor. Ein silbernes Etikett windet sich um den Hals der Flasche. Diese Flasche könnte sehr gut für die berühmten Buchstaben-Parfüme, wie auch für die floralen Düfte wie *Gardenia* benutzt worden sein. Der gleiche Lalique-Entwurf wurde dann auch von einem anderen Glashersteller in Glas aus anderer Qualität produziert. Ein sich in der Schachtel befindendes Beispiel des Dufts *Gardenia* wird hier gezeigt. Bei dem schwarz- und goldfarbenen *faux-marbre* Papier (imitierter Marmor), welches für diese Schachtel benutzt wurde, muss es sich um eine persönliche Bevorzugung des Designers gehandelt haben, da es auch in vielen anderen Präsentationen benutzt wurde. In Form einer als Urne geformten Flasche wurde eine völlig andersartige Präsentation des Parfüms *N* erstellt. Der Buchstaben-Name ist sehr auffällig auf der Seite der Flasche plaziert.

Indiscret und *Mon Image* waren möglicherweise die beiden erfolgreichsten Parfüme von Lucien Lelong. *Indiscret*, welches das französische Wort für das englische *indiscreet* (und das deutsche *indiskret*) ist, wurde in einer herrlichen mattierten Glasflasche präsentiert, von welcher man annimmt, dass die Inspiration davon ausgegangen ist, "wie eine Dame ihr Taschentuch fallen lässt". Die *Indiscret*-Flasche bezieht sich auf Lelong's Talent als grosser Couturier und ruft gleichzeitig die Sensation hervor, dass etwas enthüllt wird, irgendetwas Wunderschönes unter den vielen vielen Falten des weichen Materials. Die Graphiken der Schachtel unterstützen diese Themen in wunderschöner Form. Das Parfüm *Jabot* nimmt ebenfalls auf die Mode bezug. Die Flasche für *Jabot*, die seidene Schleife einer Dame, ist wortwörtlich eine in Glas geformte Schleife und wird in einer eleganten Hutschachtel vorgestellt.

Das Parfüm *Mon Image* (Mein Bildnis) schwört das Bildnis des jungen Narzissus herauf, und das Parfüm selbst ist eine berauschende Nachahmung des Dufts der Blume mit dem gleichen Namen. Aufgrund der Faszination des Narzissus mit seinem im Wasser widerspiegelnden Ebenbild, wird dieses Parfüm in einer einzigartigen Schachtel aus Spiegeln präsentiert. Die Flasche selbst ist von geometrischer Struktur, das Lelong Logo ist am Kopfende eingeprägt und die Flasche hat einen ausgeprägten architektonischen Aspekt.

Das Parfüm *Orgeuil* (Stolz) ist irgendwie einmalig unter den Lelong Kreationen, da es eine mit Gold umhüllte Glasflasche ist. Sie wurde zum Ende des zweiten Weltkriegs zur Feier von Frankreich's Befreiung produziert, und die Wichtigkeit des Namens ist mehr in Bezug auf Patriotismus als auf persönliche Eitelkeit zu sehen. Es ist eine Flasche, die "wir haben gesiegt" sagt und sie wird auf einem Podest aus weissem Satin in einer Schachtel aus schwarz-goldfarbenem *faux marbre* präsentiert. Viele der grossen französischen Parfümeure feierten das Ende des Krieges mit Parfüm-Kreationen, wenn auch die politische Wichtigkeit der Namen in der Zwischenzeit in Vergessenheit geraten ist: Patou *L'Heure Attendue* (Die erwartete Stunde), Guerlain *Fleur de Feu* (Blume des Feuers), Chanel *No. 46*, Schiaparelli *Le Roy Soleil* und Molyneux *Magnificence*.

Zwei Themen dominieren in den herrlichen Parfüm-Präsentationen von Lucien Lelong. Eines davon ist das Couture-Motiv, welches eine direkte visuelle Verbindung zwischen Mode und Parfüm darstellt. Das Couture-Motiv ist die Nachbildung von Stoffen, Girlanden und Federn im Medium Glas. Einige der Parfüme, die dieses Motiv benutzen sind: *Jabot*, *Les Plumes* und *Cachet*. Das andere, wiederkehrende Motiv ist das der modernen Architektur. Viele Lelong Kreationen ähneln Gebäuden oder benutzen architektonische Motive: *N*, *Mon Image*, *Balalaika*, *Murmure*, *Castel*, *Impromptu*, *Opening Night* und *Penthouse*, eine Präsentation aus vier Miniaturen. Das Lelong Logo selbst ist ein geometrischer Entwurf, basierend auf einem *L* innerhalb eines *L*'s. Wegen seiner Identifizierung einerseits und seiner wunderbaren geometrischen Symmetrie andererseits ist es ein brillantes Logo und leiht sich selbst architektonische Themen an. Eingeprägt wird es auf sehr vielen Lelong Flaschen und auf fast allen Graphiken der Parfüm-Schachteln gefunden. Parfüm-Sammler von heute und von Morgen werden immer die Fähigkeit Lelong's bewundern, die Geschmeidigkeit des Couture- mit der Strenge des Architektur-Motivs in perfekter Harmonie zueinander zu benutzen. So wie der Erfolg Lelong's in der Mode begründet war auf seine Kenntnisse bezüglich der Wichtigkeit der Stoffe für den Entwurf eines Kleides, war sein Erfolg in der Kunstfertigkeit des Parfüms nicht weniger zurückzuführen auf seine Kenntnisse in der Wichtigkeit des Entwurfs der Glasflasche, des Namens des Parfüms sowie der gesamten Präsentation in Bezug auf die blosse Identität des Duftes - und demzufolge auf seinen letztendlichen Erfolg.

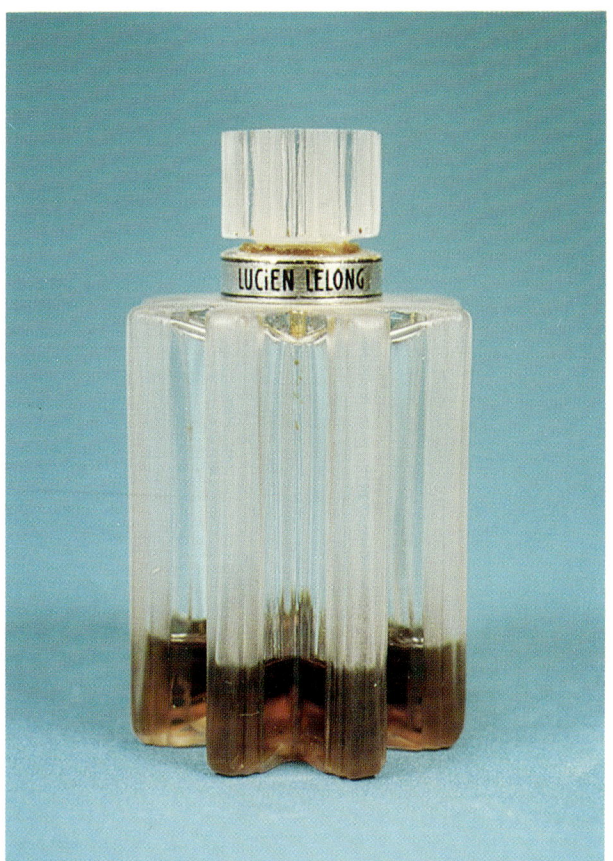

Figure 17. The Lalique perfume bottle design for *Gardenia*, signed *R. Lalique*. Collection of Randall B. Monsen and Rodney L. Baer.

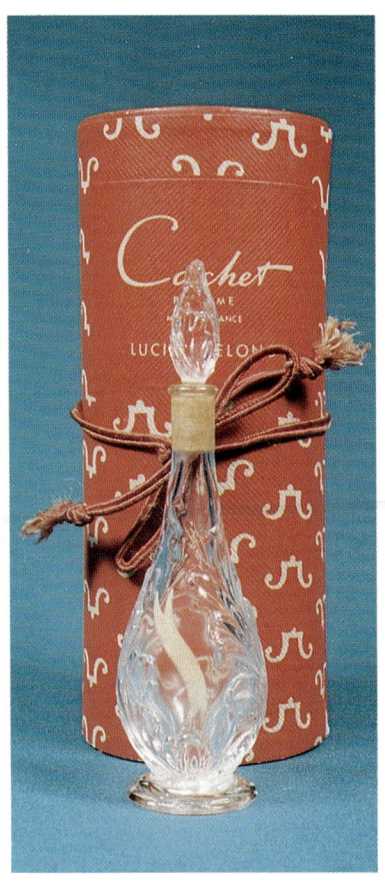

Figure 18. Lucien Lelong *Cachet,* in a bright crimson box, an uncommon color for Lelong's perfume presentations. Monsen and Baer Collection.

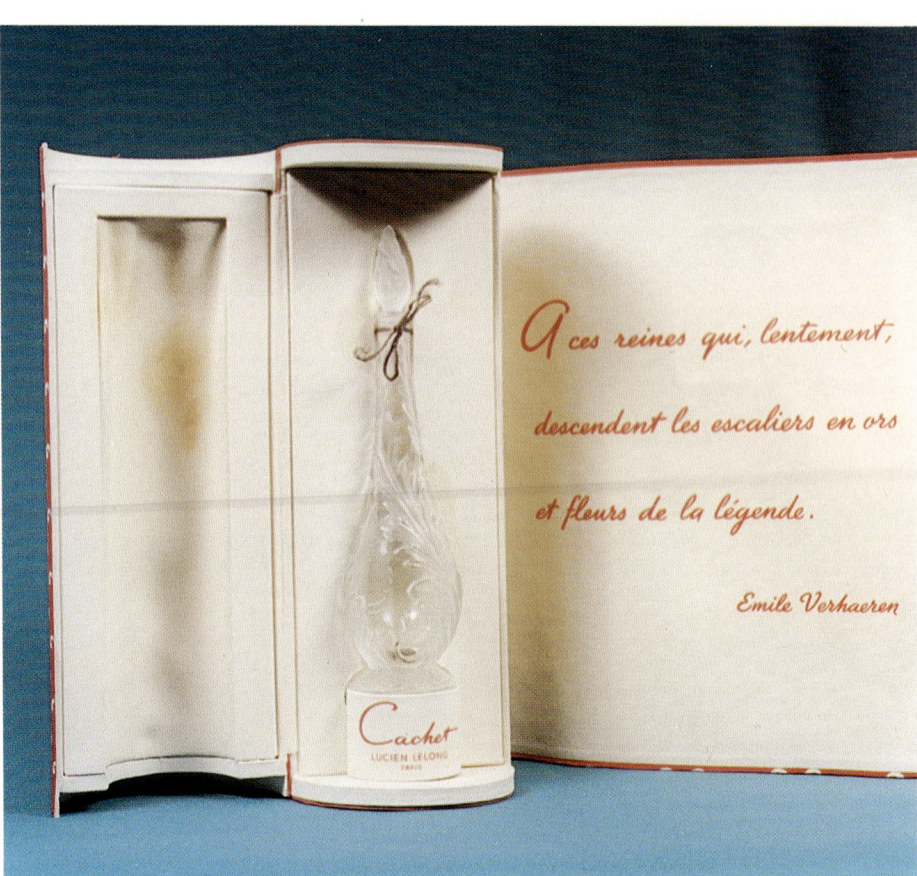

Figure 19. Lucien Lelong *Cachet.* On the inside of the long cover that wraps around the box there is a quotation by Emile Verhaeren: *A ces reines qui, lentement, descendent les escaliers en ors et fleurs de la légende* ['To the regal women who, slowly, descend the stairs in the gold and flowers of legend.']. Collection of Randall B. Monsen and Rodney L. Baer.

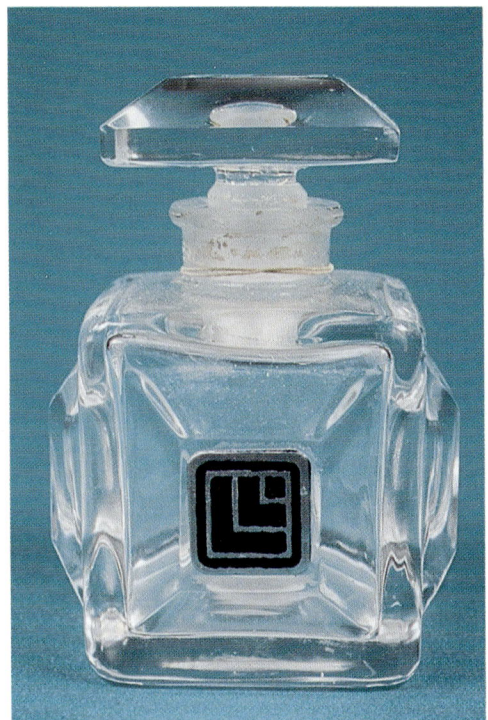

Figure 20. Lucien Lelong perfume bottle possibly used for several fragrances; the stopper bears the *LL* logo. Collection of Randall B. Monsen and Rodney L. Baer.

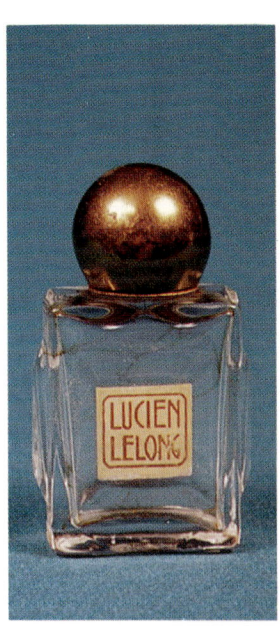

Figure 21. Lucien Lelong replica miniature of the bottle shown in Figure 20; from Lot #29, Monsen and Baer Perfume Bottle Auction VIII.

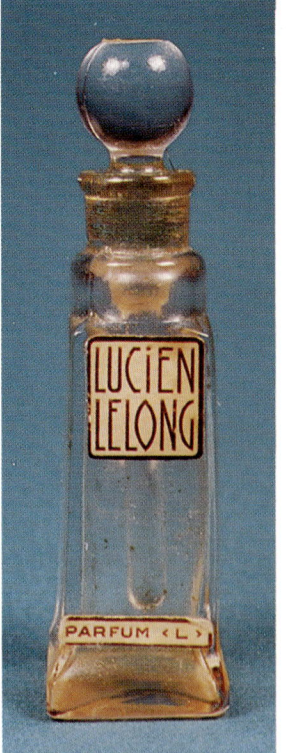

Figure 22. Lucien Lelong *L* very rare tester, from Lot #17, Monsen and Baer Perfume Bottle Auction VIII.

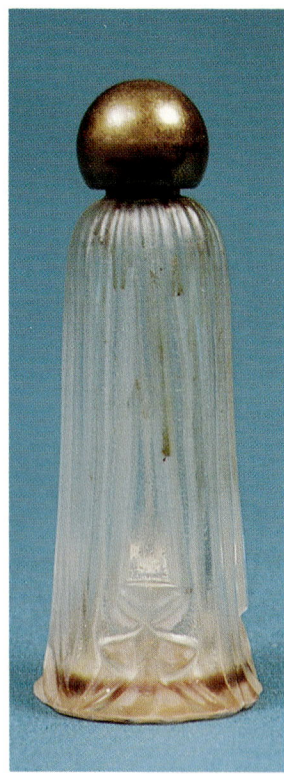

Figure 23. Lucien Lelong *Indiscret* old miniature. Monsen and Baer Collection.

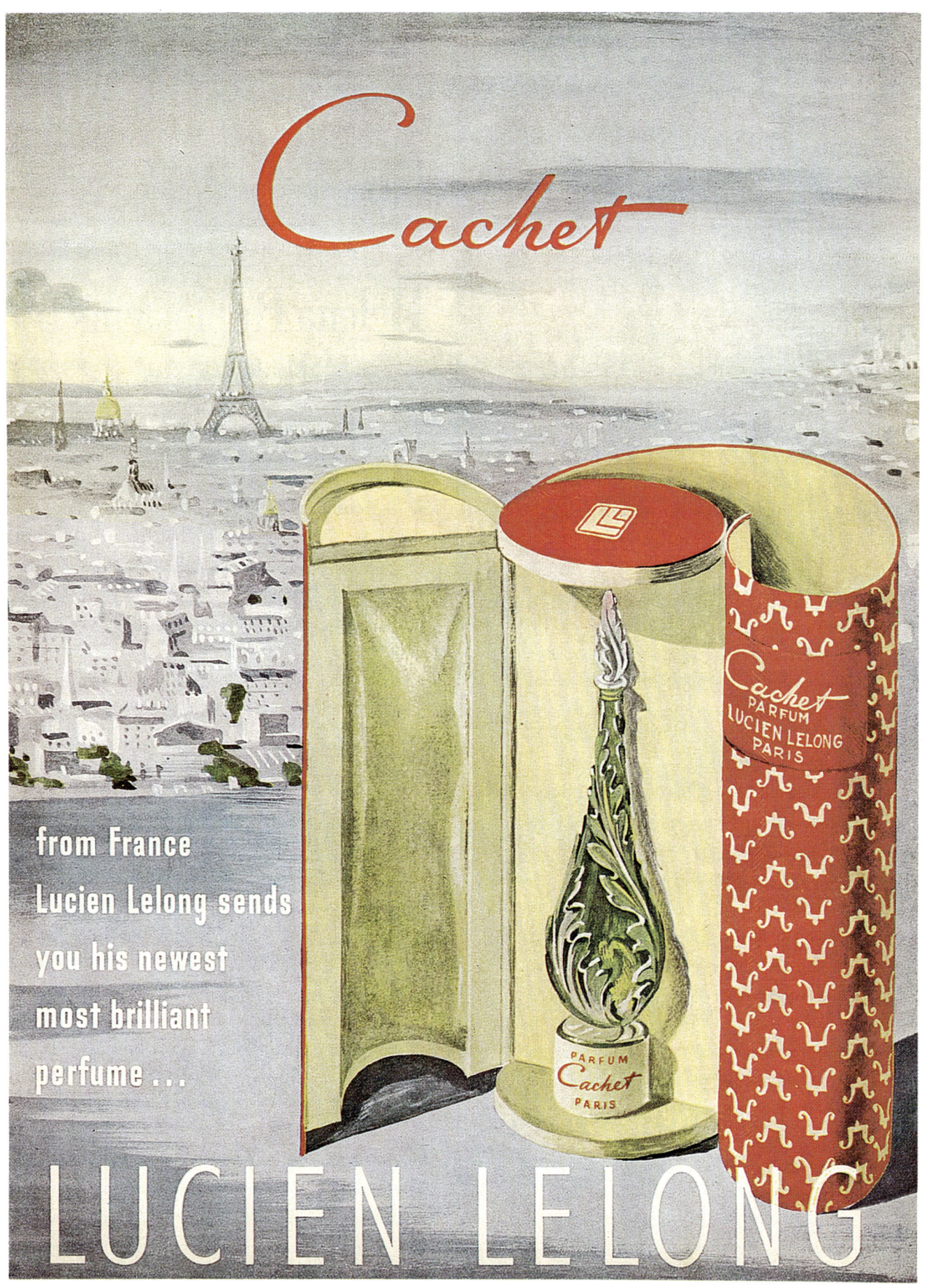

Figure 24. Lucien Lelong *Cachet,* which was presented in a unique and very beautiful box [cf. photo on the facing page]. This advertisement dates from February, 1950. Collection of Randall B. Monsen and Rodney L. Baer.

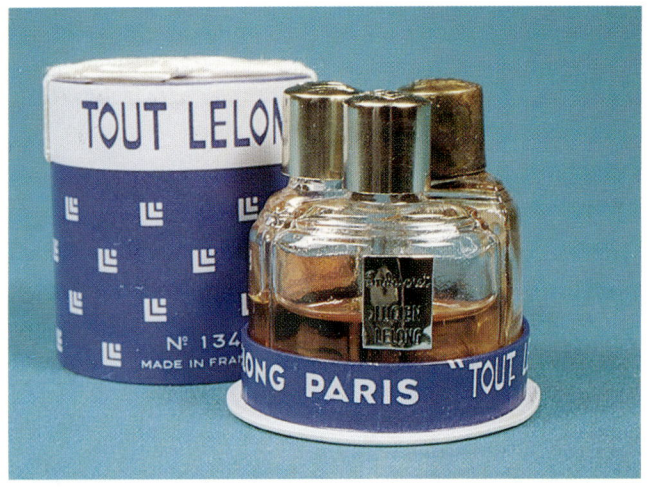
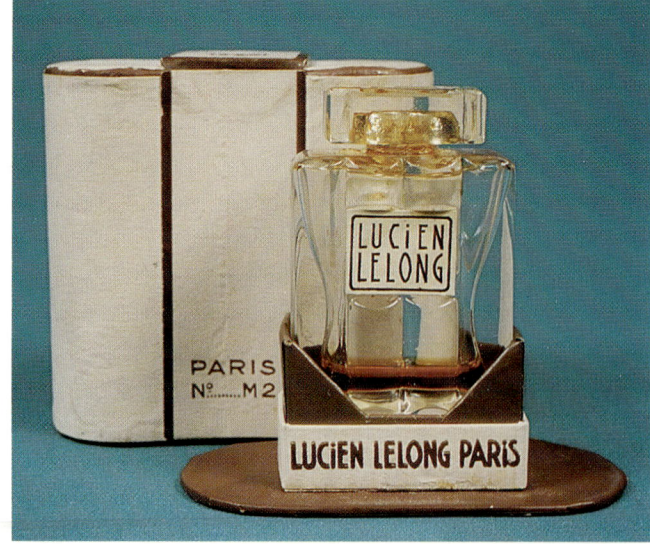
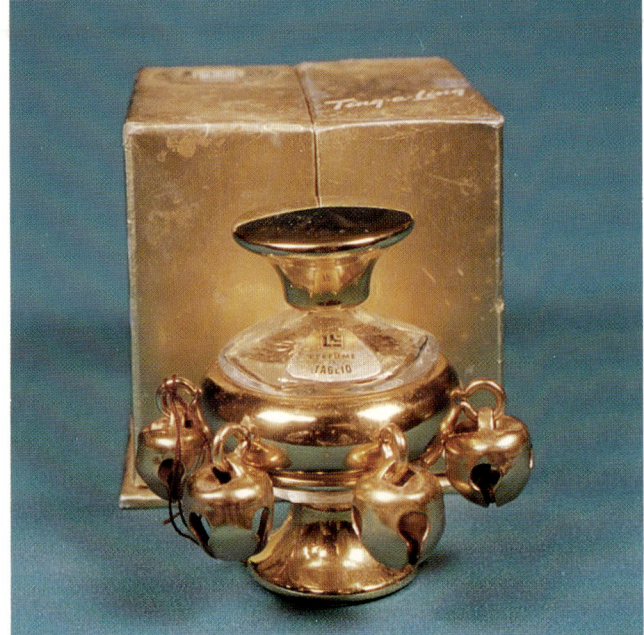
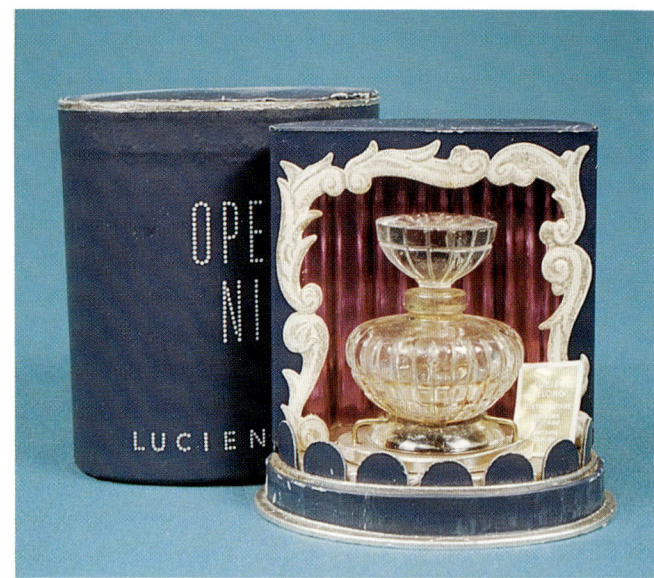
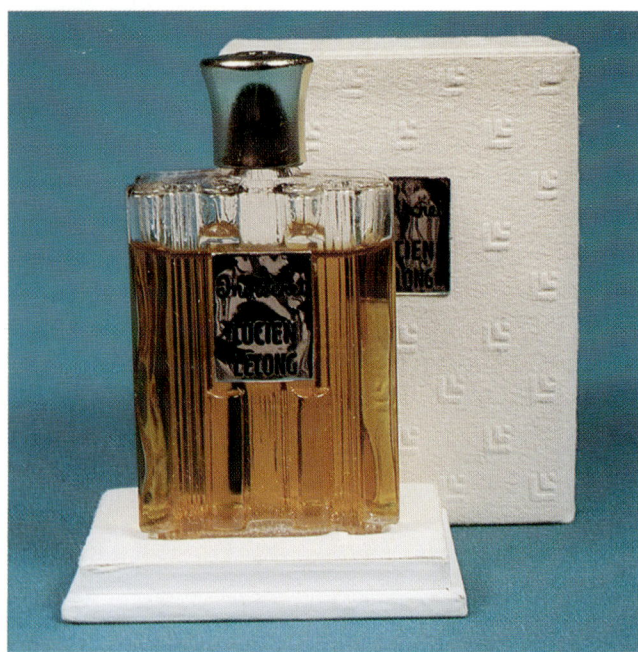
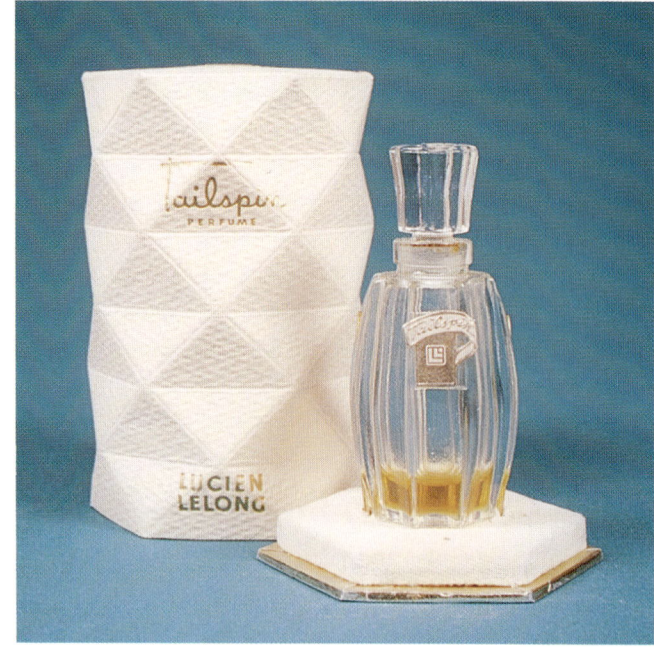

Figure 25. Upper Left: *Tout Lelong* set of three miniatures; upper right: *Murmure/Whisper*, a first size, in its box; middle left: *Ting-A-Ling* presentation of *Taglio*, in its box; middle right: *Opening Night*, in its second presentation; lower left: *Indiscret*, a rare small size in an unusual presentation; lower right: *Tailspin* in its geodesic-form box. Collection of Randall B. Monsen and Rodney L. Baer.

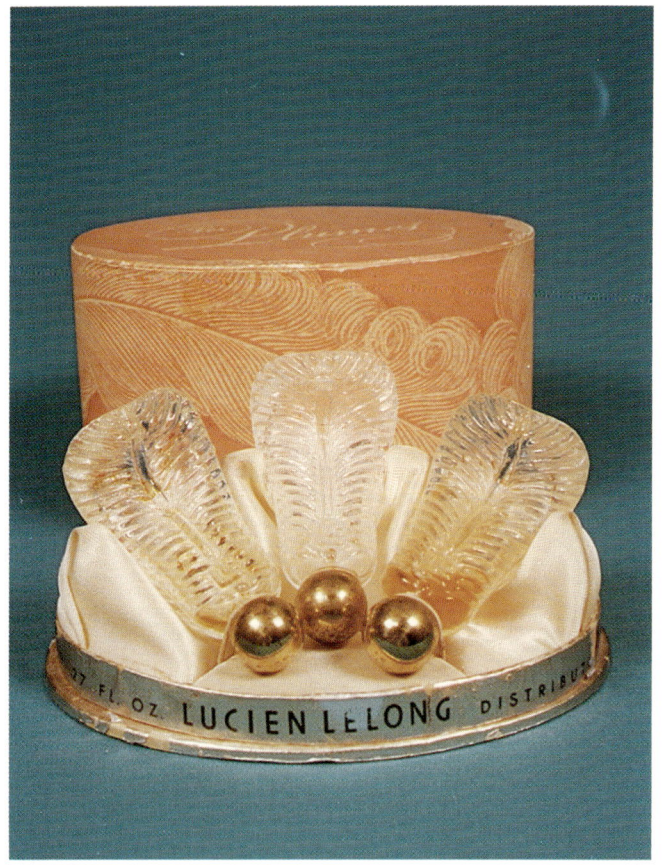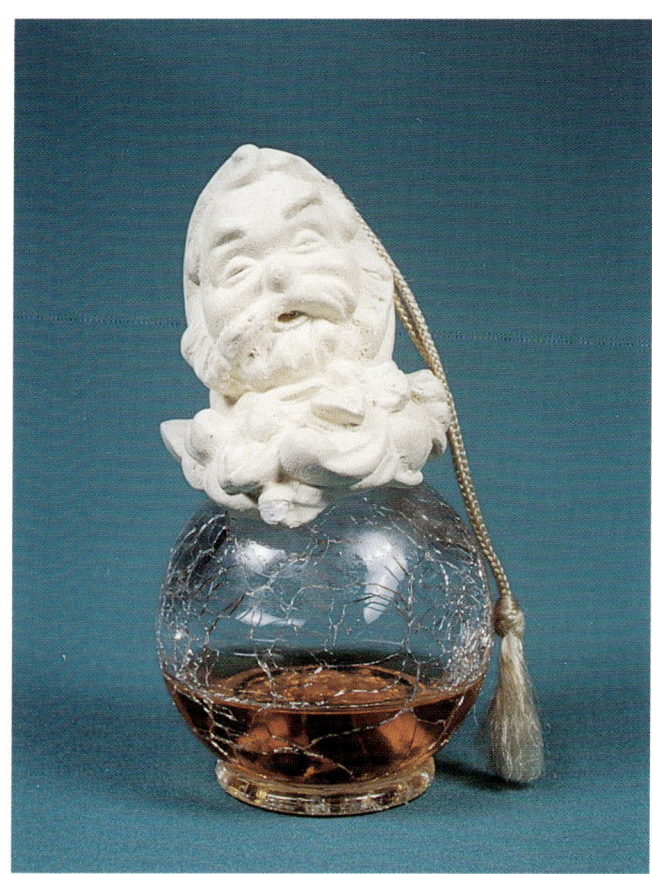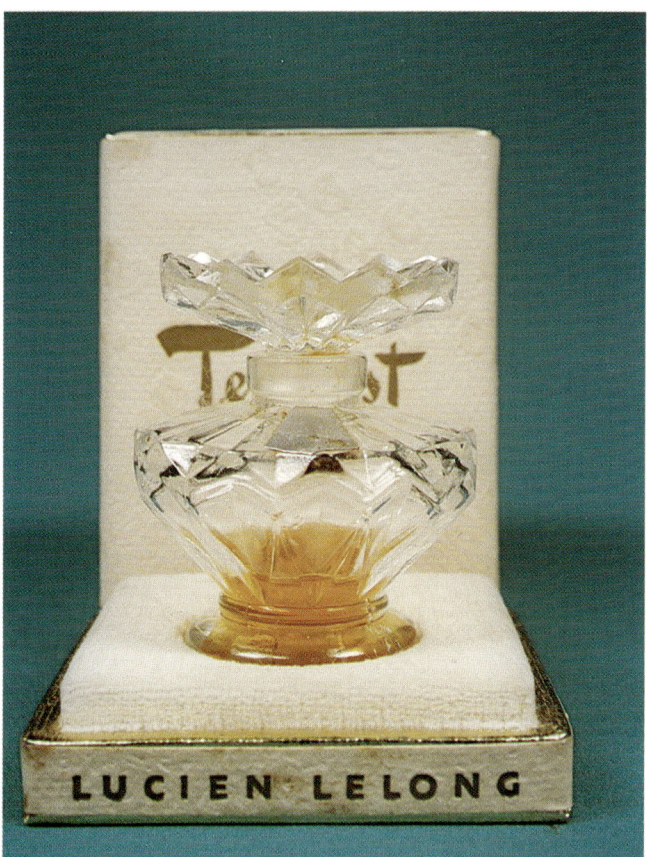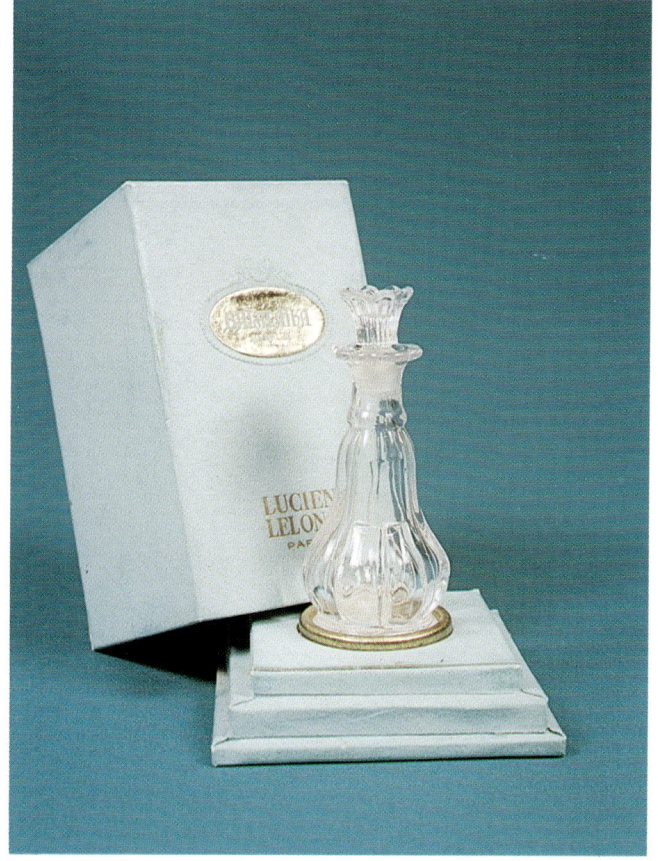

Figure 26. Upper Left: *Les Plumes* ['The Feathers'] set of three miniatures in their box; upper right: *Whisper* in the *Santa Claus* presentation which could be used as an tree ornament; lower left: *Tempest*, a bottle designed with a ruffle motif, in its box; lower right: *Balalaika* in an unusual and atypical presentation. Collection of Randall B. Monsen and Rodney L. Baer.

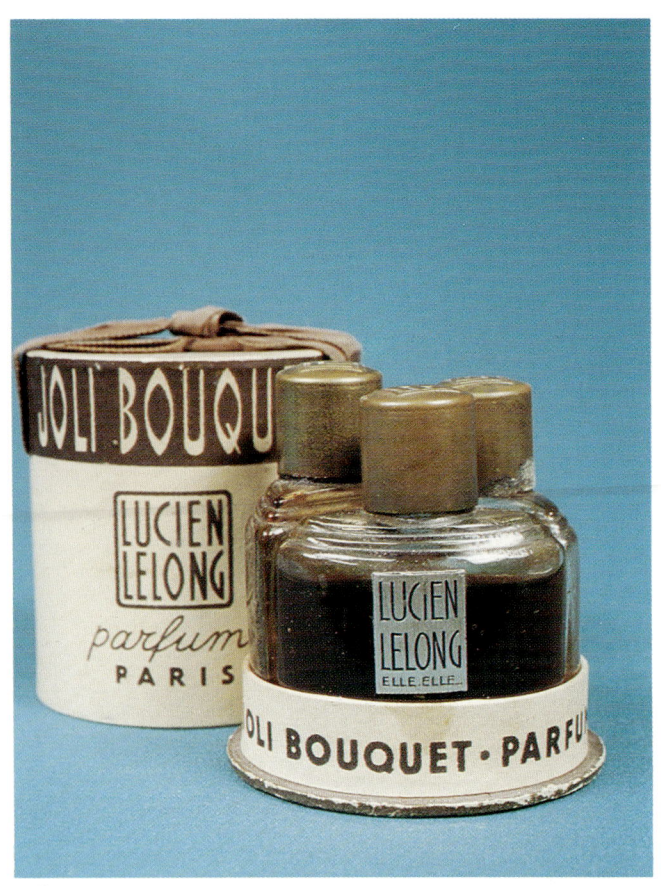
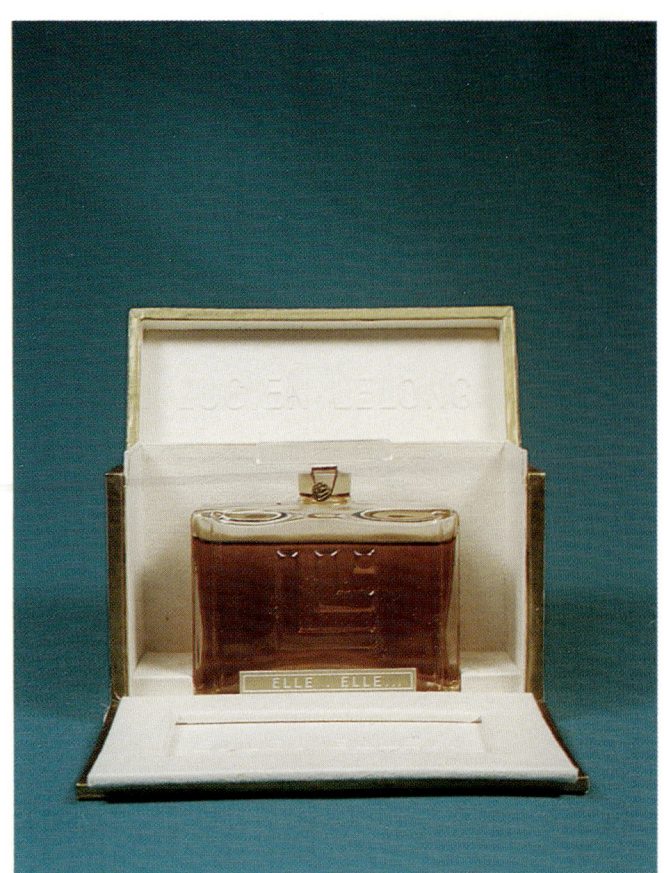
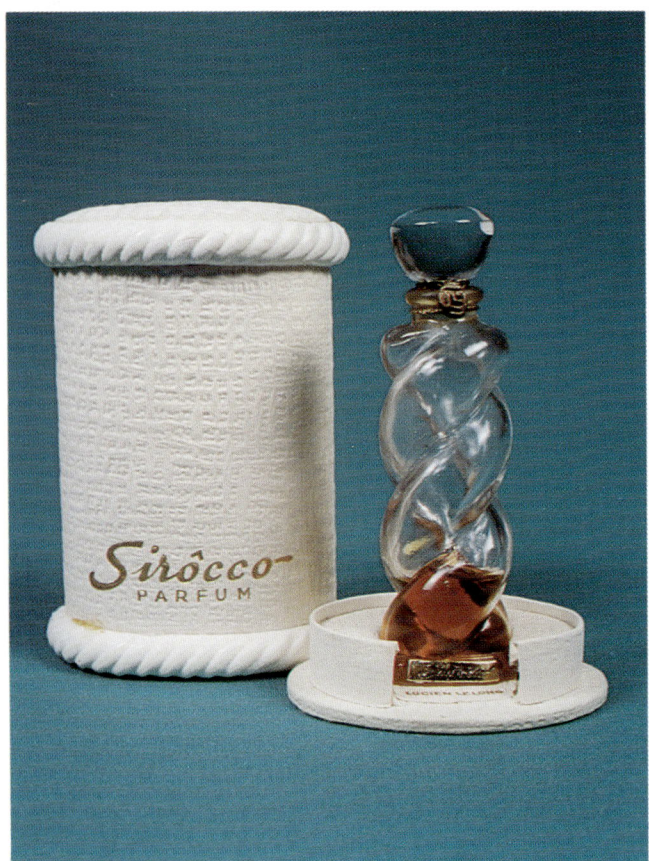
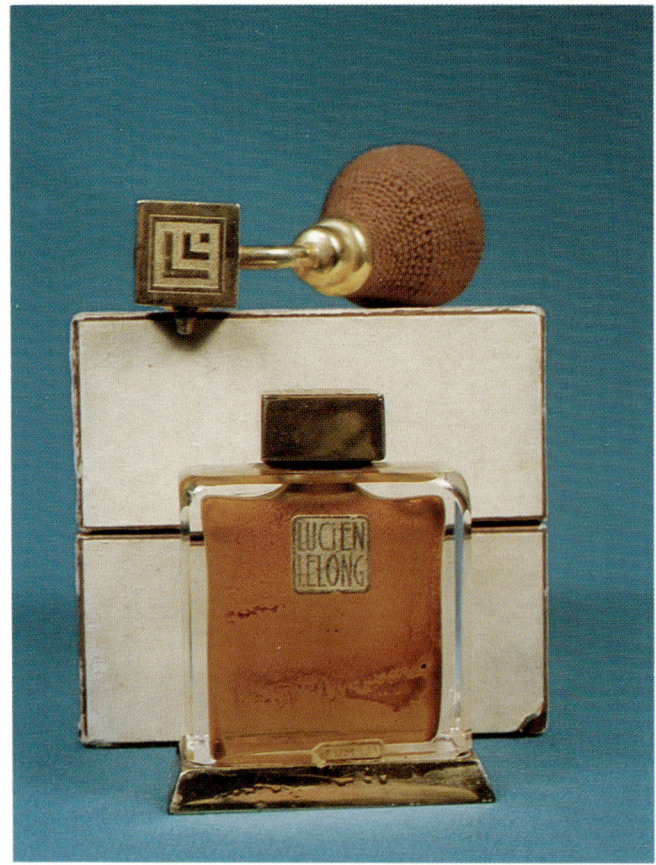

Figure 27. Upper Left: *Joli Bouquet* ['Pretty Bouquet'] set of three miniatures in their box; upper right: *Elle. Elle....* an architectural form bottle similar [but not identical] to that of *Taglio,* in its box; lower left: *Sirôcco,* a bottle designed with a rope motif, in its box; lower right: *J* in an rare crystal atomizer presentation.   Collection of Randall B. Monsen and Rodney L. Baer.

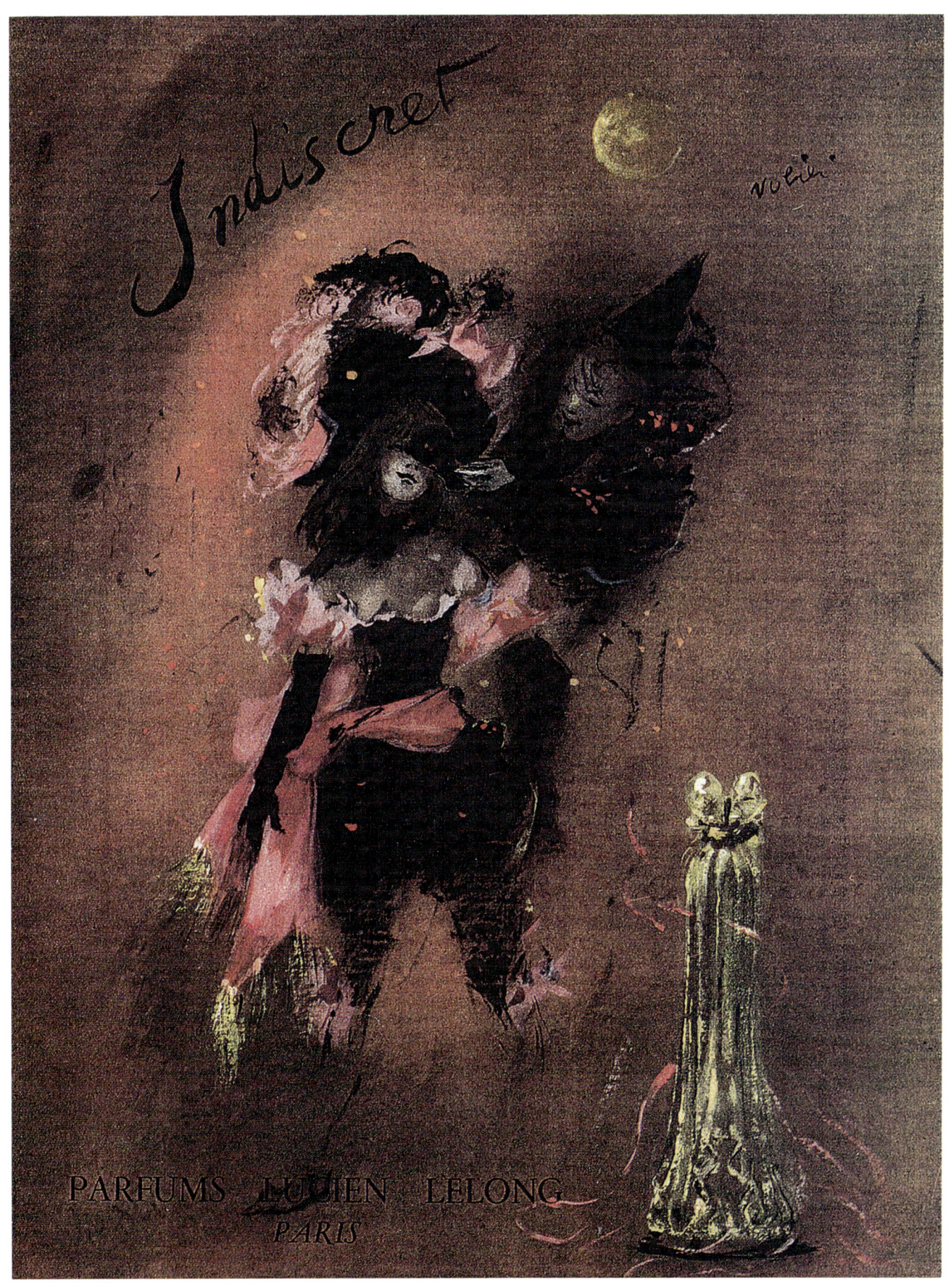

Figure 28. An example of the beautiful publicity used in the past, for *Indiscret,* circa 1947. Collection of Arnold and Lucy Neis, *Parfums Lucien Lelong.*

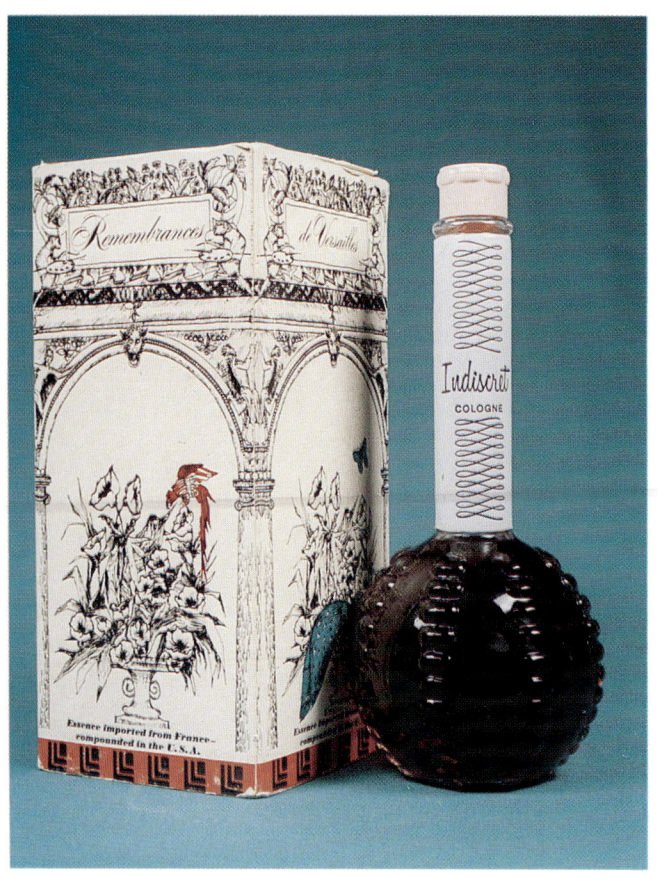
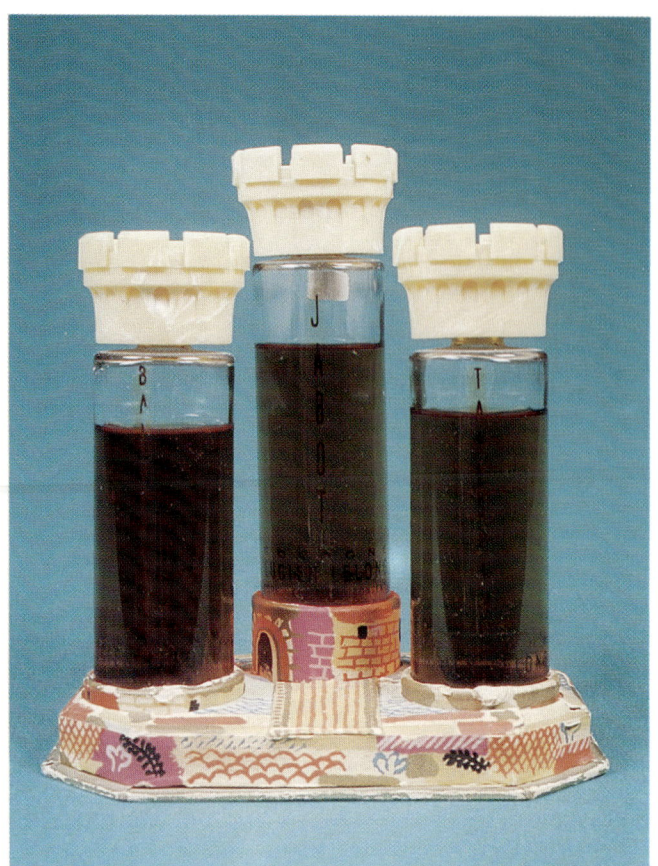
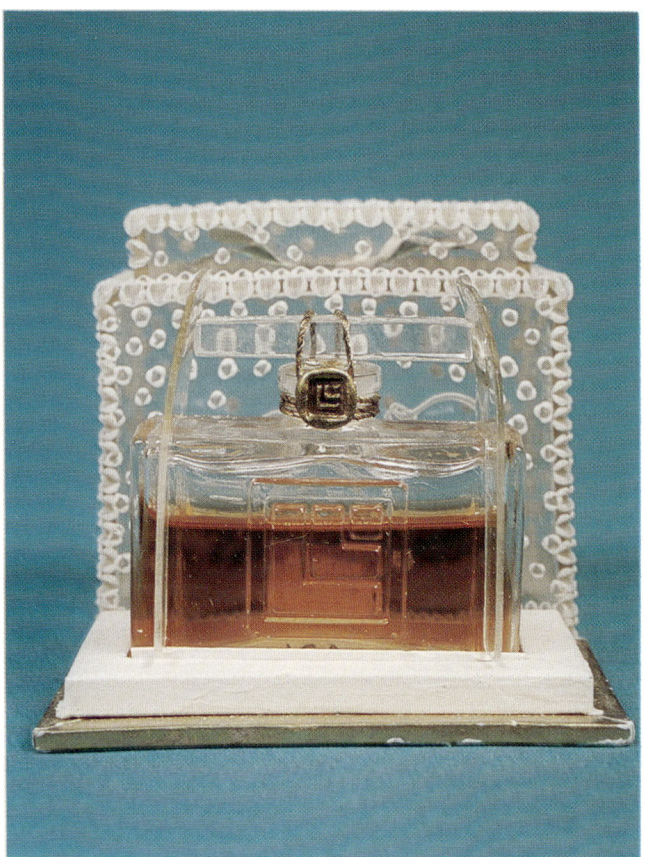
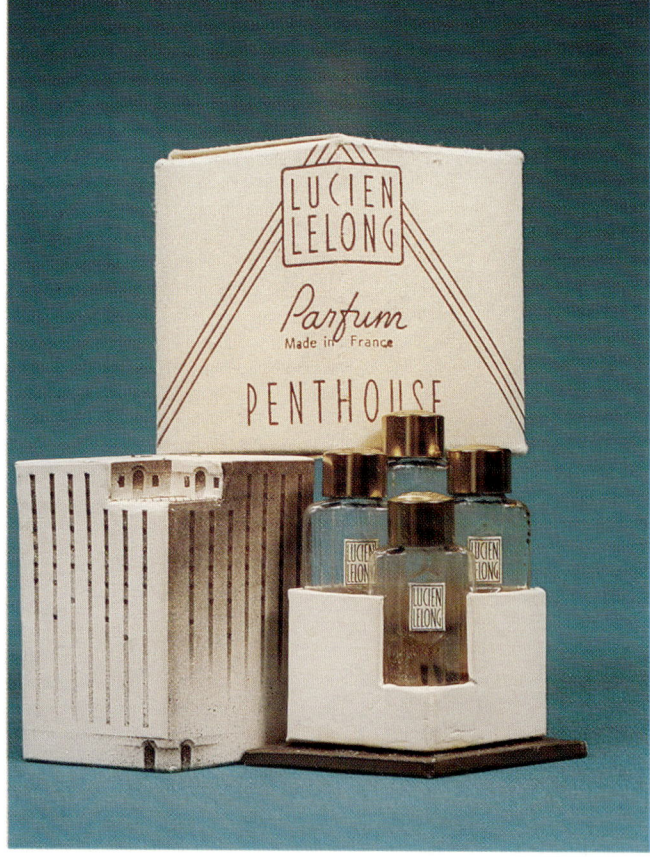

Figure 29. Upper Left: *Indiscret* cologne in the *Remembrances of Versailles* presentation; upper right: *Le Castel* a very large example, possibly for display, containing *Jabot, Balalaika, Tailspin;* lower left: *Taglio* with its unique plastic box; lower right: *Penthouse*, a very early example containing *B, C, N*, and *Whisper*.   Collection of Randall B. Monsen and Rodney L. Baer.

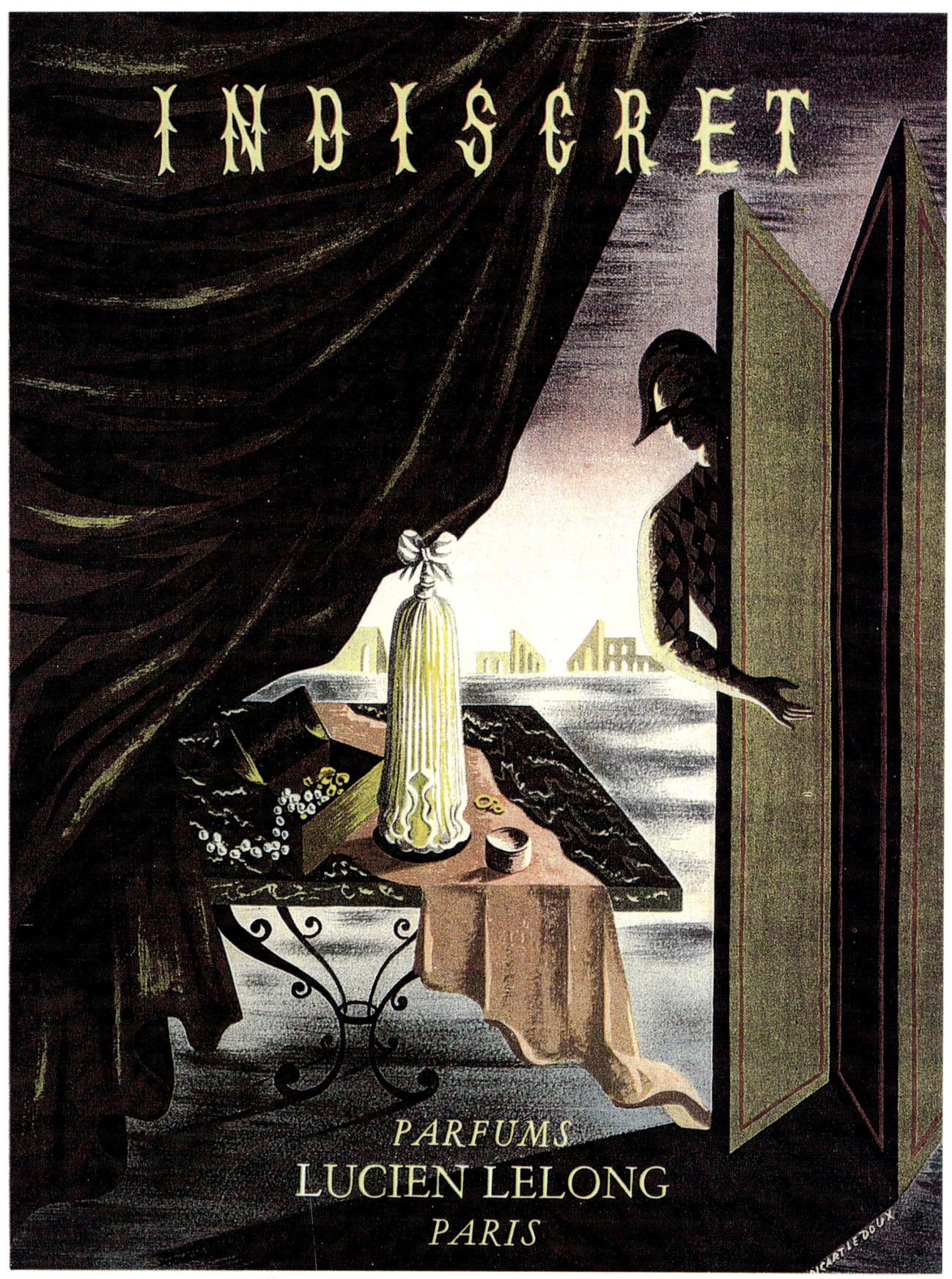

Figure 30. An example of the beautiful publicity used in the past, for *Indiscret*, circa 1947; note the influence of surrealism. Collection of Arnold and Lucy Neis, *Parfums Lucien Lelong*.

Masterpieces of Today / Chefs-d'Oeuvre d'Aujourd'hui
Christie Mayer Lefkowith

Since 1950, many small perfume companies—each with its own style of presentation—were acquired by large holding companies. This new trend intensified, especially from 1960 to 1980. Having thus lost their independence and their creative capacities, the small perfume companies had to adapt to the requirements of these large industrial groups of international scope and to produce in a more centralized and hence in a more efficient manner. The lack of skilled artisans as well as the increased cost of manpower reinforced the need to produce perfume presentations exclusively by mechanized means. Industrialization made it possible to reduce production costs, and modern life limited the demand for original and luxurious perfume presentations. Some companies even became interested in developing a somewhat industrial and uniform look. New techniques and new materials entered the production process. For example, stoppers with a plastic stem, which guaranteed firm closure, replaced ground glass stoppers. This limited the production of inventive and original presentations in the 1960's and the 1970's. Its was a sad time in the perfume industry.

However, an extraordinary presentation, as a special limited edition of 100, was created in 1969: it was *Bal à Versailles* by Jean Desprez, a return to the great French tradition of luxury perfume, comparable to the great masterpieces of the 1920's. Jean Desprez [1889-1973] descended from a family of perfumers, since his great-grandmother was Mme. Félix Millot. He worked for Les Parfums Millot, and in 1925 created *Crêpe de Chine,* one of the great successes of the century. In 1938 he founded his own perfume company and launched, in 1939, the perfumes *Grande Dame* ['Great Lady'] and *Votre Main* ['Your Hand'], named in homage to his mother, an elegant and refined woman, and a talented pianist with beautiful hands. Having taken over the Perfumery d'Orsay salon, at 17, rue de la Paix, in Paris, either in 1939 or in 1943 [there are contradictory data here], he had it decorated by his good friend, the sculptor Léon Leyritz [1888-1976] who was also a painter and a theatrical set designer. From the formation of the company, Léon Leyritz created both flacon and graphic designs for the Jean Desprez perfumes.

The perfume, *Bal à Versailles,* launched in 1962, sold first by Nieman Marcus in Dallas, met immediately with great international success. In 1969, to celebrate the triumph of *Bal à Versailles* and the prestige of Jean Desprez perfumes, Léon Leyritz created a new presentation for this perfume, as a limited edition, to be sold mainly by Nieman Marcus, at the exorbitant price of $850. Flattering articles appeared in the American press, particularly in the New York Times, and caused the limited edition to be immediately sold out—since it was recognized that this wonderful object was worthy of collecting. The flacon and its small inner stopper, both snow white, are made of Sèvres bisque porcelain. The flacon represents Janus, a mythic character, the most ancient king of Latium. The flacon is surmounted by an overcap of gold and sterling silver in the form of a crown, in the middle of which there is a jet of water, and which was produced by one of the great goldsmiths of the period. The flacon is presented in a luxurious case of red leather, engraved and gilded, with double doors lined in white silk and with a red velvet base which serves as a backdrop to emphasize the

Dès 1950, de nombreux petits parfumeurs — ayant eu chacun son propre style de présentation — furent acquis par de grands groupes. Cette nouvelle tendance ne fit que s'accentuer pendant vingt ans, au moins, surtout de 1960 à 1980. Ayant ainsi perdu leur indépendance et leurs capacités créatives, les petits parfumeurs, en général, ont dû se plier aux exigences de ces grands groupes industriels d'envergure internationale, et produire de manière plus centralisée, donc plus efficace. Le manque d'artisans habiles, ainsi que l'augmentation du coût de la main d'œuvre renforcèrent le besoin de produire des présentations de parfum exclusivement mécanisées. L'industrialisation permit de réduire les coûts de production, et la vie moderne limita la demande pour les présentations de parfum d'aspect original et luxeux. Quelques groupes s'intéressèrent même à développer un aspect uniforme et industriel. De nouvelles techniques et de nouveaux matériaux entrèrent dans le processus de production. Par exemple, les bouchons à douille plastifiée, garantissant une bonne fermeture, remplacèrent les bouchons émeri. Cela ralentit la production des présentations inventives et originales durant les années 60 et 70. Ce furent de tristes années dans la parfumerie.

Cependant une extraordinaire présentation, en édition spéciale, à tirage limité à 100 exemplaires, vit le jour en 1969: ce fut *Bal à Versilles* de Jean Desprez, un retour à la grande tradition française dans la parfumerie de luxe, comparable aux grands chefs-d'œuvre des années 20.

Jean Desprez [1889-1973] était issu d'une famille de parfumeurs puisque son arrière-grand-mère était Madame Félix Millot. Il travailla pour Les Parfums Millot, et créa en 1925 le parfum *Crêpe de Chine*, qui fut un des grands succès du siècle. En 1938, il fonda sa propre maison et lança, en 1939, les parfums *Grande Dame* et *Votre Main*, ainsi intitulés en hommage à sa mère, femme élégante et raffinée, pianiste de talent, aux très belles mains. Ayant repris le magasin de la Parfumerie d'Orsay, au 17, rue de la Paix, à Paris, soit en 1939, soit en 1943 [les informations sont contradictoires à ce sujet], il le fit décorer par son grand ami, le sculpteur Léon Leyritz [1888-1976], qui fut également peintre et créateur de décors de théâtre. Dès le départ, Léon Leyritz créa des flacons et des graphismes pour les parfums Jean Desprez.

Le parfum *Bal à Versailles*, lancé en 1962 et vendu au début par le grand magasin Nieman Marcus, à Dallas, dans le Texas, connut immédiatement un grand succès mondial. En 1969, pour marquer le triomphe de *Bal à Versailles* et le prestige des parfums Jean Desprez, Léon Leyritz créa, pour ce parfum, une présentation à tirage limité, vendue principalement par Nieman Marcus, au prix exorbitant de $850. Les articles flatteurs parus dans la presse américaine, notamment dans le New York Times, firent que, malgré son prix, l'ensemble de l'édition limitée fut immédiatement vendu — car déjà on s'était rendu compte que ce merveilleux objet était une pièce de collection.

Le flacon et son petit bouchon intérieur, tous deux d'un blanc de neige, sont en biscuit de Sèvres. Le flacon représente Janus, un personnage mythique, le plus ancien roi du Latium. Il est surmonté d'un couvre-bouchon en or fin et argent premier titre, en forme de couronne, au milieu de laquelle se trouve un jet d'eau, et qui fut produit par un des

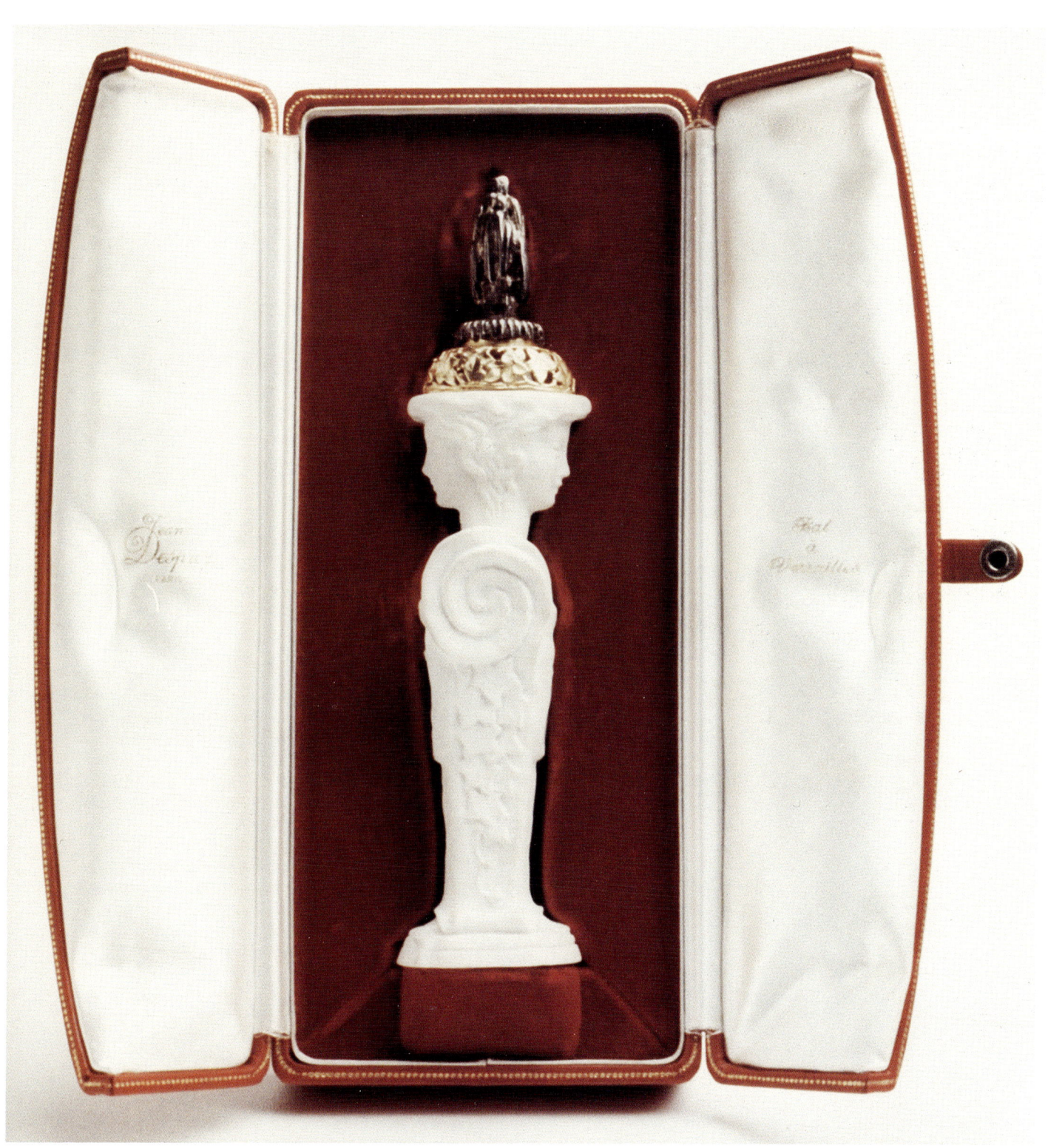

Figure 1. Jean Desprez *Bal à Versailles*, limited edition of 100. Collection of Christie and Ed Lefkowith.

white flacon. In the back, a detachable support allows the case to stand, slightly tilted backward, simulating a frame for a precious work of art.

Legend has it that Saturn, chased from the heavens by his own son Jupiter, took refuge in Latium where he was welcomed with open arms by the king, Janus. There he made peace and prosperity flourish, and full of gratitude toward king Janus, he endowed him with a wonderful capacity: the power to simultaneously see the past, as well as the future. This double ability led to his being portrayed with two faces. Janus was considered by the Romans to be a divinity and his temple in Rome was only closed in peacetime, which happened only for nine months in a thousand years. For the Romans, Janus was the first god, father of all the others, the god of dawn and of the sun, the god of open doors, the god of gushing waters, and the god of communication.

This white and sumptuous creation by Léon Leyritz represents a return toward the past through its neo-classical and neo-romantic style, so much in fashion at the end of the 1930's, when Jean Desprez founded his perfume company; it represents also a look toward the future of the perfume *Bal à Versailles*, one of the best selling perfumes worldwide. Seen from the side, the flacon is very representative of the god Janus with his two faces. But seen from the front or from the back [the two are identical], the impression is totally different, since it presents a very soft and feminine face and a woman's bust with a pearl neck-

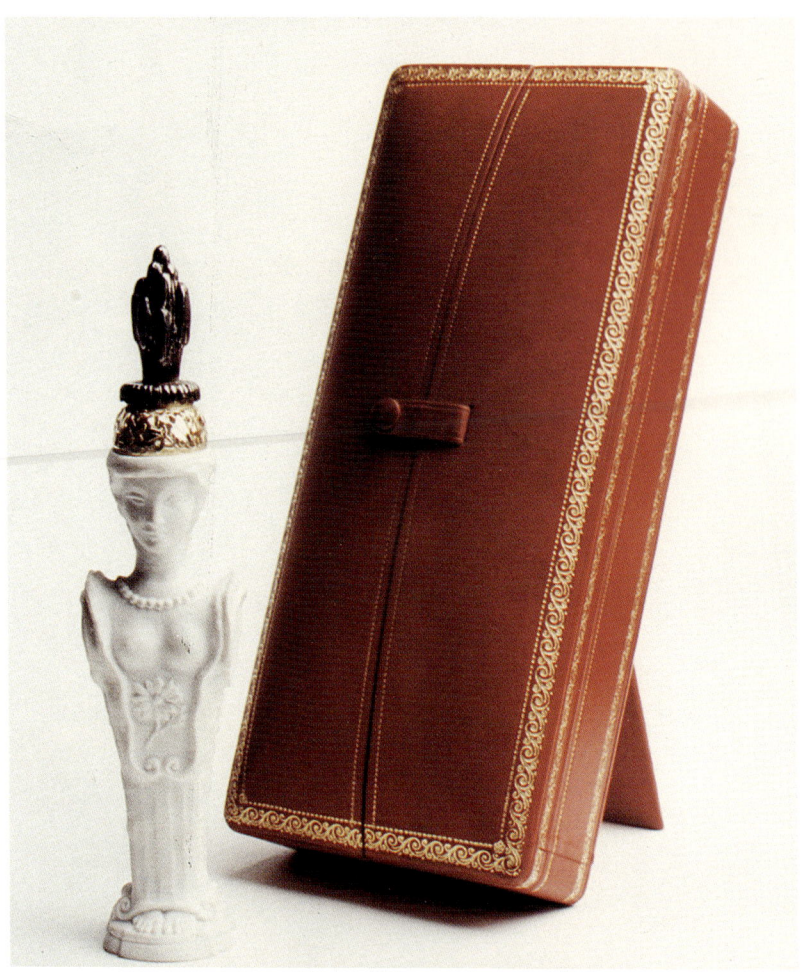

Figure 2. Jean Desprez *Bal à Versailles*, limited edition of 100. Collection of Christie and Ed Lefkowith.

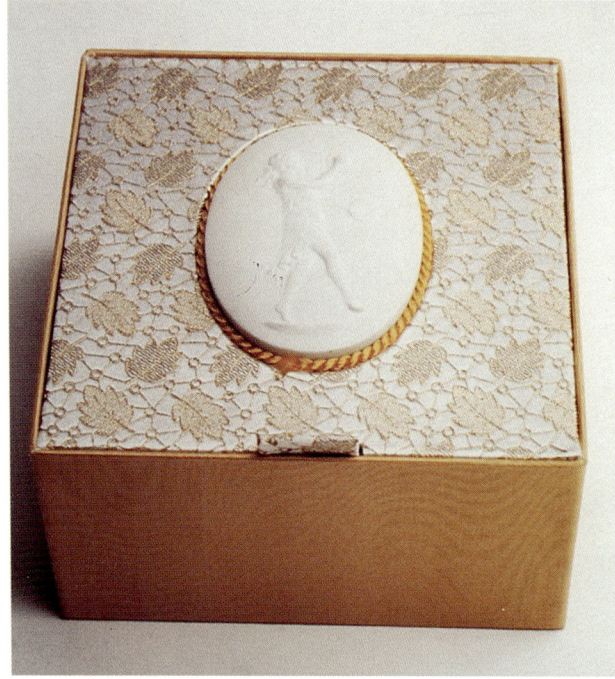

Figure 3. The powder box for Jean Desprez *Bal à Versailles*, limited edition. Collection of Christie and Ed Lefkowith.

grands orfèvres de l'époque. Le flacon est présenté dans un écrin de luxe, en cuir rouge, gravé et doré, s'ouvrant à deux battants doublés de soie blanche, avec un fond en velours rouge servant de toile de fond pour mieux faire valoir le flacon blanc. Au dos, un support détachable permet de présenter l'écrin debout, légèrement incliné vers l'arrière, tel un cadre pour un précieux objet d'art.

La légende veut que Saturne, chassé du ciel par son propre fils Jupiter, se réfugia dans le Latium où il fut accueilli à bras ouverts par le roi Janus. Il y fit fleurir la paix et l'abondance, et plein de reconnaissance envers le roi Janus, il le doua d'une merveilleuse capacité: le pouvoir de garder toujours présent à ses yeux, le passé, aussi bien que l'avenir. Cette double faculté a conduit à le représenter avec deux visages. Janus fut considéré par les Romains comme une divinité et son temple à Rome n'était fermé qu'en temps de paix, ce qui n'arriva que pendant neuf mois en mille ans. Pour les Romains, Janus fut le premier dieu, père de tous les autres, le dieu de l'aube et du soleil, le dieu des portes ouvertes, le dieu des eaux jaillissantes et le dieu de la communication. Cette blanche et somptueuse création de Léon Leyritz représente un retour vers le passé, à travers son style néoclassique et néoromatique, si en vogue à la fin des années 30, époque à laquelle Jean Desprez fonda sa parfumerie; elle représente également un regard vers l'avenir du parfum *Bal à Versailles*, un des parfums les mieux vendus au monde.

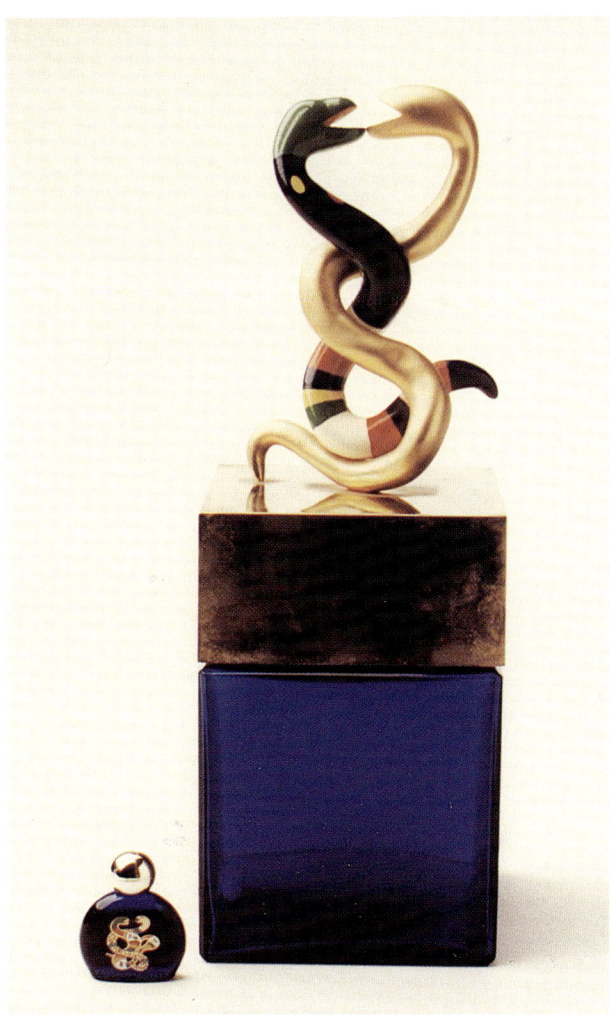

Figure 4. Niki de St. Phalle, giant factice and miniature. Collection of Christie and Ed Lefkowith.

Vu de profil, le flacon représente bien le dieu Janus aux deux visages. Mais vu de face ou de dos (les deux sont identiques), l'impression est totalement différente, car il présente un visage très doux et féminin et un buste à poitrine de femme et à collier de perles. Sous cet angle, il ressemble à une des statues sur socle qui se trouvent dans le parc du château de Versailles, mais surmontée d'une fontaine à grand jet, une de celles qui se trouvent également dans ce parc. C'est peut-être à cause de cet aspect féminin que cette présentation fut surnommée "La Janusette", un nom féminisé de Janus.

La Janusette est une rarissime présentation, un chef-d'œuvre de la parfumerie artistique de luxe. Une grande boîte à poudre carrée, recouverte de satin jaune et de soie blanche brodée d'or, est ornée d'un médaillon blanc, en biscuit de Sèvres, tel un bas-relief dépeignant un personnage de l'antiquité. Ce médaillon ressemble fort aux premiers graphismes créés pour Nina Ricci et executés en papier blanc, eux-mêmes dans le style bas-relief. Cette magnifique boîte à poudre semble être encore plus rare que la Janusette.

Cependant un vent créateur se fit sentir autour de 1980. Des signes de reprise apparurent alors dans le développement de nouvelles créations à prix modérés - ce qui n'avait pas été vu depuis les années 50.

Le parfum de Niki de Saint-Phalle est une des plus belles créations de la parfumerie de son époque, lancé en 1980, et à la portée de toutes les bourses. Niki de Saint-Phalle, scupteur de l'école française, née en 1930, vécut à New York de 1933 à 1951, ce qui explique, peut-être, son penchant pour l'art surréaliste, pour l'expressionnisme abstrait et pour l'art brut. Revenue à Paris en 1952, elle commença à peindre, et petit-à-petit, se dirigea vers la sculpture et vers un style baroque, fantastique et coloré, ce qui la fit inclure en 1961, dans l'école des "nouveaux réalistes". Elle fit beaucoup parler d'elle, et devenue une célébrité

lace. Seen from this angle it resembles one of the statues on a pedestal which are found in the park of the Château of Versailles, however surmounted by water jet fountain, one of those also found in this park. It is perhaps because of this feminine aspect, that this presentation was called La Janusette, a femininized version of the name Janus.

La Janusette is an exceedingly rare presentation, an artistic masterpiece of luxury perfume. A large square powder box, covered in yellow satin and in gold embroidered white silk, is adorned by a white medallion made of Sèvres bisque porcelain, resembling a bas-relief depicting a figure from antiquity. This medallion also strongly resembles the first graphic designs created for Nina Ricci and executed in white paper, also in the bas-relief style. This magnificent powder box seems to be even rarer that La Janusette.

A new creative wind was felt around 1980. Signs of revival appeared then in the development of new creations in the moderate price range; this had not been seen since the 1950's.

The perfume of Niki de Saint-Phalle is one of the most beautiful creations of the perfume in-

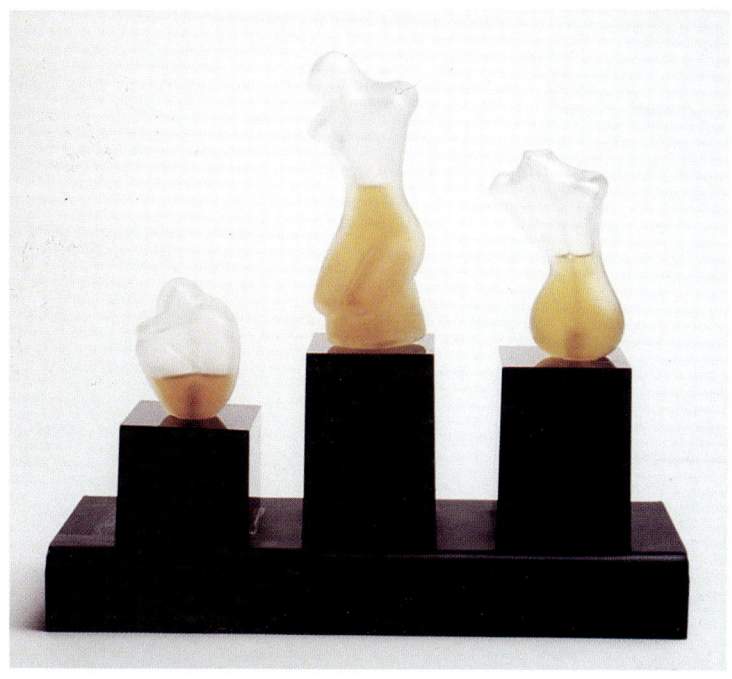

Figure 5. Jovan Sculptura set of three flacons on display stand. Collection of Christie and Ed Lefkowith.

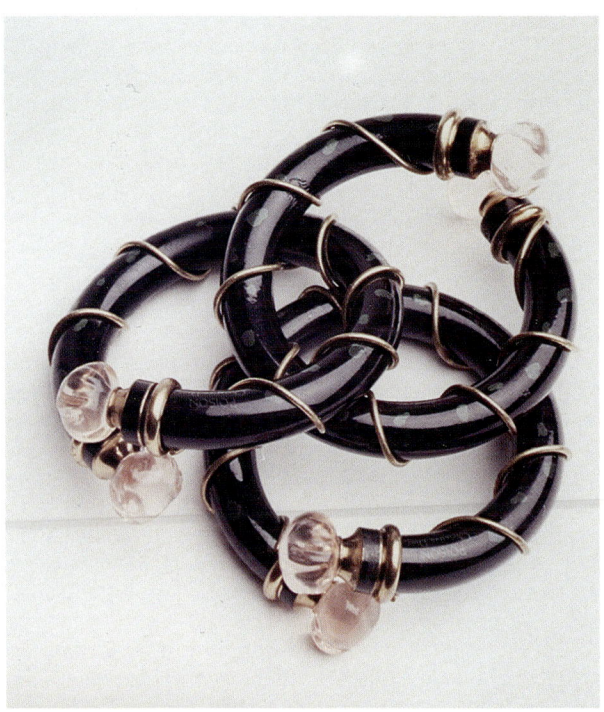

Figure 6. Christian Dior *Poison*: three flacon-bracelets. Collection of Christie and Ed Lefkowith.

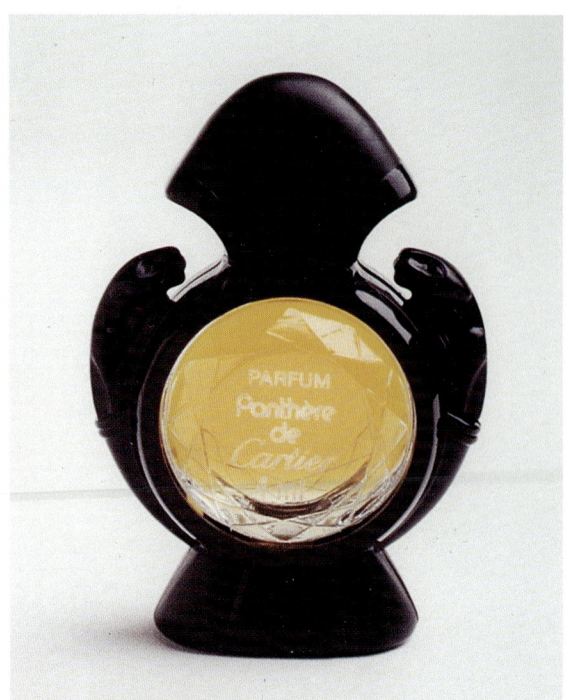

Figure 7. Cartier *Panthère* miniature. Collection of Christie and Ed Lefkowith.

dustry at that time, launched in 1980 and meant to be affordable. Niki de Saint-Phalle, a sculptor of the French school, was born in 1930 and lived in New York from 1933 to 1951, which explains, perhaps, her penchant for surrealist art, for abstract expressionism, and for *l'art brut* ['raw' and impulsive art by non-professional artists, such as psychotics, children, etc.]. Having returned to Paris in 1952, she began to paint, and gradually focused on sculpture and evolved toward a baroque, fantastic and highly colorful style, which led to her being included in 1961 in the school of the "new realists." She was much talked about and having become an artistic celebrity and a socialite, she lent her name and her talent to the creation of a perfume. This perfume is presented in a flacon and box, both decorated with a motif of intertwined and gaudy-colored serpents, symbol of *l'art brut* and of the "Cobra" spirit, an artistic movement which flourished especially in the 1960's. This presentation, which is not rare today, is nevertheless worthy of a beautiful collection.

Another beautiful presentation, created for the mass market, was *Sculptura* of Jovan, launched in 1981. There were three flacon models in frosted colorless glass, which are in fact atomizers, each presented upside down on a black plastic pedestal which hides the atomizer mechanism [this is the same principle of design as *Gardez-moi*, a Jovoy perfume of 1926, which comprises the famous black crystal Baccarat flacon in the form of a cat, presented on a base of yellow silk.] The three flacons for *Sculptura* represent three simplified sculptures of modern aspect, expressing perfectly the name of the perfume, as well as a studied elegance which was very original for its time.

In 1985, Christian Dior launched *Poison*, a heady perfume, very different from the perfumes then in fashion, and presented in a flacon of amethyst-colored glass with a colorful box. It is no more than a pretty presentation. However, a flacon-bracelet in the form of a stylized serpent, evil

artistique et mondaine, elle prêta son nom et son talent à la création d'un parfum. Ce parfum est présenté dans un flacon et dans une boîte ornés d'un motif de serpents entrelacés et bariolés, symbole de l'art brut et de l'esprit "cobra", nom d'un movement artistique qui s'épanouit surtout pendant les années 60. Cette présentation, qui n'est pas rare aujourd'hui, est pourtant digne de faire partie d'une belle collection.

Une autre belle présentation, conçue pour une grande diffusion, fut *Sculptura* de Jovan, lancée en 1981. Il y a eu trois modèles de flacons en verre incolore dépoli, qui sont en fait des vaporisateurs présentés à l'envers sur des socles en plastique noir cachant le méchanisme du vaporisateur (c'est le même principe de présentation que *Gardez-moi*, de Jovoy, de 1926, qui comprend le célèbre flacon en cristal noir de Baccarat, en forme de chat, sur socle en soie jaune). Les trois flacons *Sculptura* représentent trois sculptures simplifiées, d'aspect moderne, exprimant parfaitement le nom du parfum, ainsi qu'un effort de recherche très original pour son époque.

En 1985, les parfums Christian Dior lancèrent *Poison*, un parfum capiteux, très différent des parfums alors à la mode, et présenté dans un flacon en verre de couleur améthyste avec boîte très colorée. C'est une jolie présentation, sans plus. Par contre, un flacon-bracelet, en forme de serpent stylisé, maléfique et élégant, destiné a être offert, et non pas vendu, créé en édition spéciale limitée, fut une très belle réussite qui se situe entre le parfum et l'accessoire de mode.

Les grands créateurs font souvent allusion à leur passé, en créant des œvres d'actualité, mais qui présentent néanmoins un regard vers l'arrière. Ce fut le cas de Cartier, joailliers depuis 1847, et parfumeurs depuis 1981. En 1987, le parfum *Panthère* fut lancé dans un flacon décoré de deux panthères, allusion aux bijoux à panthères si à la mode avant la guerre. Le flacon-échantillon est particulièrement attrayant dans sa toute petite taille et très difficile à produire. C'est

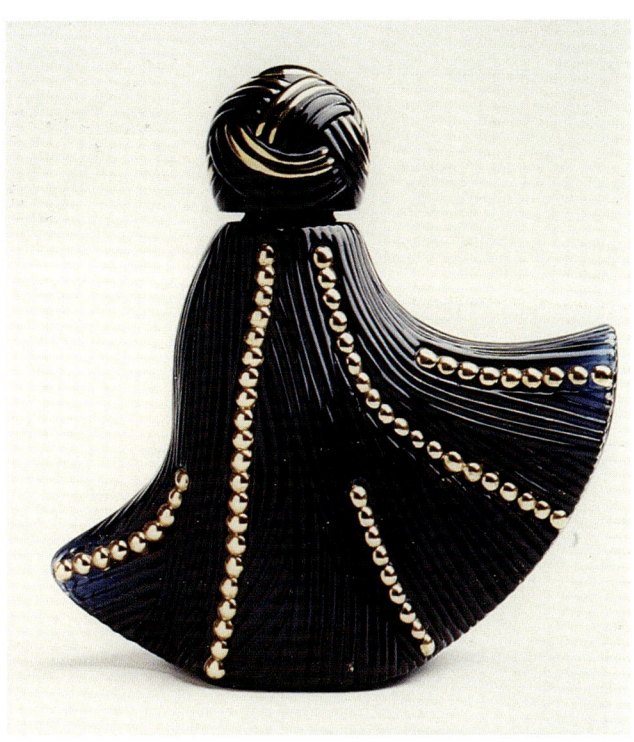

Figure 8. Isabelle Canovas giant factice. Collection of Christie and Ed Lefkowith.

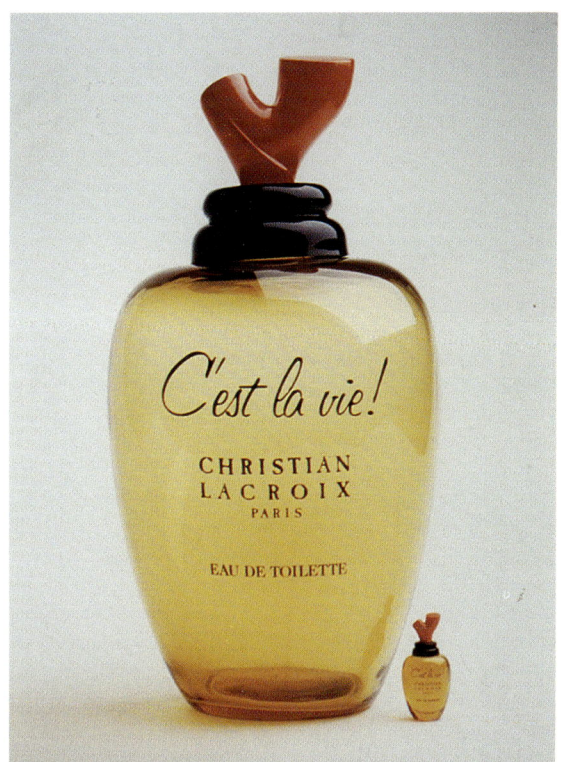

Figure 9. Christian Lacroix *C'est La Vie* giant factice and miniature. Collection of Christie and Ed Lefkowith.

and elegant, meant to be offered and not sold, was created as a special limited edition. It was a very beautiful creation, to be characterized somewhere between a perfume and a fashion accessory.

Great designers often allude to their past by creating contemporary works which nevertheless present a look backward. Such was the case of Cartier, jewelers since 1847 and perfume creators since 1981. In 1987, the perfume *Panthère* was launched in a flacon enhanced by two panthers, an allusion to the jewels with panthers so much in fashion before the war. The sample flacon is particularly appealing in its tiny size and very difficult to produce. It is one of the prettiest miniatures of the 1980's.

Isabelle Canovas, a designer of fashion accessories for *haute couture*, opened a boutique in New York more than ten years ago, on Madison Avenue near 65th Street, and launched her own perfume almost at the same time. This magnificent bottle, in dark navy blue glass with gilding, represents a leather tassel with small gilded chains which often decorated the purses and belts of her boutique, symbolic of the Isabelle Canovas style. The giant bottle, with its real glass stopper [without plastic inside], is of exceptional quality and was usually located in the display window of the boutique. Isabelle Canovas went bankrupt during the Gulf War, and this wonderful flacon, unique in this size, is possibly the only memento remaining of this boutique which was like none other.

Christian Lacroix, the brilliant couturier, made his debut at Jean Patou. His avant-garde style, poles apart from the Patou style, was very well-noted in the press and soon after, he founded his own couture house. His Provençal origins and his love of Spain are found in his fashion style and in the flacon for his perfume *C'est La Vie!!*, launched in

une des plus jolies miniatures des années 80.

Isabelle Canovas, une créatrice d'accessoires de mode pour la haute couture, ouvrit une boutique à New York, il y a plus de dix ans, sur Madison Avenue près de la 65ème rue, et lança son parfum presque en même temps. Le magnifique flacon, en verre bleu marine trés foncé et doré, représente un gland en cuir, à chaînettes dorées, qui ornait souvent les sacs et les ceintures de la maison, symbole du style Isabelle Canovas. Un flacon géant, à vrai bouchon en verre (sans plastique intérieur), et de qualité exceptionnelle, se trouvait d'habitude dans la vitrine de la boutique. Isabelle Canovas fit faillite pendant la guerre du Golf, et ce merveilleux flacon, unique dans cette taille, est peut-être le seul temoignage qui reste de cettte boutique qui ne ressemblait à aucune autre.

Christian Lacroix, ce grand couturier de génie, débuta chez Jean Patou. Son style d'avant-garde, aux antipodes du style Patou, fut très remarqué dans la presse, et peu après, il fonda sa propre maison de couture. Ses origines provençales et son amour de l'Espagne se retrouvent dans son style de mode et dans le flacon de son parfum, *C'est La Vie!*, lancé en 1989. Dessiné par Elisabeth Garouste et Mattia Bonetti, deux artistes qui ont fait équipe pour créer des accessoires d'intérieur et des objets d'art très variés, ce flacon est un mélange complexe d'allusions. Il ressemble à un coeur humain, et son bouchon pourrait bien être le départ de deux artères - symboles de la vie. Le bouchon ressemble également à une branche de corail - symbole de soleil et de chaleur, reflétant les origines du sud de Christian Lacroix. Le parfum ne connut pas un grand succès, donc cette présentation n'est pas facile à trouver aujourd'hui. C'est une vraie création moderne, qui ne ressemble à aucune autre, une très belle pièce de collection.

1989. Designed by Elisabeth Garouste and Mattia Bonetti, two artists who teamed up to create interior accessories and all kinds of art objects, the flacon is a complex mixture of allusions. It resembles a human heart, and its stopper could very well be the point of departure of two arteries — symbols of life. The stopper also resembles a coral branch — symbol of the sun and of warmth — and thus reflecting Christian Lacroix's southern origins. The perfume was not a great success, and therefore this presentation is not easy to find today. It is truly a modern creation which resembles none other, a very beautiful piece to collect.

Also in 1989, Boucheron, the great jewelers of the Place Vendôme, launched their own perfume *Boucheron*. The flacon, shaped like a ring mounted with a sapphire, is sumptuous and sober, just like a jewel by Boucheron.

Jean-Paul Gaultier is the *enfant terrible* of high fashion, imaginative, daring, and mischievous. His creations are always featured in the press, although they are not always wearable. In 1993, the perfume *Jean-Paul Gaultier* was launched. This bust-shaped flacon is reminiscent of Schiaparelli's *Shocking bust-sh*aped flacon. But the resemblance is only superficial, since the Schiaparelli presentation is romantic, refined, precious, and very feminine. The style of the Jean-Paul Gaultier presentation is hard, impersonal, and in the industrial style for mass consumption, as well as with the unisex and metallic aspect of science fiction. The large size of this presentation displays a disquiet-

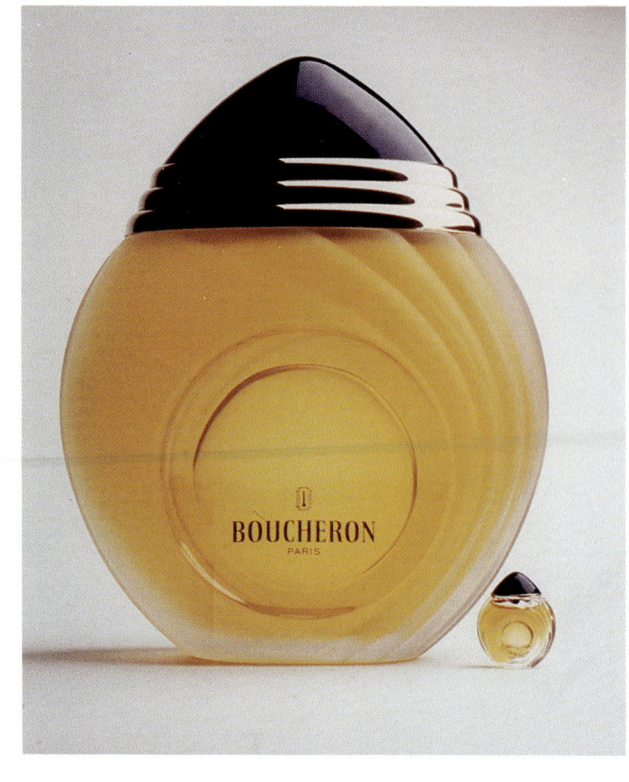

Figure 10. Boucheron giant factice and miniature. Collection of Christie and Ed Lefkowith.

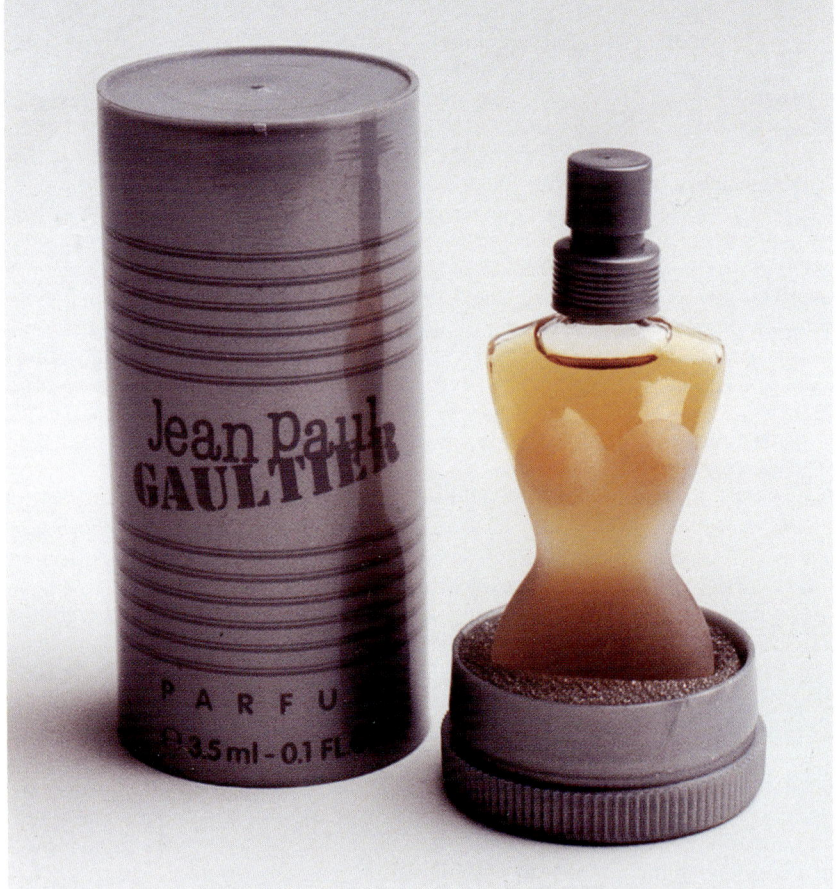

Figure 11. Jean-Paul Gaultier miniature. Collection of Christie and Ed Lefkowith.

En 1989 également, Boucheron, le grand joaillier de la Place Vendôme, lança son premier parfum *Boucheron*. Le flacon, en forme de bague sertie d'un saphir, est somptueux et sobre, tel un joyaux de la maison Boucheron.

Jean-Paul Gaultier est l'enfant terrible de la couture, plein d'imagination, d'audace et d'espièglerie. Ses créations sont toujours mises en vedette par la presse, bien que pas toujours portables. En 1993, le parfum *Jean-Paul Gaultier* fut lancé. Ce flacon-buste fait souvent penser au flacon-buste *Shocking* de Schiaparelli. Mais cette ressemblance n'est que superficielle. Tandis que la présentation de Schiaparelli est romantique, raffinée, précieuse et très feminine, la présentation de Jean-Paul Gaultier est dure, impersonnelle et de style industriel pour grande consommation, avec ce côte unisexe et métallique de science fiction. Dans sa grande taille cette présentation offre une présence inquiétante. Dans sa toute petite taille la présentation-échantillon est amusante et pleine

ing presence. The tiny sample size is amusing and full of humor. This presentation is certainly of our time, and therefore it is quite an artistic success.

In 1994, Nina Ricci launched *Deci-Delà* ['Here and There'], a perfume and a line of products whose name brings to mind the name of one of the first perfumes of Jeanne Lanvin *Comme Ci - Comme Ça* ['So-So']. The avant-garde presentation was designed by Garouste and Bonetti, and the flacon is particularly attractive in bright orangey rose glass, decorated with the biomorphic shapes of microscopic organisms which themselves possess a certain beauty. The asymmetrical stopper resembles a primitive underwater creature, or simply a pebble. The matching box completes the presentation, and the entire line of products is presented with this theme. *Deci-Delà* is a very beautiful creation by Garouste and Bonetti, two innovative and original artists.

The twentieth century has been the grand century of perfume, even if at times, masterpieces have been rare. A renaissance in the art of the presentation has been felt since the beginning of the 1980's, and this century, which is rapidly coming to a close, will nevertheless finish brilliantly, and this thanks to Baccarat, whose extraordinary creations for the perfume industry, spanning more than one hundred years, do not cease to astonish, and are the delight of collectors today. This year Baccarat launches a perfume, its own perfume, an event in the perfume industry. This perfume, the first of a trilogy of perfumes [the two others will be launched in 1998 and in 1999 respectively] is called *Une Nuit étoilée au Bengale* ['A Starry Night in the Bengal'], the first chapter of a legend, *Les Contes d'Ailleurs* ['Tales from Afar'] of Baccarat. *Une Nuit étoilée au Bengale* will only be presented as a limited edition of 1500, to be sold only by Baccarat.

This new creation recalls a tradition in the perfume industry, lacking today, a tradition which brought together in close collaboration and, as of the beginning of the project, the perfume company, the 'nose,' the designer, the glass producer, the printer and the box manufacturer. All these artists worked in unison and without financial constraints to produce something more than a perfume to be marketed, but instead to create a complex work of art likely to arouse intense pleasure and total escape.

This sensual and mysterious perfume with oriental notes, created by Christiane Nagel, is identified by a name which perfectly expresses the lyrical mixture of its rare ingredients, and is presented in a flacon of midnight blue crystal like a heart-shaped teardrop, whose stopper of celestial green crystal seems to jet out of the flacon like a magic exhalation. The flacon is suspended from an arch of clear crystal studded with gilded stars which rests upon the stepped pedestal of a sumptuous box thus completing the staging of the perfume. This presentation, designed by Federico Restepo, is surrounded by a legend of Hindu inspiration, whose text supports the visual aspect and the olfactive sensation of the perfume. Yet these legendary sources of inspiration and this return to a mythic era have done nothing to impede the creation of a work of art of singular and flagrant modernism, which, like every viable work of art, can do no less than express the spirit of its time.

d'humour. Cette présentation est bien de notre temps, donc tout à fait réussie.

En 1994, Nina Ricci lança *Deci-Delà*, un parfum et une ligne de produits dont le nom rappelle celui d'un des premiers parfums de Jeanne Lanvin, *Comme Ci - Comme Ça*. La présentation d'avant garde a été dessinée par Garouste et Bonetti, le flacon étant particulièrement attrayant en verre rose orangé vif, à décor de formes biomorphiques, qui rappellent ces vies microscopiques non dépourvues de beauté. Le bouchon asymétrique ressemble à un animal primitif sous-marin, ou tout simplement à un caillou. La boîte assortie complète la présentation, et toute la gamme de produits est présentée sur ce même thème. Deci-Delà est une très belle création de Garouste et Bonetti, deux artistes novateurs et originaux.

Le XXème siècle a été le grand siècle de la parfumerie, même si, pendant un certain temps, les chefs-d'œuvre se sont faits rares. Une renaissance dans l'art de la présentation s'est fait ressentir depuis le début des années 80 et, ce siècle qui va bientôt s'achever, finira tout de même en beauté — et ceci grâce à Baccarat, dont les extraordinaires créations pour la parfumerie ne cessent d'étonner depuis plus de cent ans, et font la joie des collectionneurs d'aujourd'hui. Car Baccarat lance cette année un parfum, son parfum, un événement dans la parfumerie. Ce parfum, le premier d'une trilogie de parfums (les deux autres seront lancés en 1998 et 1999 respectivement), s'intitule *Une Nuit étoilée au Bengale*, le chapitre premier d'une légende, *Les Contes d'Ailleurs,* de Baccarat. *Une Nuit étoilée au Bengale* ne sera présenté qu'en édition limitée et numérotée, tirée à 1500 exemplaires, en vente chez Baccarat, exclusivement.

Cette nouvelle création remonte vers une tradition, aujourd'hui disparue, une tradition dans la parfumerie qui réunissait en collaboration étroite, et dès le départ d'un projet, le parfumeur, le nez, l'artiste concepteur, la cristallerie, l'imprimerie et la cartonnerie. Tous ces créateurs travaillaient, en unisson, sans contraintes financières, pour produire beaucoup plus qu'un parfum à commercialiser, mais pour créer une œuvre artistique complexe, capable de susciter un plaisir intense et une évasion totale.

Ce parfum, sensuel et mystérieux, aux notes orientales, créé par Christiane Nagel, identifié par un nom qui exprime parfaitement le mélange lyrique de ses rares ingrédients, est présenté dans un flacon en cristal bleu-nuit, tel une goutte en forme de coeur, dont le bouchon en cristal d'un vert astral semble jaillir du flacon, tel un effluve magique. Ce flacon est suspendu à une arche en cristal incolore, constellée d'or qui repose sur le socle à gradins d'un somptueux coffret complétant ainsi la mise en scène du parfum. Cette présentation, conçue par Federico Restepo, est entourée d'une légende d'inspiration indoue, dont le texte sert de support à l'aspect visuel et à la sensation olfactive du parfum. Ces sources d'inspiration légendaires et ce retour aux temps mythiques n'ont pas empêché, bien au contraire, la création d'une œuvre d'art d'un modernisme flagrant et singulier, qui comme toute œuvre d'art valable ne peut qu'exprimer l'esprit de son temps.

Correspondence for the author can be addressed to:
Christie M. Lefkowith, FDR Station, PO Box 5200, New York, N.Y. 10150-5200.

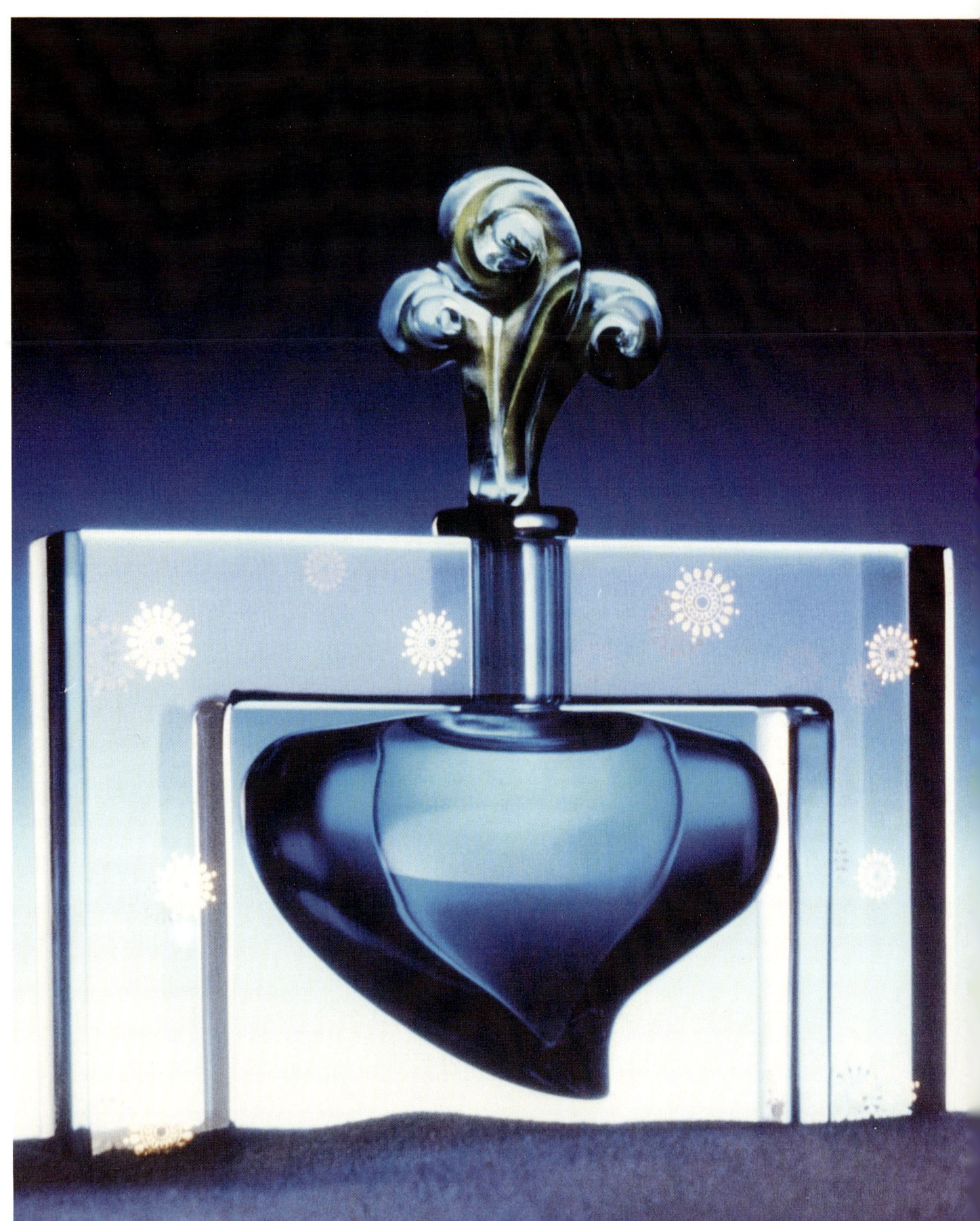

Figure 12. Baccarat *Une Nuit étoilée au Bengale*. Courtesy of Compagnie des Cristailleries de Baccarat.

Meisterwerke der heutigen Zeit

Seit 1950 wurden viele kleine Parfümfirmen, jede mit eigenem Stil der Präsentation, von grossen Konglomeraten gekauft. Diese neue Richtung behauptete sich mehr und mehr, besonders zwischen 1960 und 1980. Da diese Parfümfirmen dadurch ihre Unabhängigkeit und ihre kreative Kapazität verloren hatten, mussten sie sich den Bedürfnissen grosser industrieller Gruppen von internationalem Einfluss beugen und in einer mehr zentralisierten und somit einer leistungsfähigeren Weise produzieren. Der Mangel an befähigten Kunsthandwerkern, wie auch die erhöhten Handwerkskosten, verstärkten das Bedürfnis, völlig mechanisierte Parfüm-Präsentationen herzustellen. Industrialisierung erlaubte eine Herabsetzung der Produktionskosten und modernes Leben schränkte originelle und luxuriöse Parfüm-Präsentationen ein. Neue Techniken und neue Materialien drangen in den Produktionsprozess ein. Zum Beispiel entstanden Stöpsel mit einer Plastikspitze, die einen dichten Verschluss garantierten und Mattglasstöpsel ersetzten. Dies begrenzte die Produktion schöpferischer und origineller Präsentationen in den 60er und den 70er Jahren. Es war eine traurige Zeit für die Parfüm-Industrie.

Dennoch wurde in 1960 eine extraordinäre Präsentation in einer speziell limitierten Auflage von 100 Stück erschaffen: *Bal à Versailles* von Jean Desprez. Eine Rückkehr zur grossen französischen Tradition luxuriöser Parfüme, vergleichbar mit den grossen Meisterwerken der 20er Jahre. Jean Desprez (1889-1973) stammte aus einer Familie von Parfümherstellern ab, da seine Urgrossmutter Mme. Félix Millot war. Er arbeitete für Les Parfums Millot und erschuf in 1925 *Crêpe de Chine*, einer der grossen Erfolge des Jahrhunderts. In 1938 gründete er sein eigenes Haus und brachte in 1939 die Parfüme *Grande Dame* und *Votre Main* (Deine Hand) heraus, beide benannt in einer Hommage an seine Mutter, eine elegante und gebildete Dame und eine Pianistin mit wunderschönen Händen. Nachdem er den Laden der Parfümerie d'Orsay in der Rue de la Paix No. 17 in Paris entweder in 1939 oder in 1943 übernommen hatte (es bestehen diesbezüglich widersprüchliche Daten), liess er ihn von seinem guten Freund, Léon Leyritz (1888-1976) dekorieren. Leyritz war auch ein Maler und Gestalter von Bühnendekorationen und entwarf von Beginn an sowohl Flasche als auch das graphische Design der Jean Desprez Parfüme.

Das Parfüm *Bal à Versailles*, in 1962 herausgebracht und zuerst von Nieman Marcus in Dallas verkauft, erfreute sich sofort eines internationalen Erfolges. Um diesen Erfolg von *Bal à Versailles* und das Prestige der Jean Desprez Parfüme zu kennzeichnen, erschuf Léon Leyritz in 1969 eine limitierte Präsentation davon, die hauptsächlich von Nieman Marcus zu einem exorbitanten Preis von $850 verkauft wurde. Schmeichelhafte Artikel in der amerikanischen Presse, besonders in der New York Times, erwirkten, dass die limitierte Edition sofort ausverkauft war, da es ersichtlich war, dass dieses wunderbare Objekt wert war gesammelt zu werden. Die Flasche und ihr kleiner innerer Stöpsel, beide schneeweiss, sind aus unglasiertem weissen Porzellan von Sèvres. Die Flasche verkörpert Janus, einen mythischen Charakter, den ältesten König Latiums. Sie ist mit einer Kappe aus feinem Gold und Sterling Silber verziert, geschaffen von einem der grossen Juweliere dieser Zeit, und ist in Form einer Krone gehalten, in deren Mitte sich ein Wasserstrahl befindet. Die Flasche wird in einem luxuriösem Etui aus rotem Leder präsentiert, verziert und vergoldet. Es lässt sich durch zwei Türen öffnen, die in weisser Seide ausgeschlagen sind, im Kontrast zu rotem Samt als Hintergrund, der auch die weisse Flasche hervorhebt. Am hinteren Teil des Etuis ist eine bewegliche Stütze angebracht, die es erlaubt die Schachtel aufzustellen, etwas nach hinten abgeschrägt, ähnlich eines Rahmens für ein kostbares Kunstwerk.

Die Legende erzählt, dass Saturn, von seinem eigenen Sohn Jupiter aus den Himmeln vertrieben, Zuflucht in Latium nahm, wo er von König Janus mit offenen Armen empfangen wurde. Dort fand er Frieden und Wohlergehen und voller Dankbarkeit gegenüber König Janus beschenkte er ihn mit einer wunderbaren Eigenschaft: Die Kraft mit seinen Augen gleichzeitig die Vergangenheit wie auch die Zukunft zu sehen. Diese doppelte Fähigkeit führte dazu, dass er mit zwei Gesichtern dargestellt wird. Janus wurde von den Römern als eine Gottheit betrachtet, und sein Tempel in Rom war nur zu Friedenszeiten geschlossen, was nur einmal für einen Zeitraum von neun Monaten innerhalb tausend Jahren der Fall war. Für die Römer war Janus der erste Gott, Vater aller anderen, der Gott der Morgendämmerung und der Sonne, der Gott der offenen Türen, der Gott der strömenden Wasser und der Gott der Kommunikation.

Diese prächtige weisse Kreation von Léon Leyritz verkörpert eine Rückkehr zu der Vergangenheit. Über ihren neoklassizistischen und neoromantischen Stil hinaus (der zum Ende von 1930 so sehr in Mode war, der Ära in der Jean Desprez sein Parfümhaus gegründet hatte), vertritt sie auch einen Blick hin in die Zukunft des Parfüms *Bal à Versailles*, eines der best verkauften Parfüme der Welt. - Von der Seite her gesehen, stellt die Flasche sehr gut den Gott Janus mit zwei Gesichtern dar. Aber von vorne oder von hinten gesehen (beide Seiten sind identisch), ist der Eindruck völlig anders, da sie ein sehr weiches und feminines Gesicht und eine Damenbüste mit einer Perlenkette zeigen. Aus diesem Blickwinkel ähnelt sie einer der Statuen auf Podesten, wie man sie im Park des Schlosses von Versailles findet, aber bedeckt mit Wasserstrahlen, wie es auch im Park der Fall ist. Möglicherweise wurde die Präsentation aus diesem femininen Aspekt heraus bald *La Janusette* genannt, die feminine Form von Janus.

La Janusette ist eine ausserordentlich rare Präsentation, ein Meisterwerk der artistischen Parfüm-Industrie de Luxe. Eine grosse, viereckige Puderdose ist überzogen mit gelbem Satin und weisser Seide und dekoriert mit einem weissen Medaillon aus unglasiertem weissen Porzellan von Sèvres; wie ein Basrelief, das eine Person des klassischen Altertums darstellt. Dieses Medaillon ähnelt sehr stark den ersten graphischen Entwürfen, die für Nina Ricci in weissem Papier, ebenfalls im Basrelief-Stil, geschaffen und ausgeführt wurden. Diese prachtvolle Puderdose scheint noch rarer zu sein als *La Janusette*.

Ein neuer kreativer Wind war um das Jahr 1980 herum spürbar. Zeichen der Wiederbelebung waren in der Entwicklung neuer Kreationen in moderater Preisgruppe sichtbar, was seit den 50er Jahren nicht mehr der Fall war.

Das Parfüm von Niki de Saint-Phalle, auf allen Märkten in 1980 herausgebracht, ist eines der allerschönsten Kreationen der Parfüm-Industrie dieser Zeit. Niki de Saint-Phalle, eine Bildhauerin der französischen Schule, wurde 1930 geboren und lebte in New York von 1933 bis 1951, was vielleicht ihre Neigung für surrealistische Kunst, abstrakten Expressionismus und *l'art brut* erklärt. Nachdem sie in 1952 nach Paris zurückgekehrt war, begann sie zu malen und entwickelte sich Schritt für Schritt hin zur Bildhauerei und zu einem barocken, fantastischen und sehr farbenfreudigen Stil, was dazu führte, dass sie in 1961 in die Schule der *neuen Realisten* aufgenommen wurde. Es wurde sehr viel über sie geredet und da sie eine künstlerische und weltliche Berühmtheit geworden war, borgte sie ihren Namen und ihr Talent der Parfümkreation. Dieses Parfüm ist in einer Flasche und Schachtel präsentiert, die beide mit einem Motiv von lebhaft gefärbten, ineinander verwundenen Schlangen dekoriert sind, Symbole der *l'art brut* und des *Kobra-Geistes*, einer künstlerischen Bewegung, die besonders in den 60er Jahren florierte. Diese Präsentation, welche heute nicht leicht rar werden kann, ist nichtsdestotrotz ein wetvoller Teil einer eindrucksvollen Sammlung.

Eine weitere wunderschöne Präsentation war *Sculptura* von Jovan, in 1981 herausgebracht und für den Massenmarkt hergestellt. Es gab drei Modelle für Flaschen in mattiertem Glas, die eigentlich Zerstäuber sind, auf einem Podest aus schwarzer Plastik, das den Metallteil des Zerstäubers verbirgt, auf den Kopf gestellt. (Es handelt sich hierbei um dasselbe Prinzip der Präsentation wie *Gardez-moi* von Jovoy, 1926, der berühmten schwarzen Kristallflasche von Baccarat in der Form einer Katze auf einem Sockel aus gelber Seide.) Die drei Flaschen für *Sculptura* stellen drei vereinfachte Skulpturen modernen Erscheinungsbildes dar, die den Namen des Parfüms vorbildlich erläutern, wie auch eine durchdachte Eleganz, die für diese Zeit sehr einzigartig war.

Christian Dior brachte in 1985 ein *starkes* Parfüm heraus, das sich von den in Mode befindlichen Parfümen sehr unterschied. Es wurde in einer Flasche in tieffarbenem violett und einer passenden Schachtel präsentiert. Es ist eine schöne Darstellung, nicht mehr. Als Kontrast wurde eine Armspangenflasche in einer limitierten Auflage hergestellt, als Geschenk gedacht und nicht zum Verkauf bestimmt. Sie hatte die Form einer stilisierten Schlange, boshaft und elegant. Dies war eine sehr schöne Kreation, einzuordnen irgendwo zwischen einem Parfüm und einem Mode-Accessoire.

Mit Kreationen von zeitgenössischen Arbeiten, die nichtsdestotrotz einen Blick zurück darbieten, machen grosse Designer oft Anspielungen auf ihre Vergangenheit. Bei Cartier war dies der Fall. Juweliere seit 1847 und Parfümschöpfer seit 1981. Das Parfüm *Panthère* wurde in 1987 in einer mit zwei Panthern dekorierten Flasche herausgebracht; Anspielung auf den Schmuck mit Panthern, der vor dem Krieg so sehr in Mode war. Die Musterflasche ist in ihrer sehr winzigen Grösse besonders ansprechend und sehr schwierig herzustellen. Sie ist eine der schönsten Miniaturen der 80er Jahre.

Isabelle Canovas, eine Schöpferin von Mode-Accessoires der Haute Couture, eröffnete vor über zehn Jahren eine Boutique in New York auf der Madison Avenue in der Nähe der 65. Strasse und brachte ihr eigenes Parfüm fast zur gleichen Zeit heraus. Diese prächtige Flasche aus dunklem, marineblauem Glas mit Vergoldung verkörpert eine lederne Quaste mit Goldkordeln, die häufig Handtaschen und Gürtel ihrer Boutique dekorierte, symbolisch für den Isabelle Canovas Stil. Die gigantische Flasche mit Vergoldung und möglicherweise einzigartig, mit einem echten Glas Stöpsel (ohne Plastik) und von ausserordentlicher Qualität, war meistens im Schaufenster ihrer Boutique ausgestellt. Isabelle Canovas meldete während des Golfkrieges Bankrott an und diese wunderbare Flasche, einzigartig in ihrer Grösse, ist möglicherweise der einzig verbliebene Beweis dieser Boutique, die wie keine andere war.

Christian Lacroix, der inspirierte Modeschöpfer, gab sein Debut bei Jean Patou. Sein avant-garde Stil, im Gegensatz zum Patou-Stil, wurde von der Presse sehr gut kommentiert und bald danach gründete er sein eigenes Modehaus. Seine provencialischen Ursprünge und seine Liebe für Spanien kann man in seinem Modestil und in der Flasche seines Parfüms *C'est La Vie!!* finden, das in 1989 herauskam. Von Garouste und Bonetti entworfen (zwei Künstlern, die ein Team formten um Innen-Accessoires und mannigfaltige Kunst-Objekte zu kreieren), ist die Flasche eine Mischung von komplexen Allusionen. Sie ähnelt einem menschlichen Herz, und ihr Stöpsel könnte sehr wohl der Anfang zweier Arterien sein - Symbole des Lebens. Er ähnelt auch einem Korallenzweig - Symbol der Sonne und der Wärme, nahe zu Christian Lacroix's südlicher Abstammung. Das Parfüm war kein grosser Erfolg, und deshalb findet man es heute nicht leicht. Es ist wahrhaftig eine moderne Kreation, die keiner anderen ähnelt, eine sehr schöne Flasche für eine Sammlung.

Ebenfalls in 1989 brachte Boucheron, der grosse Juwelier des Place Vendôme, das eigene Parfüm *Boucheron* heraus. Die Flasche in Form eines Ringes mit einem Saphir gefasst ist kostspielig und solide, genau wie ein Juwel der Boucheron-Niederlassung.

Jean-Paul Gaultier ist das *enfant terrible* der hohen Mode. Voller Erfindungskraft, Verwegenheit und Ausgelassenheit, sind seine Kreationen immer ein Treffer bei der Presse, auch wenn sie nicht immer tragbar sind. Das *Parfüm Jean-Paul Gaultier* kam 1993 heraus. Diese als Büste geformte Flasche erinnert an die ihr ähnelnde von Schiaparelli *Shocking*. Aber diese Ähnlichkeit ist nur oberflächlich, da Schiaparelli's Präsentation romantisch, vornehm, edel und sehr feminin ist. Der Stil der Jean-Paul Gaultier Präsentation ist hart, unpersönlich und in einem unisex und metallenen Aspekt des Science-Fiction-Stils und in der industriellen Art des Massenverbrauchs gehalten. In der grossen Ausführung hat diese Darstellung eine beunruhigende Präsenz. In ihrer sehr kleinen Mustergrösse ist sie amüsierend und voller Humor. Diese Präsentation ist ganz bestimmt aus unserer Zeit und somit ist sie ein wahrhafter künstlerischer Erfolg.

Deci-Delà (Hier und Dort) wurde von Nina Ricci in 1994 herausgebracht, ein Parfüm und eine Produktionslinie, dessen Name den eines der ersten Parfüme von Jeanne Lanvin *Comme Ci - Comme Ça* (Wie Dies oder Das) in Erinnerung bringt. Die avant-garde Präsentation wurde von Garouste und Bonetti entworfen. Die Flasche war besonders attraktiv in hell orangenem Rosetten-Glas, dekoriert mit biomorphischem Netzwerk, das an mikroskopische Organismen erinnert, die selbst nicht ohne Schönheit sind. Der asymmetrische Stöpsel ähnelt einer primitiven Unterwasser-Kreatur, oder einfach einem Kieselstein. Die passende Schachtel vervollständigt die Präsentation und die komplette Linie der Produkte ist in diesem Thema dargestellt. *Deci-Delà* ist eine wunderschöne Kreation von Garouste und Bonetti, zwei innovative und originelle Künstler.

Das 20. Jahrhundert war das grösste Jahrhundert für Parfüm, wenn auch die Meisterwerke während einiger Perioden selten waren. Die Renaissance der Kunst der Präsentation ist seit Beginn der 80er Jahre spürbar und dieses Jahrhundert, welches rapide seinem Ende zugeht, wird nichtsdestotrotz in Schönheit enden. Dank an Baccarat, dessen extraordinäre Kreationen für die Parfüm-Industrie über mehr als einhundert Jahre nicht aufhören zu erstaunen und welche die Wonne der heutigen Sammler sind. In 1997 brachte Baccarat sein eigenes Parfüm heraus, ein Ereignis in der Parfüm-Industrie. Dieses Parfüm, als erstes einer Trilogie von Parfümen (die beiden anderen erscheinen in 1998 bzw. 1999) wird *Une Nuit Etoilée au Bengale* (Eine sternenbeleuchtete Nacht in den Bengalen) genannt, das erste Kapitel einer Legende *Les Contes d'Ailleurs* (Geschichten aus der Ferne) von Baccarat. *Une Nuit étoilée au Bengale* wird nur in einer limitierten Edition von 1,500 Stück erscheinen und nur von Baccarat verkauft werden.

Diese neue Kreation ruft eine Tradition in der Parfüm-Industrie zurück, an der es heute mangelt; eine Tradition, welche die Parfüm-Firma, die "Nase", den Designer, den Glashersteller, den Drucker und den Hersteller der Schachtel von Anfang an in enger Kollaboration zusammenbrachte. Alle diese Kunsthandwerker arbeiteten im Gleichklang und ohne finanzielle Einschränkungen um etwas herzustellen, das mehr als nur ein Produkt, sondern stattdessen ein komplexes Kunstwerk war, das fähig sei Freude und totale Entrückung zu erwecken.

Dieses sinnliche und mysteriöse Parfüm mit orientalischem Einschlag, von Christiane Nagel erschaffen, wird durch seinen Namen, der sehr genau seine lyrische Mischung und seltenen Inhaltsstoffe erklärt, identifiziert. Die Flasche ist aus mitternachtsblauem Kristall, geformt als herzförmige Träne, und ihr Stöpsel aus astral-grünem Kristall scheint wie ein magischer Strom aus der Flasche zu entweichen. Die Flasche hängt an einem Bogen aus goldverziertem Kristall und sitzt auf einem stufenförmigen Podest, dessen Schachtel die Bühne für das Parfüm bildet. Diese Präsentation, von Federico Restopo entworfen, ist umringt von einer hindustanisch inspirierten Legende, dessen Text die visuellen Aspekte und die geruchsinnlichen Sensationen des Parfüms unterstützen.

Diese legendären Quellen der Inspiration und diese Rückkehr zu einer mythischen Ära, konnten dennoch die Kreation von Kunstwerken eines einzigartigen und offenkundigen Modernismus nicht verhindern, der, wie jedes lebensfähige Werk der Kunst, nichts weniger tun kann als den Geist seiner Zeit auszudrücken.

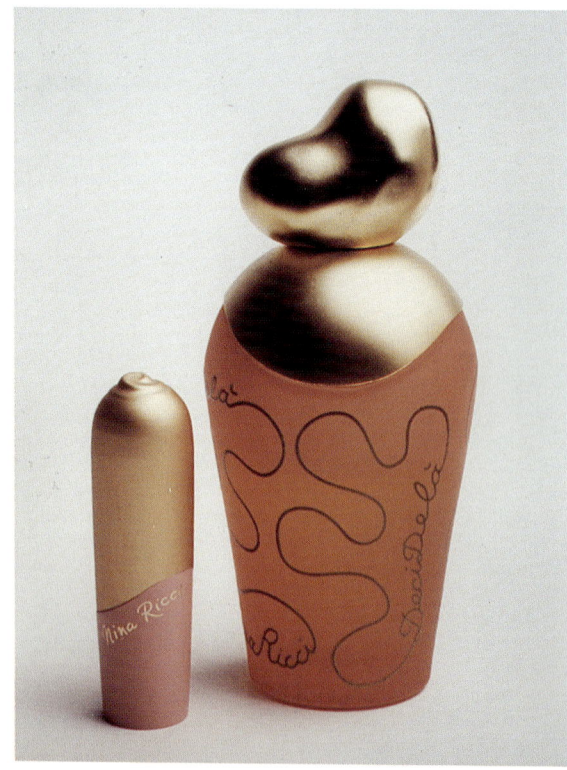

Figure 13. Nina Ricci *Deci-Delà,* with lipstick. Collection of Christie and Ed Lefkowith.

AUCTION LOTS
MINIATURES
SAMPLES
FLACONS DE SAC
FIRST SIZES
COMPACTS
SOLIDS

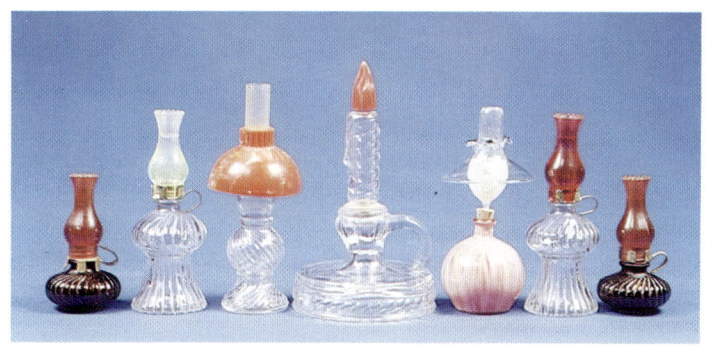

Lot #1. Collection of seven novelty perfumes shaped as lamps: two of amber glass with red plastic shades, 2.5" [6.4 cm]; one molded as a candle and mounted in a glass candleholder, 4.5" [11.4 cm]; two molded of clear glass, one with a red shade, one with a yellow one, each 3.6" [9.1 cm]; one molded of clear glass with a marbelized red plastic shade, 4.2" [10.7 cm]; one of blown glass with a glass shade, 3.6" [9.1 cm]; all empty, of American manufacture. Seven items. Est. $50.00-$100.00.

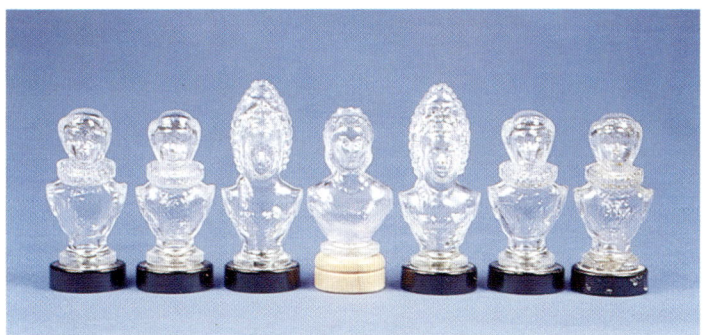

Lot #2. Collection of seven small glass bottles mounted on plastic or wood bases, each molded as a bust of a 17th or 18th century European lady, height of the tallest 3.8" [9.7 cm], all empty. Seven items. Est. $50.00-$75.00.

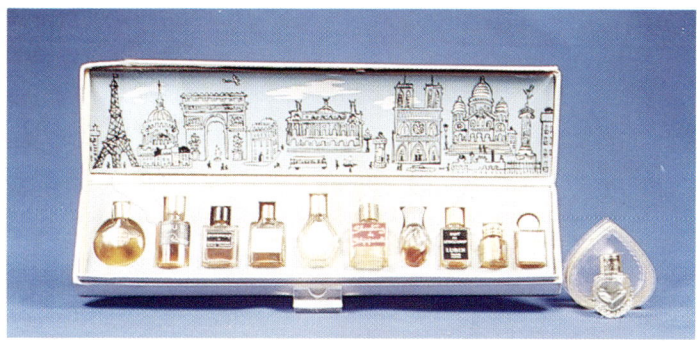

Lot #3. Les Parfums de Paris Set #1 Opera with ten glass miniatures: Worth *Je Reviens*, Dana *Tabu*, Balenciaga *Quadrille*, Raphael *Réplique*, D'Albret *Ecusson*, Schiaparelli *Shocking*, Révillon *Carnet de Bal*, Lubin *Nuit de Longchamp*, Le Galion *Bourrasque*, Lucien Lelong *Indiscret*, in their white box which is worn; Nina Ricci *Coeur-Joie* glass mini heart-shaped bottle with gold cap, in its plastic box with label around the sides. 11 minis total. Est. $150.00-$200.00.

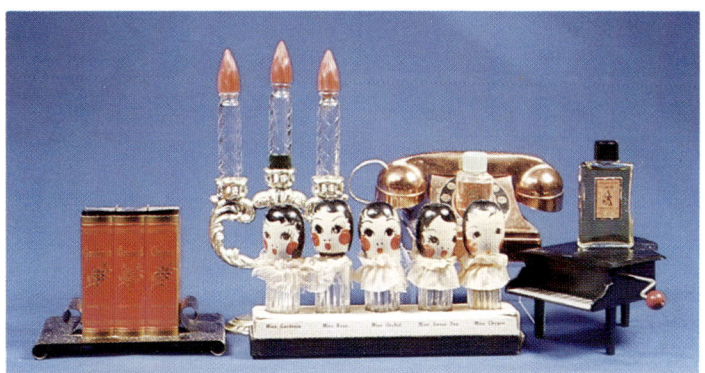

Lot #4. Lot of 5 novelty perfumes: Cardinal *Book of Perfume Bouquet*, *Gardenia*, *Chypre* glass book-shaped minis with black caps, in a metal bookcase holder; Karoff *Floral Quints Miss Rose*, etc., glass bottles with wood caps, cover lacking; Charles V *Cheval Bleu* glass mini in a piano music box; Candelabra set of three glass candle minis in a plastic candelabra; B. Ansehl *Number Please* glass mini in a plastic telephone. Five items. Est. $100.00-$150.00.

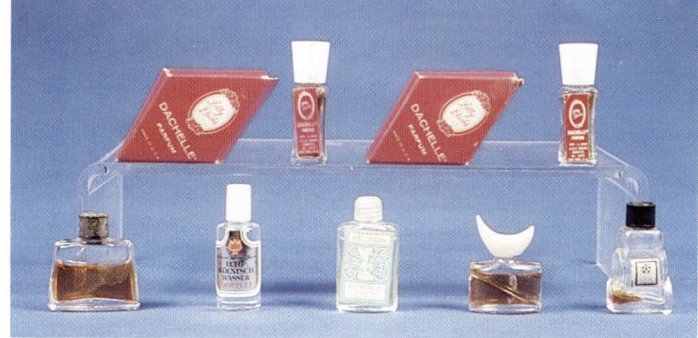

Lot #5. Lot of 7 minis: Ciro *New Horizons*; Lily Daché *Dachelle*, two examples, each in its red box; *Echt Kölnisch Wasser*; Fuller Brush *Beckon*; J.-M. Sinan *Sinan*; unidentified perfumer *OK*. Seven items. Est. $100.00-$150.00.

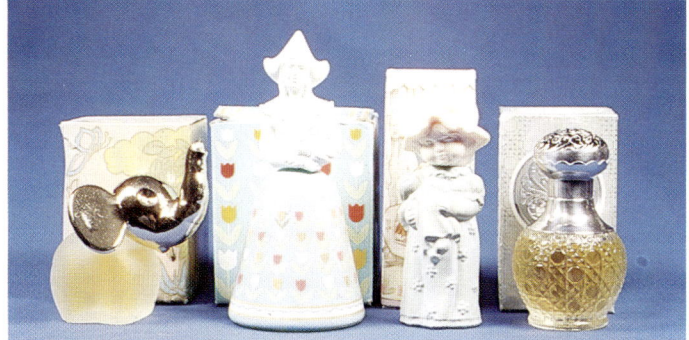

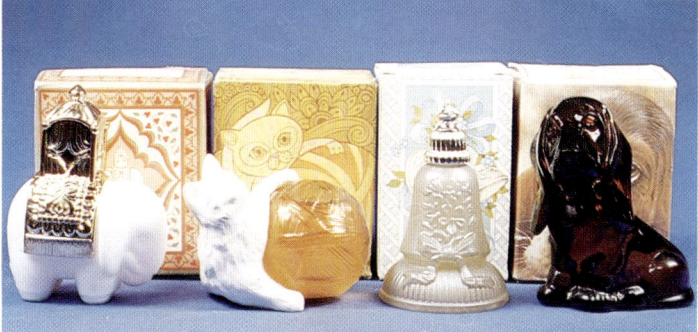

Lot #6. Lot of 8 Avon perfumes in their original boxes, various heights: *Brocade, Charisma Joyous Bell, Charisma Royal Elephant, Imperial Garden Cologne Good Luck Elephant, Moonwind Dutch Maid, Occur! Little Dream Girl, Sonnet Kitten Petite, Sweet Honesty Baby Basset*. Eight items. Est. $75.00-$150.00.

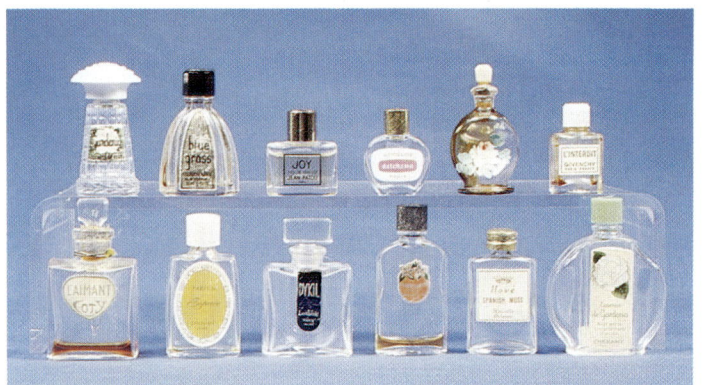 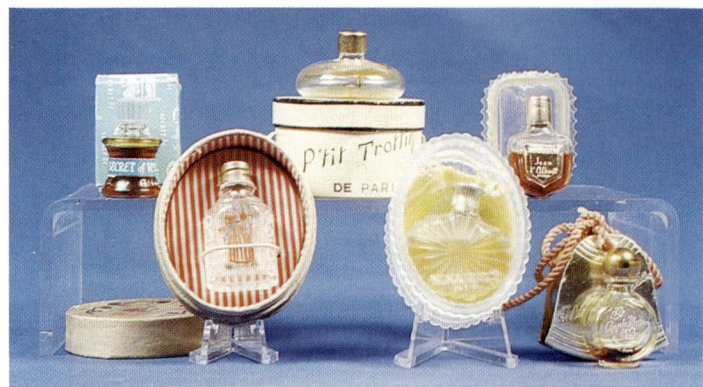

Lot #7. Lot of 18 minis: Elizabeth Arden *Blue Grass;* Bo-Kay *Orange Blossom;* Cheramy *Espace, Essence de Gardenia;* Coty *L'Aimant* glass tester; d'Albret *Ecusson* in its plastic case; Cecile D'Avril *Hey-Day;* Duchess of Paris *Gardenia;* Givenchy *L'Interdit;* Hové *Spanish Moss;* Lenthéric *Dykil* [glass stopper]; Moehr *Mimosa* in its *P'tit Trottin* hatbox, Patou *Joy;* Révillon *Detchema;* Ricci *L'Air du Temps* frosted sunburst, signed *Lalique,* in its plastic case; Helena Rubenstein *Apple Blossom* in its bell box; Shulton *Early American* in its box; Weil *Secret of Venus* in its box. 18 items. Est. $255.00-$510.00.

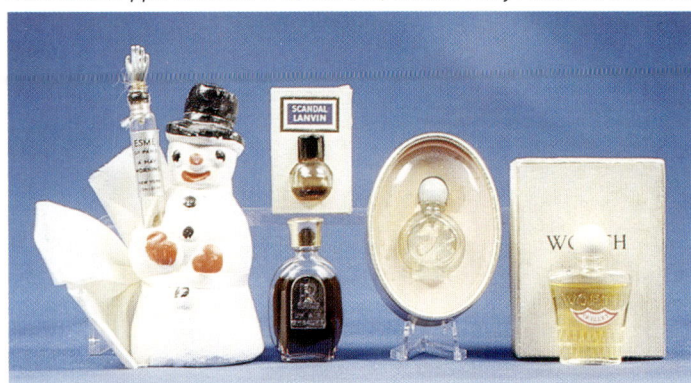 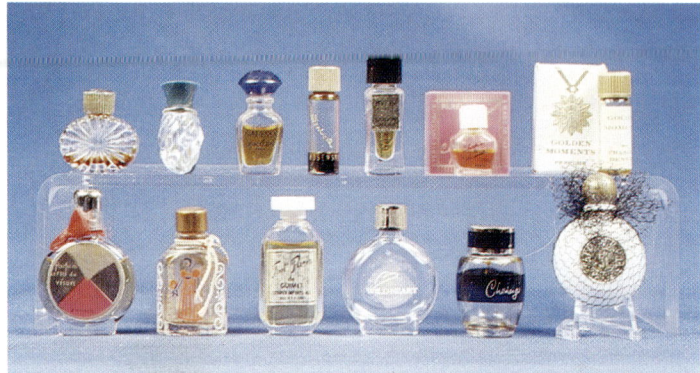

Lot #8. Lot of 18 minis: Frances Denney *Chenango, Golden Moments,* in its box; Esmé of Paris *A May Morning,* in a snowman holder; Guerlain *Nahema;* Guimet *Tout Paris;* Lanvin *My Sin, Scandal,* in its box; Révillon *Carnet de Bal;* Revlon *Wildheart;* Ricci *L'Air du Temps;* Rigaud *Un Air Embaumé;* Rochas *La Rose;* Rosenstein *Odalisque;* Helena Rubenstein *Heaven Sent,* in its oval box; Schiaparelli *Shocking* in plastic cube; Shulton *Early American;* unidentified maker *Le Feu de Vésuve;* Worth *Oeillet* in its box. 18 items. Est. $270.00-$540.00.

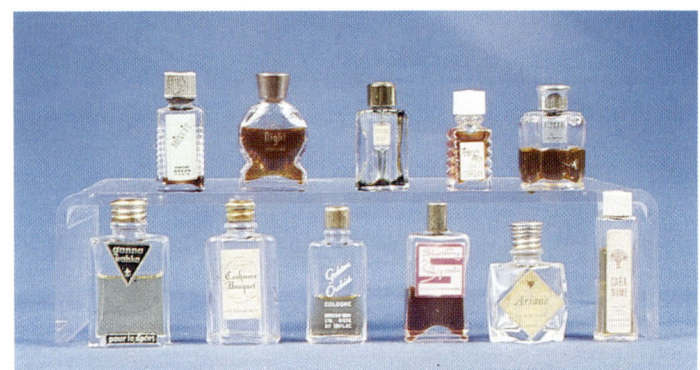 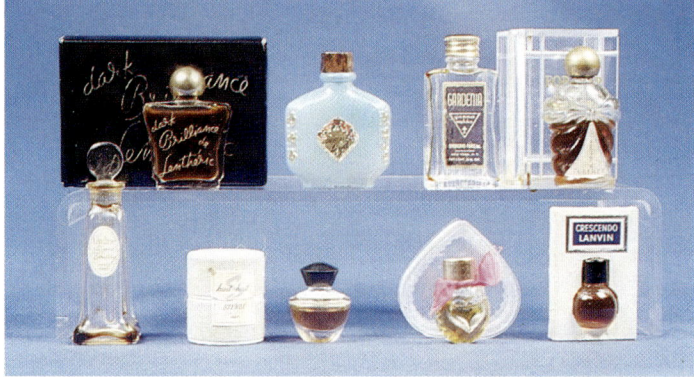

Lot #9. Lot of 19 minis: Cara Nome *Cara Nome;* Colgate *Cashmere Bouquet;* Corday *Toujours Moi;* Dana *Emir;* Kay Daumit [Kathryn] *Forever Amber* in its lucite case; Dorothy Gray *Golden Orchid;* Heim *Ariane;* Lanvin *Crescendo* in its box; Lazell *Sweet Pea;* Lelong *Opening Night;* Lenthéric *Dark Brilliance* in its box; Countess Maritza *Silent Night;* Odéon *Minuit;* Ricci *Coeur-Joie* in its plastic case; Schiaparelli *Shocking;* Sterlé *Huit-Huit* in its box; Suzanne Thierry *Ondine* glass tester; Ganna Walska *Pour le Sport, Gardenia.* 19 items. Est. $275.00-$475.00.

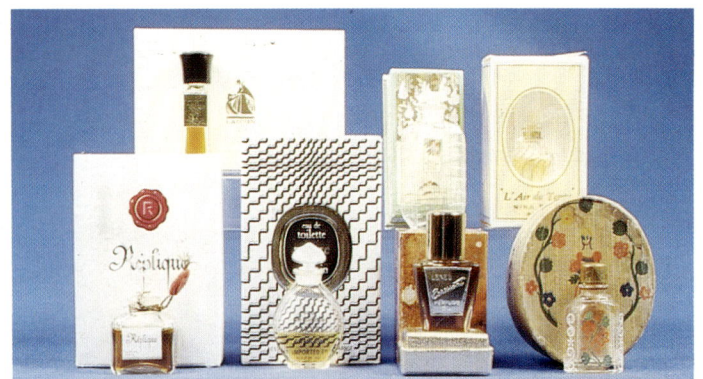 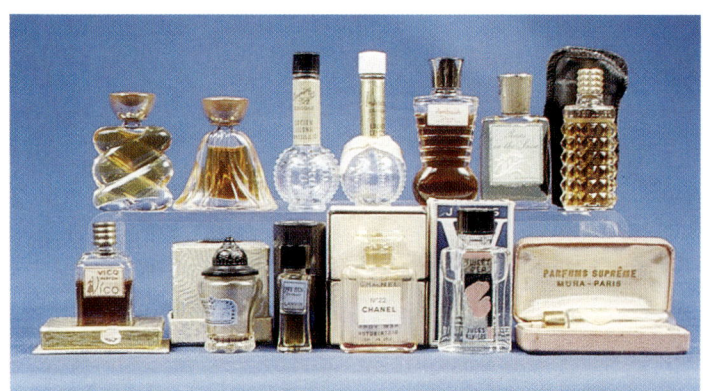

Lot #10. Lot of 20 glass minis with caps, various sizes: Chanel *#22* in box; Cheramy *April Showers* in box; Dana *Ambush, Roses in the Snow;* Duchess of Paris *Infatuation* in box; Guerlain *Parure* in box; Lanvin *Crescendo* in box, *My Sin* in box; Lelong *Indiscret* [2 diff.], *Opening Night, Sirôcco;* Lenel *Caressant* in box; Lubin *Nuit de Longchamp* in pouch; Mura *Rare Orchid* in pink box; Raphael *Réplique* in box; Ricci *L'Air du Temps* single dove in box; J. Riviere *Sweet Pea* in box; Shulton *Old Spice* in box; Vicq *Vicq* parfum. 20 items. Est. $100.00-$200.00.

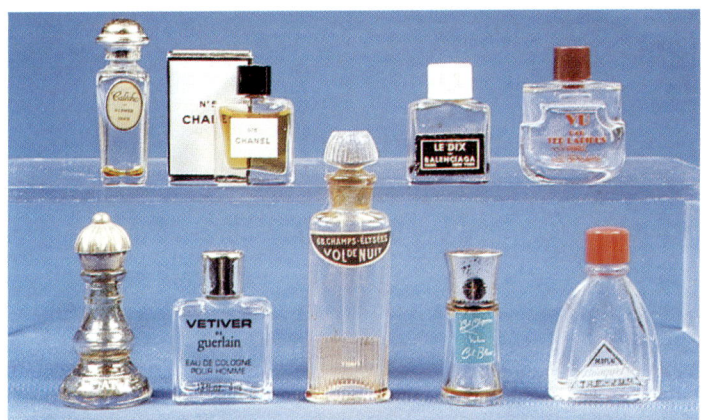
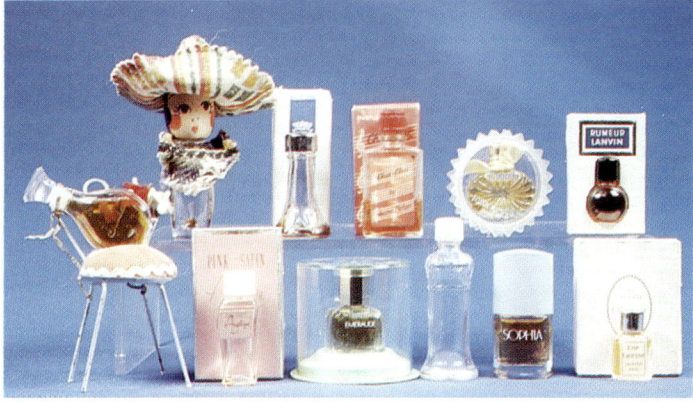

Lot #11. Lot of 20 minis: Angelique *Pink Satin* in its box; Balenciaga *Le Dix*; Ceil Chapman *Ceil Bleue*; Chanel *No. 5* in its box; Mary Chess *Strategy*; Coty *Emeraude* in its plastic case; *Sophia*; Guerlian *Vetiver* and *Vol de Nuit* rare glass tester; Hermès *Calèche*, Houbigant *Chantilly* on its chair, Karoff *Buckarette*, Lanvin *Rumeur*; Ted Lapidus *Vu*; Lily Bermuda *Jasmin*; Matchabelli *Spring Fancy*; Obéron *Une Caresse*; André Philippe *Cha-Cha* in its red box; Ricci *L'Air du Temps* in its plastic case; Tré-Jur *Bouquet*. Twenty minis. Est. $300.00-$500.00.

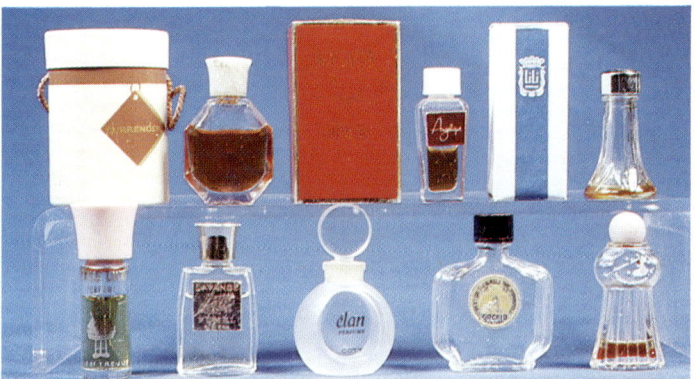
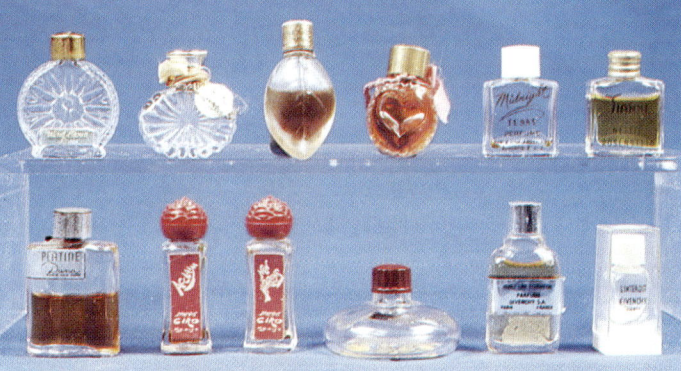

Lot #12. Lot of 20 minis: Angelique *Red Satin* in its box; Bordighera; Ciro *Acclaim, New Horizons, Surrender* in its box; Coty *Elan*; Dana *Platine*; Funel *Lavande*; Givenchy *Gentleman, L'Interdit* in its plastic case; Lili Bermuda *Easter Lily* in its box; Renaud *Orchid*; Ricci *Coeur-Joie, Fille d'Eve, L'Air du Temps*; Rosenstein *Tianne*; Helena Rubenstein *Heaven Sent*; Tré-Jur *Little Lulu*; Tussy *Midnight*; unidentified perfumer *Wind Blown Roses*. Twenty items. Est. $300.00-$600.00.

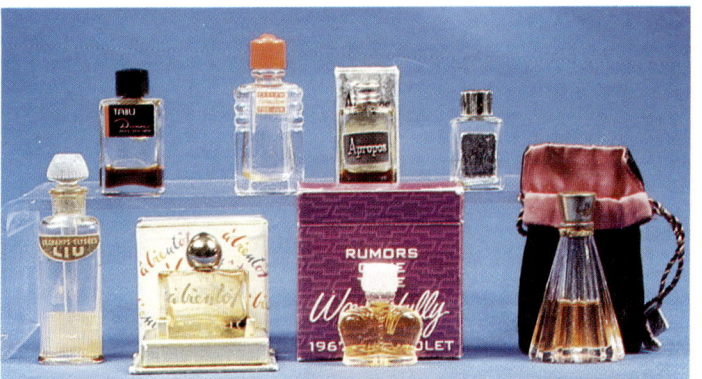
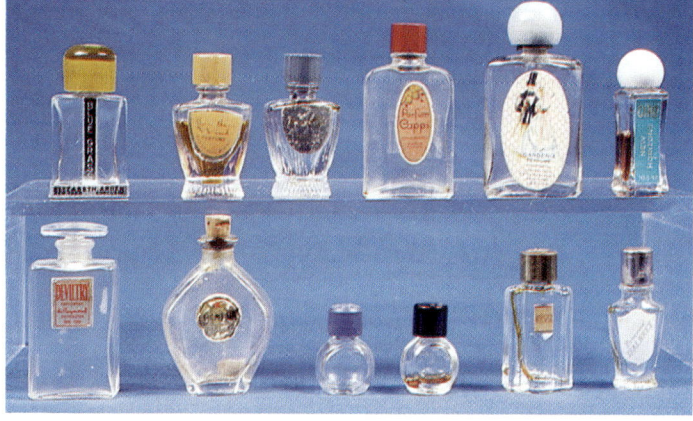

Lot #13. Lot of 20 minis: Elizabeth Arden *Blue Grass*; Bourjois *On the Wind, Moon Tide*; Cheramy *Parfum Cappi*; Churchill *Gardenia*; Ciro *New Horizons*; d'Albret *Princesse*; Dana *Tabu*; De Raymond *Deviltry* with glass stopper; D'Orsay *Intoxication* in its black bag; Guerlian *Liu* rare glass tester; Jergens *Ben-Hur*; Lanvin *Arpège, Crescendo*; Lelong *Whisper*; Lenthéric *A Bientôt* in its box; Matchabelli *Cachet* and *Prophecy* in its box [1967 Chevrolet]; Tré-Jur *Carnation*; unidentified perfumer *Apropos*. 20 items. Est. $400.00-$700.00.

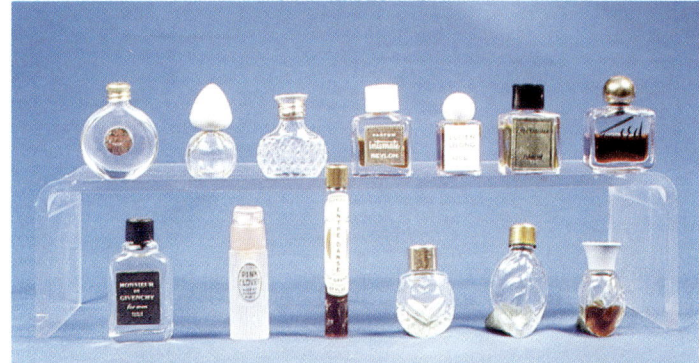
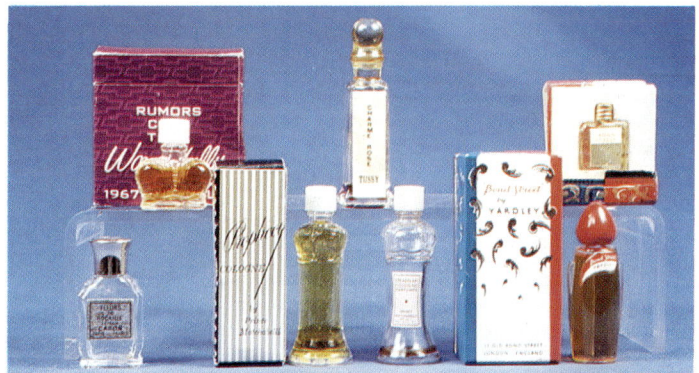

Lot #14. Lot of 20 minis: Harriet Hubbard Ayer *Pink Clover*; Caron *Fleurs de Rocaille*; Grandee *Entre Danse*; Lenthéric *Tweed*; Givenchy *Monsieur*; Lelong *Indiscret*; Matchabelli *Prophecy* cologne in its box and *Prophecy* crown in its box [both Chevrolet], *Stradivari*; Révillon *Carnet de Bal*; Revlon *Intimate*; Ricci *Capricci, Coeur-Joie, Fille d'Eve*; Tuvaché *Nectaroma*; Tussy *Charme Rose* glass tester; Worth *Je Reviens*; Yardley *Bond Street* in its very rare tiny matchbook box and a different bottle, *Lotus*, also in its box. 20 items. Est. $300.00-$600.00.

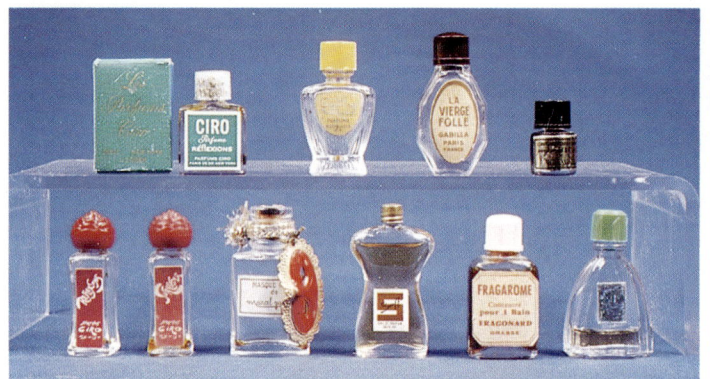 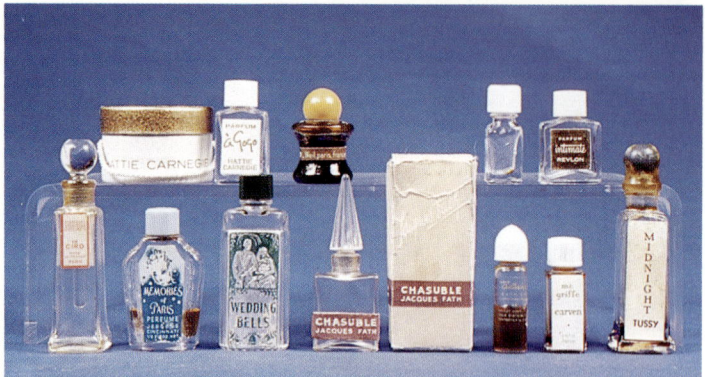

Lot #15. Lot of 21 minis: Bourjois *On The Wind*; Hattie Carnegie *A Gogo*, in hatbox; Carven *Ma Griffe*; Ciro *Surrender* [2 diff., one a tester], *Reflexions* [2 diff., one with box]; Marie Earle/Rallet *Ballerina* bath oil; Jacques Fath *Chasuble* with glass stopper and box; Fragonard *Fragarome Lavande*; Gabilla *La Vierge Folle*; Marcel Guerlain *Masque Rouge*; Jergens *Memories of Paris*; Lenthéric *Tweed*; Revlon *Intimate*; Schiaparelli *Snuff*; Mary Sherman bath oil; Tré-Jur *Gardenia Bouquet*; Tussy *Midnight* glass tester; unidentifed perfumer *Wedding Bells*; Weil *Bamboo* bath oil. Total of 21 minis. Est. $500.00-$600.00.

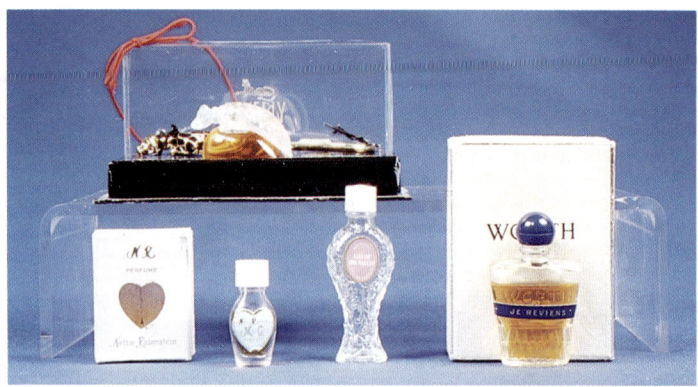 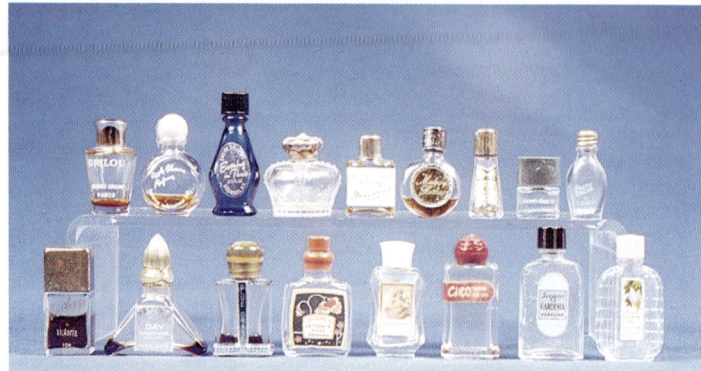

Lot #16. Lot of 21 minis: Elizabeth Arden *Blue Grass*, *Night and Day*; Bourjois *Evening in Paris*; Cheramy *April Showers*; Ciro *Danger*; Colgate *La France Rose*; Coventry *Imperial Carnation*; Garmella *Lavanda Montanino*; Gourielli *Lily of the Valley*; Griffe *Grilou*; Gale Hayman *Beverly Hills*, in its box with key chain; Jergens *Gardenia*; Leigh *Poetic Dream*; Lenthéric *12*; Molyneux *Le Numéro Cinq*; Pele *Ginger*; Rochas *Madame Rochas*; Rosenstein *Mlle. Ghe* in its box; Helena Rubenstein *Apple Blossom*; Victoria *Vice Versa*; Worth *Je Reviens*, in its box. Total of 21 items. Est. $315.00-$630.00.

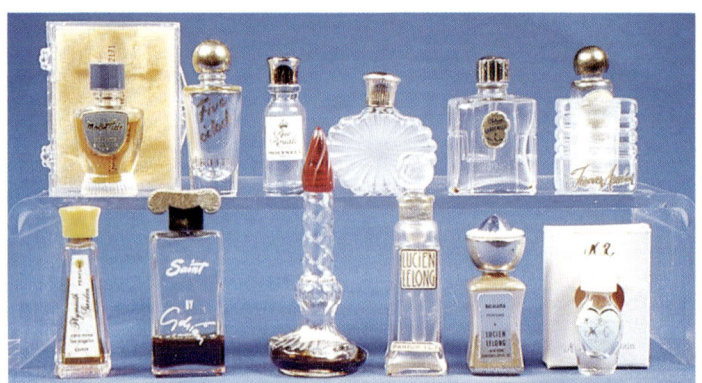 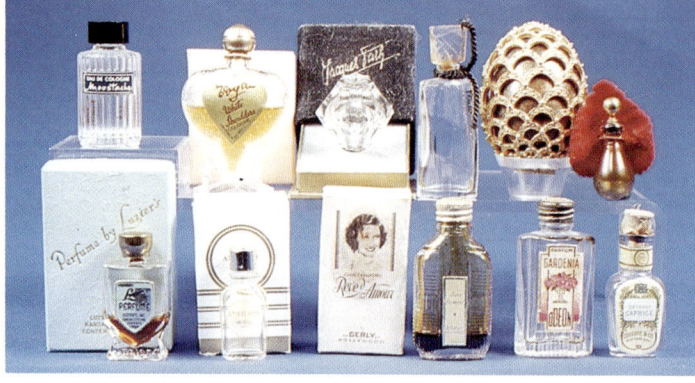

Lot #17. Lot of 22 minis: Adrian *Saint*; Bourjois *Moon Tide* in its box [Ford cars]; Cara Nome *Plymouth Garden*; Colgate *Caprice*; Evyan *White Shoulders* in box; *Fath de Fath* in box; Gerly *Reve d'Amour* [for Joan Crawford], in box; Gourielli *Five O'Clock*; Kathryn *Forever Amber* in lucite holder; Lelong *Balalaika*, *Parfum L* glass tester; Luzier *Poppaea* in its box; Bob Mackie *Mackie*; Molyneux *Rue Royale*; Mosell glass mini in a metal egg, Odeon *Gardenia*; Palmer *Gardenglo*; Ricci *L'Air du Temps* sunburst signed *Lalique*; Rochas *Moustache*; Rosenstein *Mlle. Ghe* in its box; Schiaparelli *Sleeping*; Weil *Antilope* in its box. 22 items. Est. $330.00-$660.00.

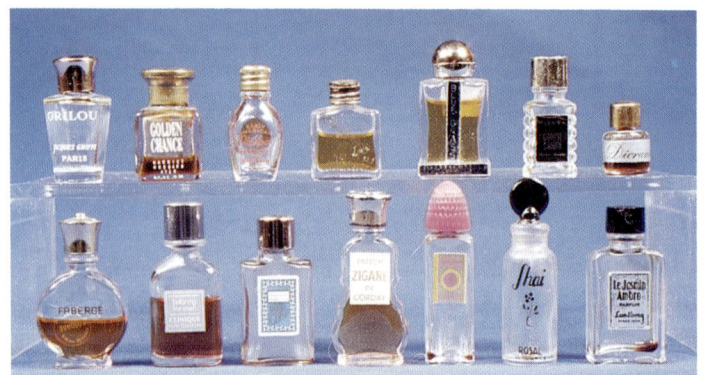 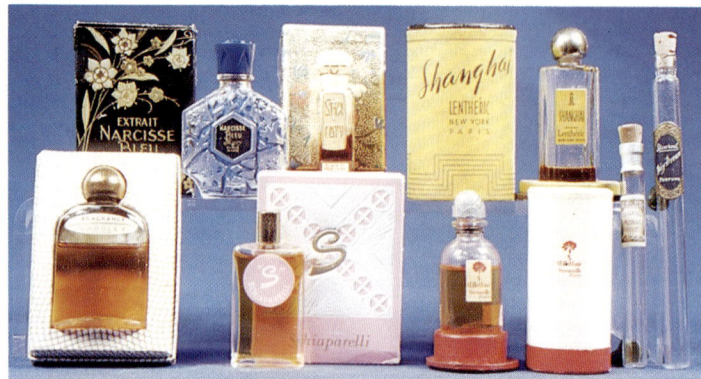

Lot #18. Lot of 22 minis: Elizabeth Arden *Blue Grass*; Harriet Hubbard Ayer *Golden Chance*; Clinique *Tailoring for Men*; Colgate *Monad Violet* vial; Corday *Zigane*; Corse-Salomé *Ylanga*; Coty *Styx* in its box; Dior *Diorama*; Fabergé *Woodhue*; Fragonard *Belle de Nuit*; Grenoville *Oeillet Fané* in its box; Griffe *Grilou*; Hudnut *Yanky Clover*; Lenthéric *Shanghai* in its box; Lundborg *Le Jasmin Ambré*; Mury *Narcisse Bleu* in its box; Rosal *Shai*; Rosenstein *Odalisque*; Schiaparelli *S* in its box; Shulton *Old Spice*; Stearns *Daydream* vial; Yardley *Fragrance*. Total of 22 minis. Est. $330.00-$660.00.

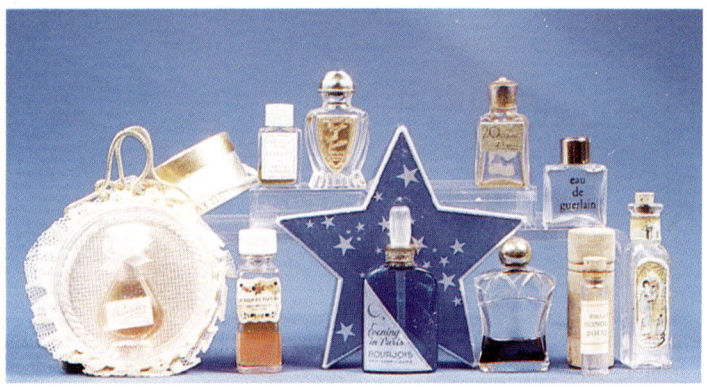
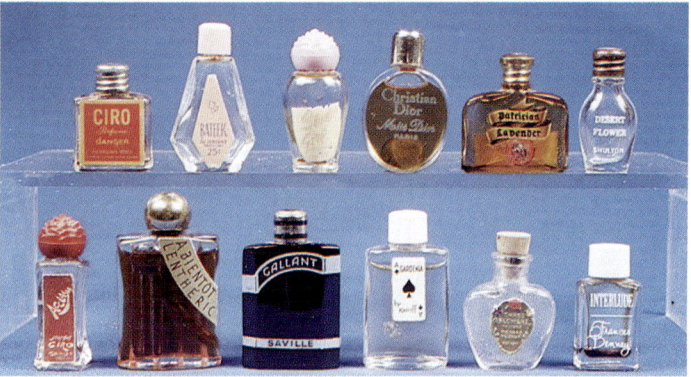

Lot #19. Lot of 22 minis: Bourjois *Evening in Paris* in its blue star box; Hattie Carnegie *Carnegie Pink* in its hatbox; Ciro *Acclaim, Danger*; Dana *20 Carats*; Frances Denney *Interlude*; Dior *Miss Dior*; Evyan *White Shoulders*; Dorothy Gray; Guerlain *Eau*; Hollywood Perfumes *Studio Girl*; Houbigant *Chantilly* in its plastic case, *Quelques Fleurs* tester; Hudnut *Three Flowers*; Jergens *Bateek*; Karoff *Gardenia*; Lazell *Massatta*; Leigh *Desert Flower*; Lenthéric *A Bientôt*; Rieger *Honolulu Bouquet* in its wood case; Saville *Gallant*; unidentified perfumer *Patrician Lavender*. Total of 22 minis. Est. $330.00-$660.00.

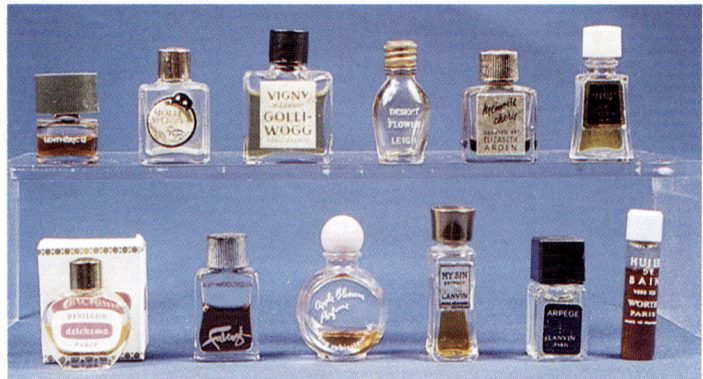
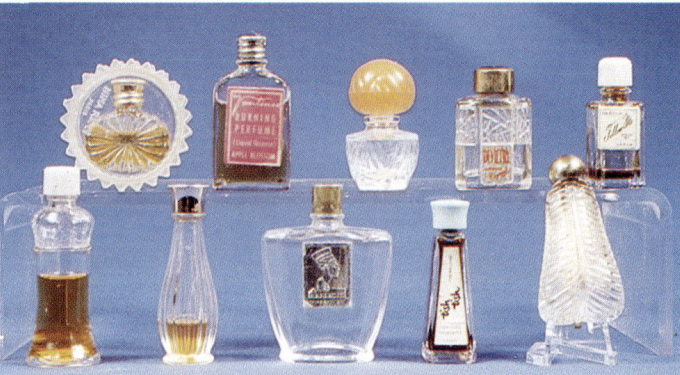

Lot #20. Lot of 22 minis: Elizabeth Arden *Mémoire Chérie*; Cara Nome *Tish Tish*; Chabrawichi *Nefertiti*; Coty *Paris*; de Raymond *Deviltry*; Fabergé *Aphrodisia, Fleurs du Monde*; Lanvin *Arpège, My Sin*; Leigh *Desert Flower*; Lelong *Jabot* dress clip; Lenthéric *12*; Matchabelli *Incanto*; Révillon *Carnet de Bal, Detchema* in its box; Ricci *L'Air du Temps* in plastic case; Rubenstein *Apple Blossom*; Vantine's *Burning Perfume*; Varva *Follow Me*; Vigny *Golliwogg*, two diff.; Worth *Vers Toi* bath oil. Total of 22 minis. Est. $220.00-$330.00.

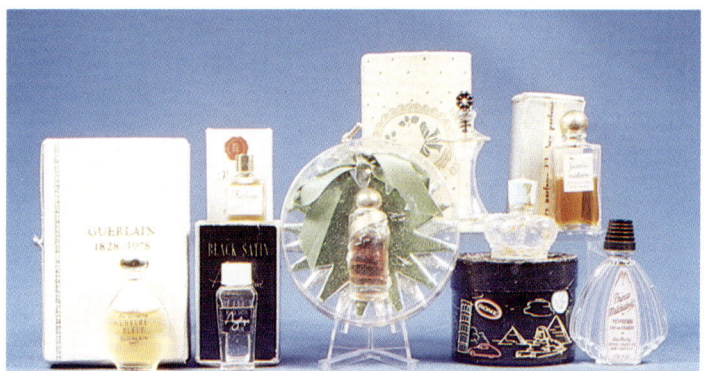
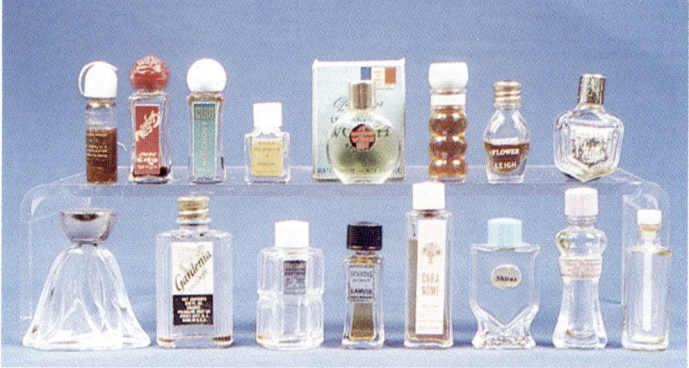

Lot #21. Lot of 24 minis: Angelique *Black Satin* in box; Ciro *Reflexions*, 2 diff.; Colgate *Gardenia*; d'Albret *Ecusson*; Marie Earle/Rallet *Ballerina*; de Rauch *Belle*; Goya *Gardenia*; Guerlain *L'Heure Bleue* in box [1978]; Isabey *Jasmin* in box; Langlois *Cara Nome*; Lanvin *Scandal*; Leigh *Desert Flower*; Lelong *Opening Night*; Lenthéric *Confetti* in box; Luzier *Shiraz*; Matchabelli *Duchess of York, Potpourri* crown in box, *Potpourri* cologne; Raphael *Réplique* in box; Old South *Woodland Spice* in box; Shulton *Desert Flower*; Lucretia Vanderbilt *Concentrated Perfume*; Worth *Je Reviens* in box. 24 items. Est. $240.00-$360.00.

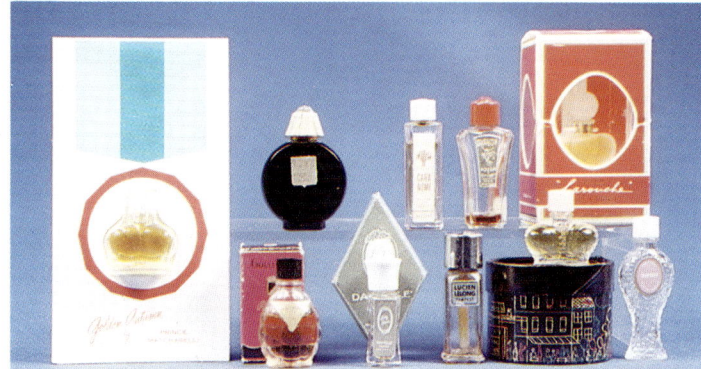
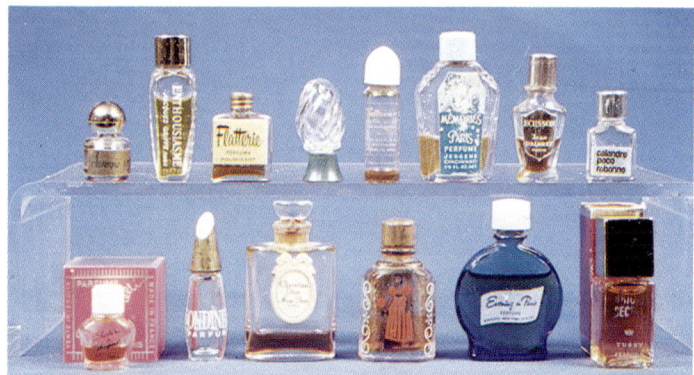

Lot #22. Lot of 24 minis: Auvergne *After Five*; Bourjois *Evening in Paris*; Lilly Daché *Dachelle* in box; D'Albret *Ecusson*; Dior *Miss Dior*; Marie Earle/Rallet *Ballerina*; Gourielli *Daphne*; Griffe *Enthousiasme*; Houbigant *Flatterie*; Jergens *Memories of Paris*; Langlois *Cara Nome*; Lelong *Tempest* tester; Matchabelli *Added Attraction* in hatbox, *Golden Autumn*; Paquin *Ever After*; Révillon *Carnet de Bal*; Paco Rabanne *Calandre*; Ricci *Farouche* in box; Roger & Gallet *Fleurs d'Amour*; Schiaparelli *Shocking* in plastic cube; Shulton *Early American*; Suzanne Thierry *Ondine*; Tussy *Bright Secret*; Vigny *Golliwogg* in box. 24 minis total. Est. $360.00-$720.00.

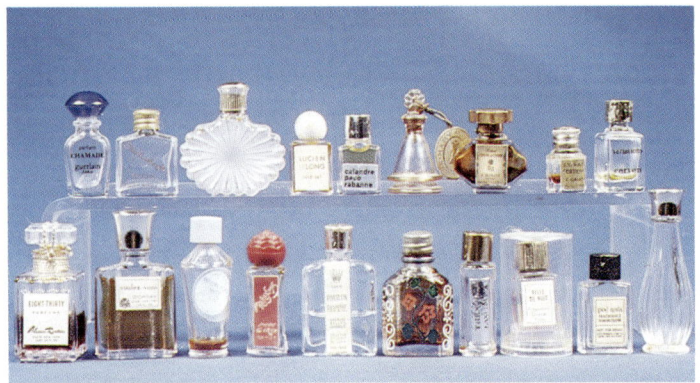 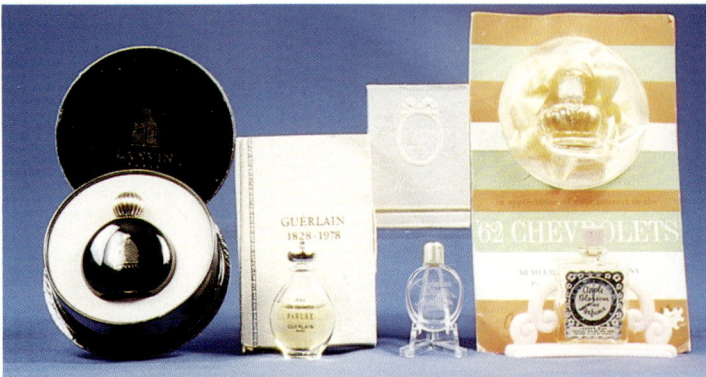

Lot #23. Lot of 24 minis: Caron *Pour Un Homme*; Carven *Variations*; Ciro *Reflexions*; Mary Chess *White Lilac*; Dior *Miss Dior* in box; D'Orsay *Voulez-Vous*; Fragonard *Belle de Nuit* in box; Gourielli *Moon Light Mist*; Guerlain *Chamade, Parure* in box; Lancôme *Trésor*; Lander *Apple Blossom Time* in plastic holder; Lanvin *Arpège* in black box; Le Galion *Sortilège*; Lelong *Indiscret*; Matchabelli *Golden Autumn* [1962 Chevys]; Millot *Crêpe de Chine*; Paco Rabanne *Calandre*; Maurice Rentner *Eight-Thirty*; Edith Rehnborg *Poé Rava*; Révillon *Carnet de Bal*; Ricci *L'Air du Temps*; Rosenstein *Odalisque*; Shulton *Early American*. Est. $360.00-$720.00.

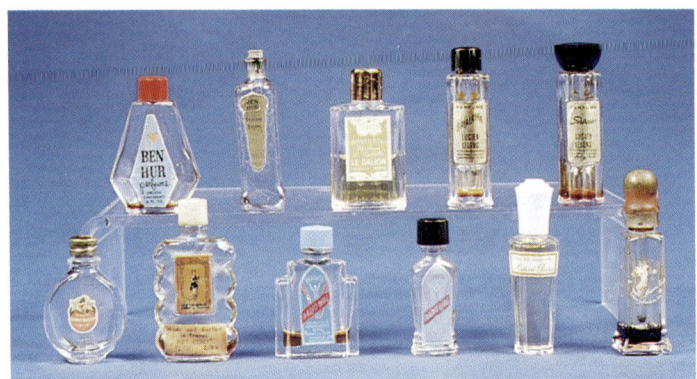 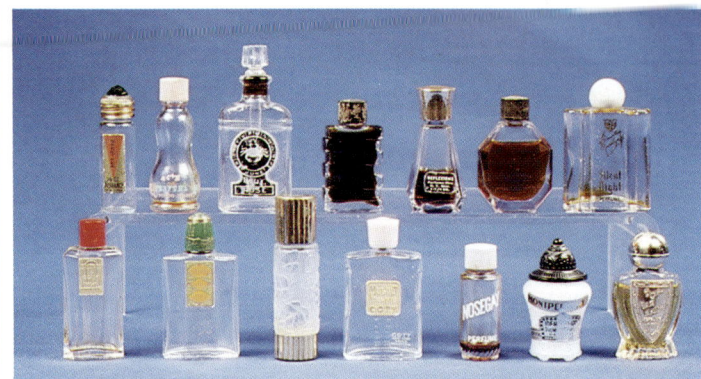

Lot #24. Lot of 25 glass minis with caps, various sizes: Alfrance *Sweet Pea;* Avon *Young Hearts;* Barée *Rose;* Ciro *Danger, Reflexions, Surrender;* Countess Martiza *Silent Night;* Coty *L'Aimant, Emeraude, L'Origan, Muguet des Bois;* Dorothy Gray *Nosegay;* Duchess of Paris *Infatuation;* Evyan *White Shoulders;* Jergens *Ben Hur* [2 diff.]; Le Galion *Sortilège;* Lelong *Balalaika, Sirôcco;* unidentified maker *Orange Blossom;* Piver *Pompeia;* Belco *Radio Girl* [2 diff.]; Rochas *Mme. Rochas;* Rubenstein *Heaven Sent* tester. Total of 25 items. Est. $175.00-$275.00.

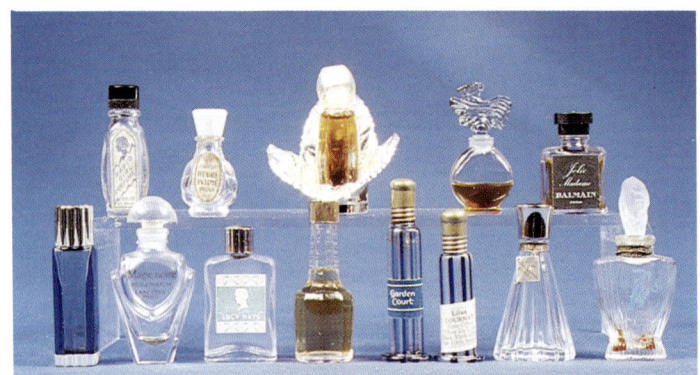 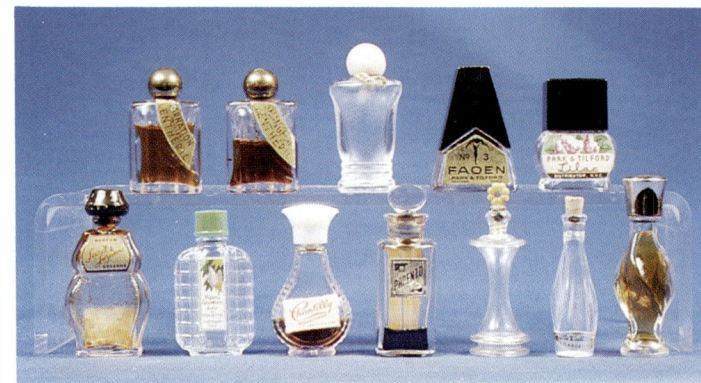

Lot #25. Lot of 25 glass minis with caps, various sizes: Avon *Lucy Hays;* Balmain *Jolie Madame;* Belco *Radio Girl;* Cheramy *April Showers;* D'Orsay *Divine, Intoxication;* B. Gould *Skylark;* D. Gray *Nosegay;* Guerlain *Parure;* Houbigant *Chantilly* [2 diff.]; Lancôme *Magie Noire;* Lavaliere *Gardenia;* Lenthéric *Carnation, Shanghai;* Lournay *Lilas;* Nelson *Garden Court;* Parento tester; Park & Tilford *Faoen, Lilac;* Suzanne *Secret de S.;* Vigny *Heure Intime;* Worth *Je Reviens;* 2 unidentified. 25 items. Est. $175.00-$275.00.

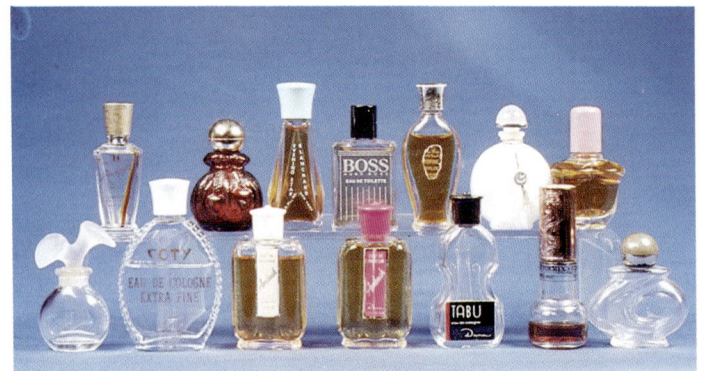 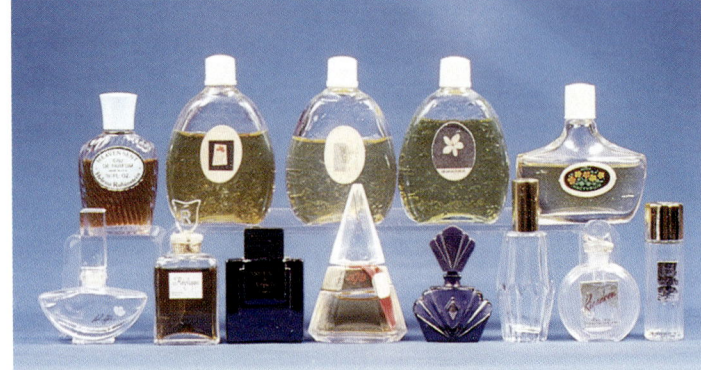

Lot #26. Lot of 27 minis: Elizabeth Arden *Blue Grass*; Avon *Moonwind*; Blanchard *Evening Star*; Hugo Boss *Boss*; Bourjois *On the Wind* [label worn]; Cacharel *Anaïs-Anaïs*; Charles of the Ritz *Enjoli*; Chloé; Coty *Eau*; Dana *Ambush* [2 diff.], *Tabu*; Fabergé *Cologne for Men*; Galanos *Eau*; Le Galion *Sortilège*; Hayman *273*; Houbigant *Chantilly*; Paveau *Rigadoon*; Raphael *Réplique*; de la Renta *Ruffles*; Rubenstein *Heaven Sent*; Elizabeth Taylor *Passion*; Van Cleef & Arpels; four Russian perfumes *Fialka, Nasturtsia, Rusalka, Siren*. 27 items. Est. $125.00-$250.00.

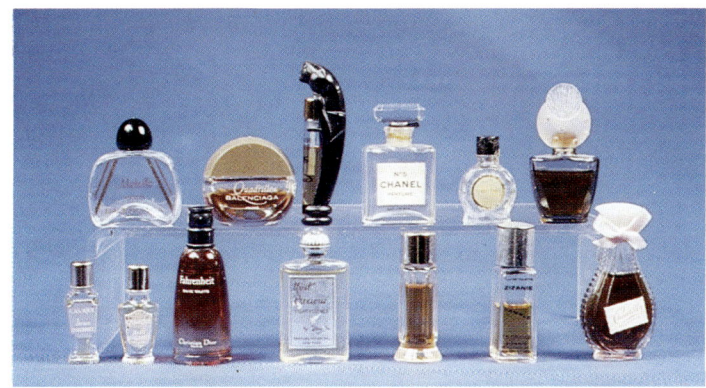 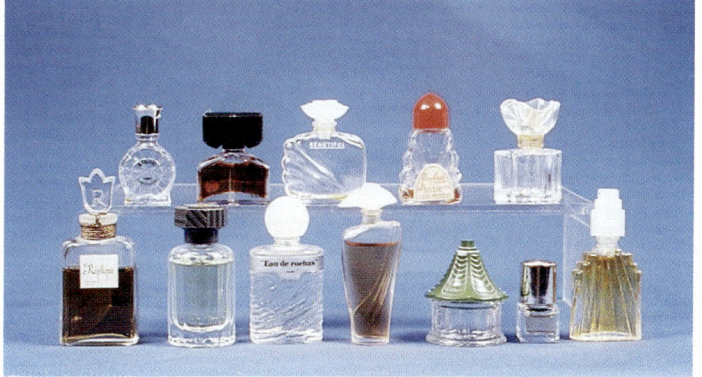

Lot #27. Lot of 25 miniatures: Balenciaga *Michelle, Quadrille;* Cartier *Panthère;* Chanel *No. 5;* Charles V *Tendre Eve;* Cher *Uninhibited;* d'Albret *Casaque* [2 diff.]; Dior *Fahrenheit;* Evyan *Most Precious;* Max Factor *Primitif;* Fragonard *Zizanie;* Houbigant *Chantilly;* Laboissiere *Lilac;* Laroche *Fidji;* Lauder *Beautiful;* Luft *May Buds;* Oscar de la Renta; Raphael *Réplique* [glass stopper]; Ricci *Club;* Rochas *Eau;* 4 unidentified bottles. Total of 25. Est. $125.00-$250.00.

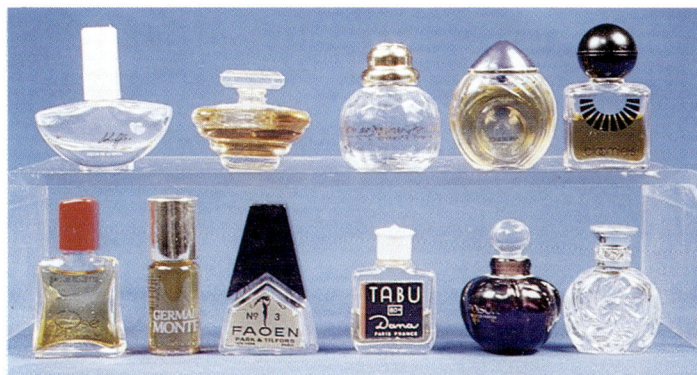 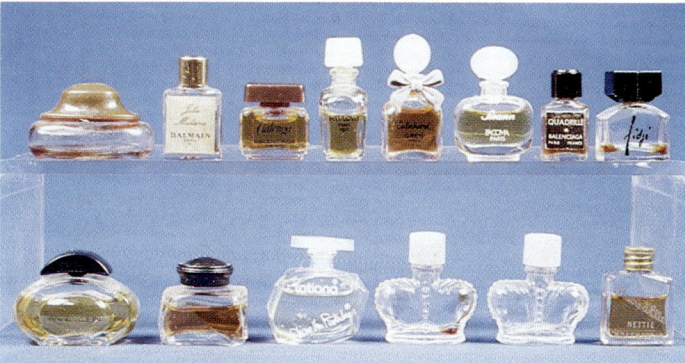

Lot #28. Lot of 25 minis: Balenciaga *Cialenga, Quadrille;* Balmain *Jolie Madame;* Bloomingdale's *Bloomies;* Boucheron; Furstenburg *Tatiana;* Dana *Tabu;* Dior *Poison;* Grès *Cabochard;* Anne Klein; Calvin Klein *Obsession;* Lancôme *Trésor;* Laroche *Fidji, J'ai Osé;* Ralph Lauren *Safari;* Matchabelli *Added Attraction, Beloved;* Germaine Monteil; Pacoma *Swann;* Park & Tilford *Faoen;* Pavlova *1922;* de la Renta *Ruffles;* Rosenstein *Fleurs d'Elle;* Rykiel *7e Sens;* Saint Laurent *Paris.* Total of 25l. Est. $125.00-$250.00.

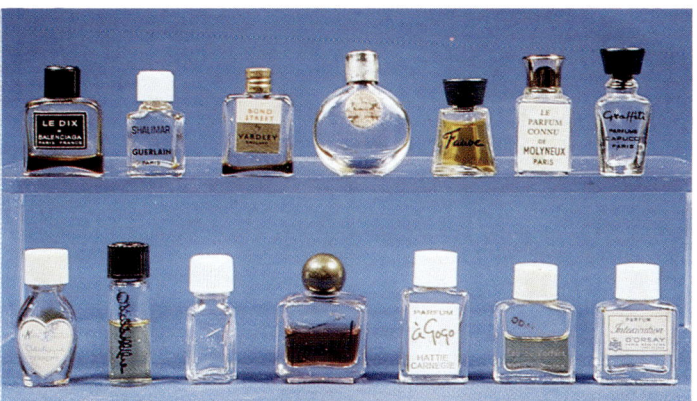 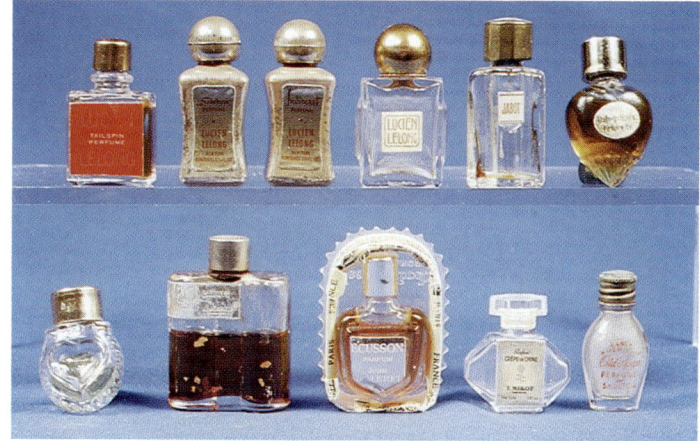

Lot #29. Lot of 25 glass minis with caps, various sizes: Avon *Unforgettable;* Balenciaga *Le Dix;* Capucci *Graffiti;* H. Carnegie *Parfum à Gogo;* D'Albret *Ecusson;* Dana *20 Carats;* D'Orsay *Intoxication;* Guerlain *Shalimar;* Lelong *Indiscret, Jabot, Sirôcco, Tailspin,* one unmarked; Lenthéric *Tweed* [2 diff.]; Millot *Crêpe de Chine;* Molyneux *Le Parfum Connu;* Ricci *Coeur Joie* single heart; Rosenstein *Odalisque* [3 diff.]; Shulton *Old Spice;* ; unidentified maker *Fauve;* Worth *Vers Toi;* Yardley *Bond Street.* Total of 25 items. Est. $150.00-$250.00.

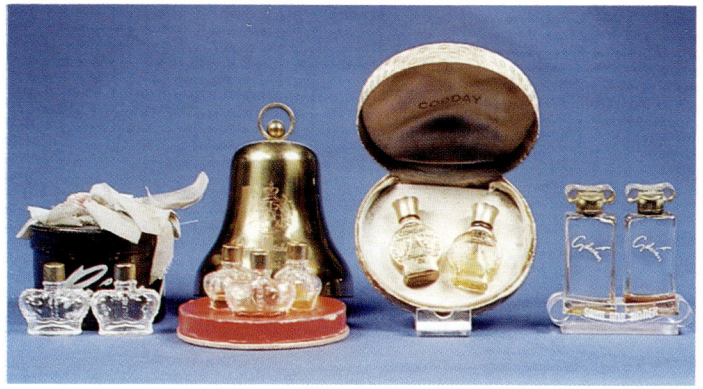

Lot #30. Adrian *Saint* and *Sinner* clear glass bottles with lucite caps, total height 2.6" [6.6 cm], empty, names in white enamel, in a lucite holder; Corday *Toujours Toi* and *Toujours Moi* ['Always Thee' and 'Always Me'] glass miniature bottles with gold caps, each 1.6" [4 cm], one enameled in gold, the other enameled with gold letters, empty, in their fabric box [heavily stained]; Matchabelli *Katherine the Great, Duchess of York, Ave Maria,* clear glass miniature crowns with gold caps, 1.3" [3.4 cm], emtpy, gold labels on bottoms, in a brass bell presentation decorated with Prince Matchabelli coat of arms; Matchabelli *Duchess of York* pair of clear glass miniature crowns with gold caps, 1.3" [3.4 cm], emtpy, gold labels on bottoms, in their black hatbox presentation. Total of four items. Est. $300.00-$400.00.

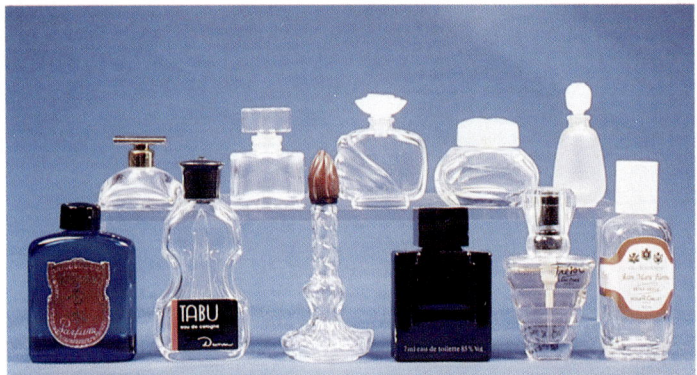
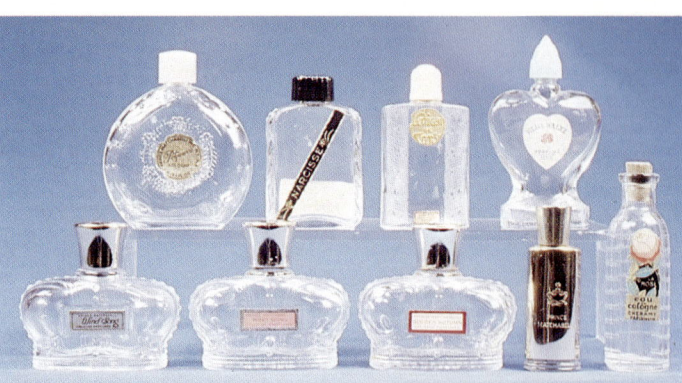
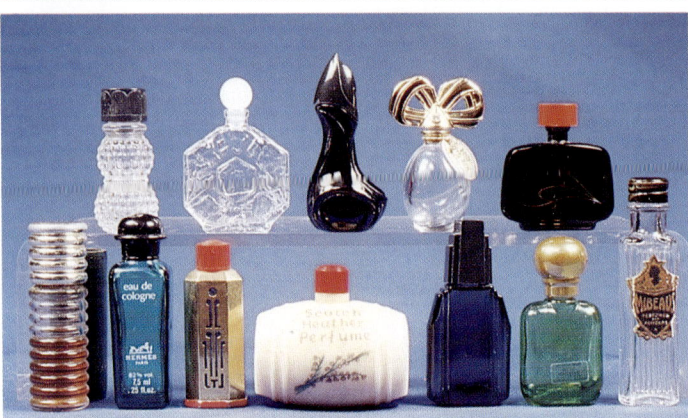

Lot #31. Lot of 32 minis: Brosseau *Ombre Rose*; Cheramy *La Rose*; Coty *L'Origan*; Dana *Tabu*; Elizabeth Taylor *White Diamonds*; Federal *Narcisse*; Hermès *Eau*; Donna Karan *Parfum*; Lancôme *Trésor*; Estée Lauder *Beautiful, Knowing, Private Collection, Spellbound, White Linen*; Lauren *Polo*; Matchabelli *Golden Autumn, Potpourri, Windsong* [2 diff.], one unlabeled; Maxim's Mibeaus *Mon Ami*; Patou *Joy*, Roger & Gallet *Farina*; Schiaparelli *Sleeping* [no label], unidentified makers *Blue Waltz, L'Orient, Privé, Scotch Heather*; two unmarked bottles; Van Cleef & Arpels *Eau*. Thirty-two items total. Est. $100.00-$200.00.

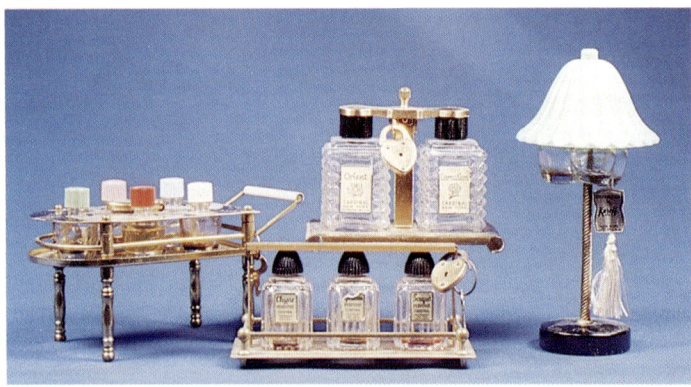
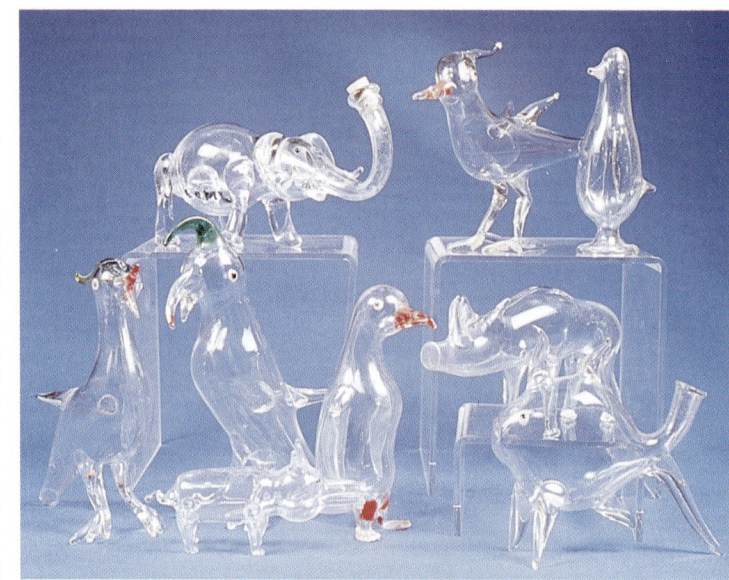

Lot #32. Karoff *Morning, Noon, Nite Aromalite* ["Three Scentamental Perfumes"] clear glass minis with violet caps in their lamp holder, with label; Cardinal *Chypre, Bouquet, Gardenia* three clear glass bottles with green plastic caps, with labels [one label torn], in their metal holder with lock and key; Stuart *Perfumador* metal tea cart with five glass minis with colored plastic caps, locked in the cart with a padlock and with a key; Cardinal *Orient* and *Carnation* in a locked metal holder. Four items. Est. $50.00-$100.00.

Lot #33. Lot of 9 blown glass bottles in the shape of various animals: several varieties of birds [including a penguin], an elephant, a rhinocerous, a pig, and a goldfish; various heights. Nine items. Est. $100.00-$150.00.

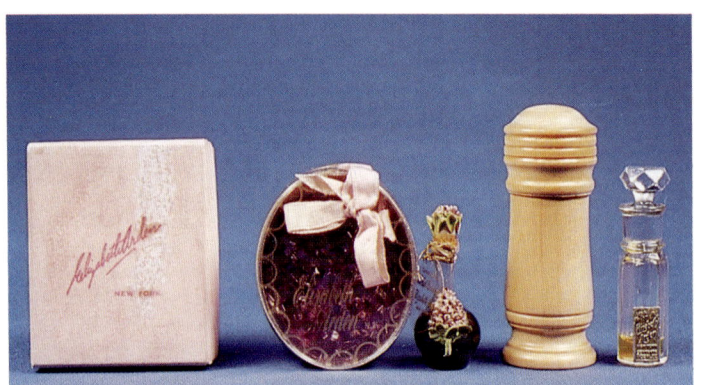
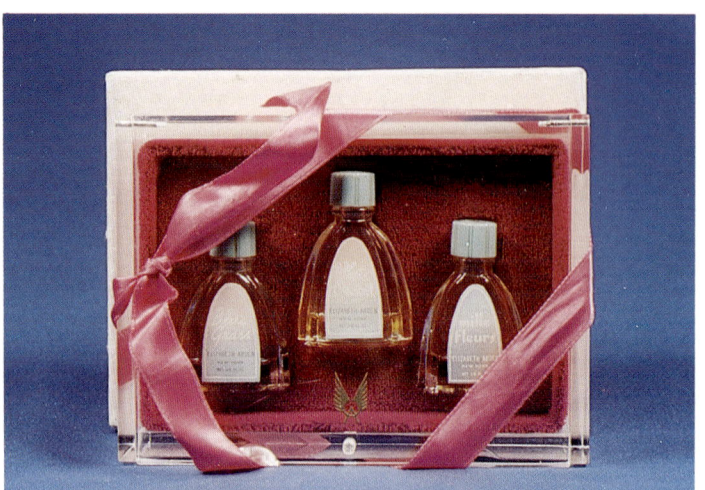

Lot #34. Elizabeth Arden *Blue Grass, White Orchid, Mille Fleurs* set of three clear glass miniature bottles with aqua caps and pink and blue labels, each 1.7" [4.3 cm], in a clear lucite box with *Arden* emblem and label, in its pink box; *Violet Essence* clear glass bottle and decorated cork stopper, 2" [5.1 cm], full and sealed, the bottle also decorated with violets, celluloid label, in its oval box and outer box; *Cupid's Breath* clear glass bottle and stopper, 2.4" [6.1 cm], gold label, empty, in its wood box with label underneath. Total of three items with five minis. Est. $450.00-$600.00.

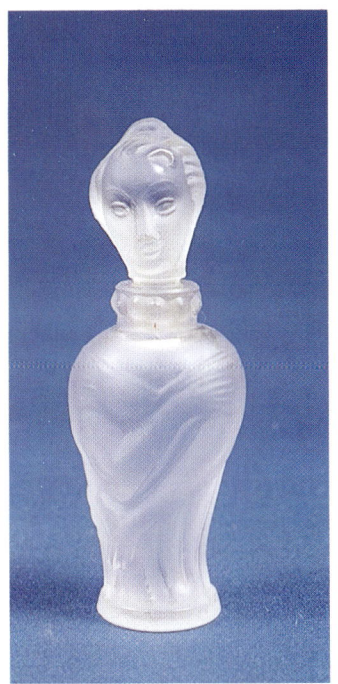

Lot #35. Elizabeth Arden *Mémoire Chérie* ['Cherished Memory'] frosted glass bottle and stopper in the form of a woman, 3" [7.6 cm], empty, probably a first size. Est. $250.00-$350.00.

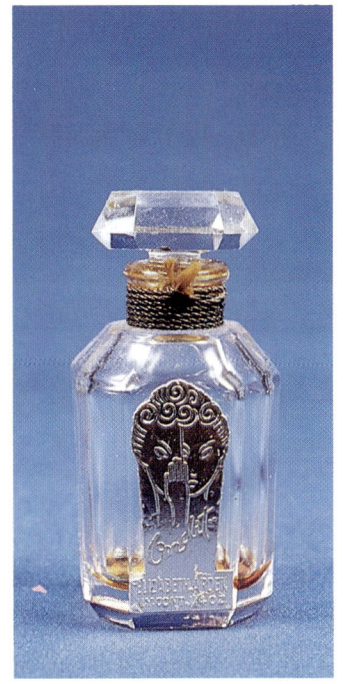

Lot #36. Elizabeth Arden *On Dit* ['So They Say'] clear glass bottle and stopper, 2" [5.1 cm], both bottle and stopper molded with multiple facets, empty, gold label on front depicting two women whispering to each other. Est. $100.00-$150.00.

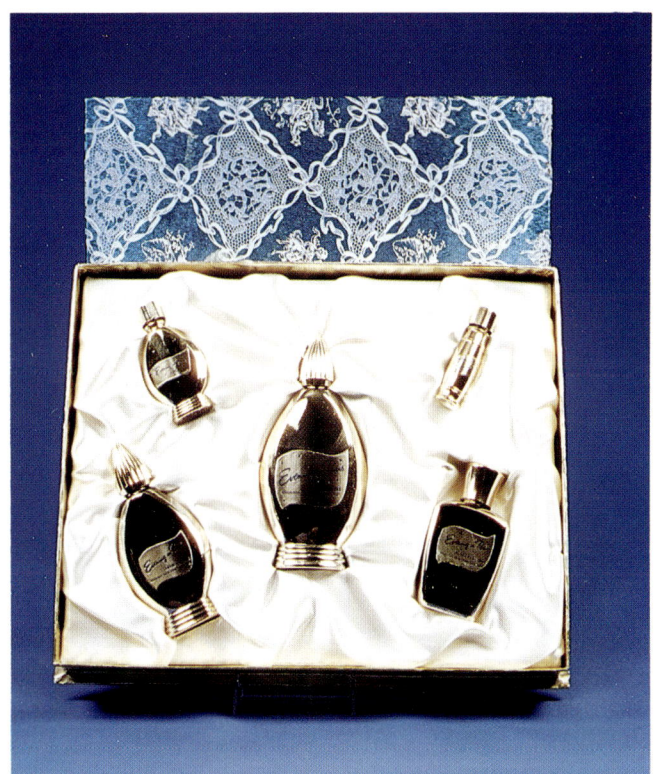

Lot #37. Bourjois *Evening in Paris* set of five glass bottles covered in gold enamel with gold caps, from 2" to 4.5" [5.1 to 11.4 cm], all with gold labels, in unused condition, in their gold and blue foil box with a lace print design [portion of paper on side edge of back is torn]. Est. $100.00-$125.00.

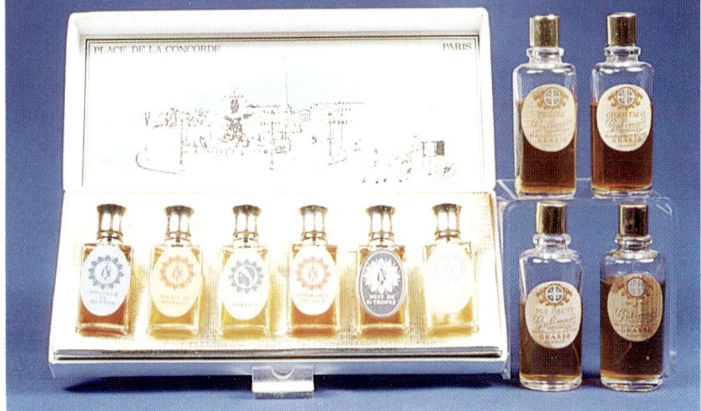

Lot #38. Berneux *Perfumes of the French Riviera: Douceur de Menton, Soleil de Monaco, Corsica, Attirance de Nice, Nuit de St. Tropez, Hiver de Cannes,* each a clear glass miniature with gold cap, full of perfume, pretty oval labels on front, in their white box; Galimard *Ma Faute, J, Peggia, Christmas* clear glass bottles with gold caps, 3" [7.6 cm], some perfume, all with labels [some stains]. Ten minis total. Est. $100.00-$150.00.

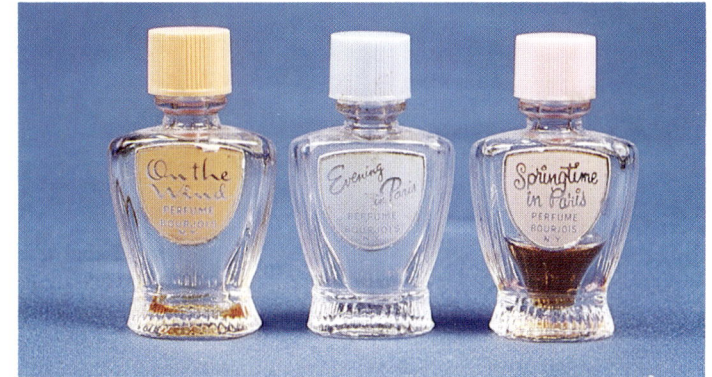

Lot #39. Bourjois *Evening in Paris, On the Wind,* and *Springtime in Paris:* three identical clear glass bottles with plastic caps, 1.7" [4.3 cm], each bottle molded with vertical ribs, all empty, blue, orange, and pink labels and correspondingly colored caps. This miniature of *Springtime in Paris* is extremely hard to find. Three items. Est. $150.00-$300.00.

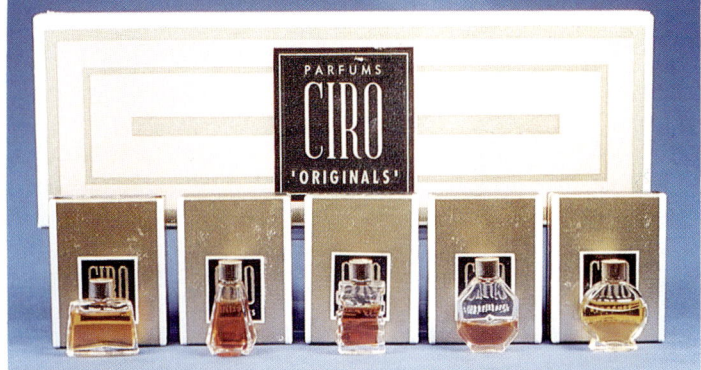

Lot #40. Ciro *Originals* set of five replica miniatures in individual boxes *Reflexions, New Horizons, Danger, Surrender, Ricochet,* various heights, unused condition, all with labels, in a presentation box. Est. $200.00-$275.00.

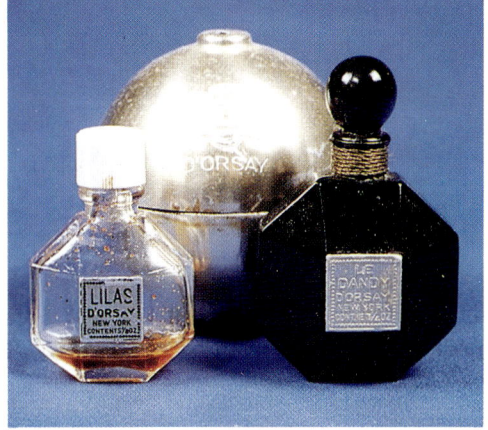

Lot #41. D'Orsay *Lilas* clear glass bottle and white cap, 1.6" [4.1 cm], an octagonal replica of the standard bottle, near empty, in a Christmas globe ornament presentation embossed with the *D'Orsay* logo; *Le Dandy* black glass bottle and stopper, 2.1" [5.3 cm], gold label, empty. Two items. Est. $75.00-$125.00.

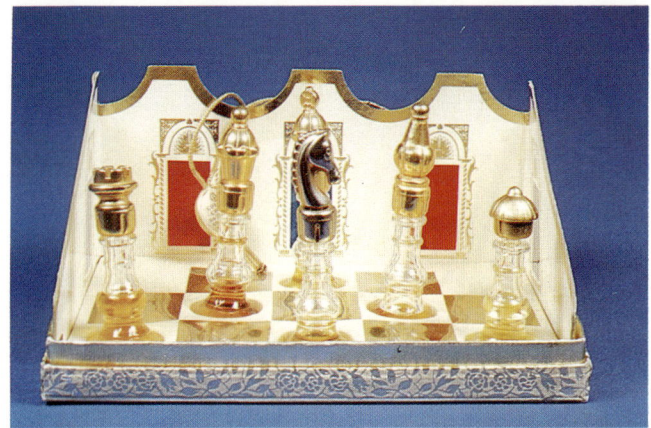

Lot #42. Mary Chess *Golden Court - Strategy* [King], *Tapestry* [Queen], *White Lilac* [Castle], *Yram* [Bishop], *Gardenia* [Knight], *Yram* [Pawn] set of six clear glass bottles and gold caps shaped as chess pieces, various heights from 2.3" to 3" [5.8 to 7.6 cm], each with some perfume, gold labels on bottom, in their chessboard holder. Est. $250.00-$300.00.

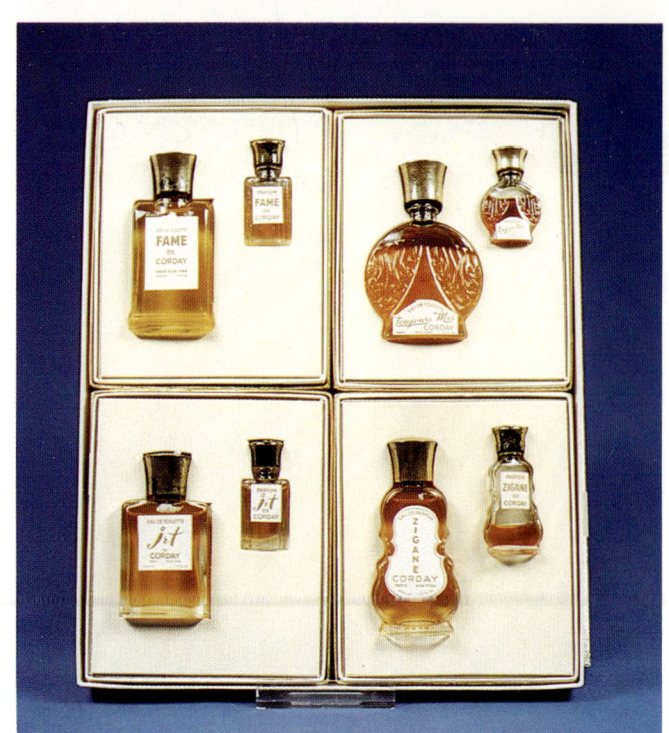

Lot #43. Corday *Her Majesty's Wardrobe of Fragrances - Fame, Jet, Toujours Moi,* and *Zigane* set of clear glass bottles with gold caps and their corresponding replica miniatures, heights from 2.6" to 3.2" [6.6 to 8.1 cm] and 1.6" to 2" [4.1 to 5.1 cm] for the miniatures; all with white and gold labels in unused condition; each pair of bottles is in its own gold box, all fitted into a larger box [with outer box], with a small advertising pamphlet "Look, Mommy, French Perfumes!" Est. $150.00-$225.00.

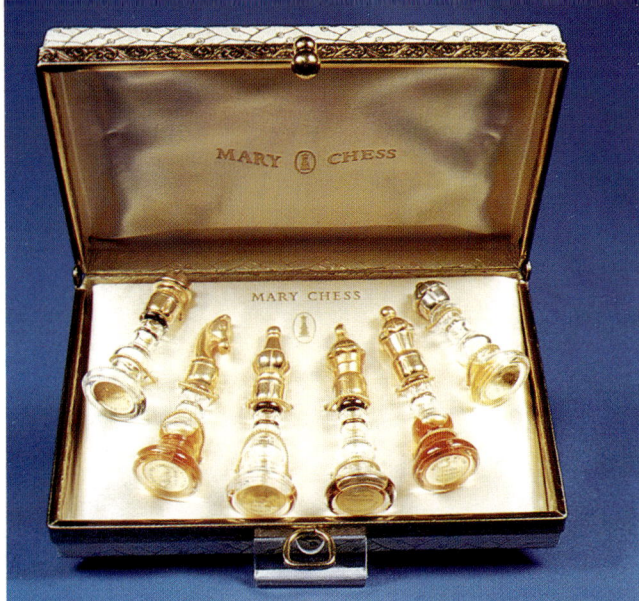

Lot #44. Mary Chess *Gardenia* [King], *Yram* [Queen], *Carnation* [Castle], *Strategy* [Bishop], *Tapestry* [Knight], *White Lilac* [Pawn] set of six clear glass bottles and gold caps shaped as chess pieces, various heights from 2.3" [5.8 cm] to 3" [7.6 cm], each with some perfume, gold labels on bottom, in their gold purse-form box. Est. $400.00-$500.00.

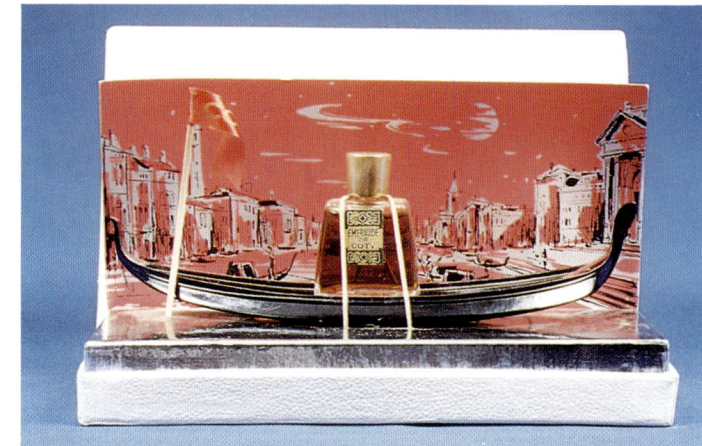

Lot #45. Coty *Emeraude* clear glass bottle with gold cap, 1.8" [4.5 cm], full, green and gold label, in a Venetian gondola set against a backdrop of Venice with a flag marked *Coty*, in its cream box. Est. $200.00-$300.00.

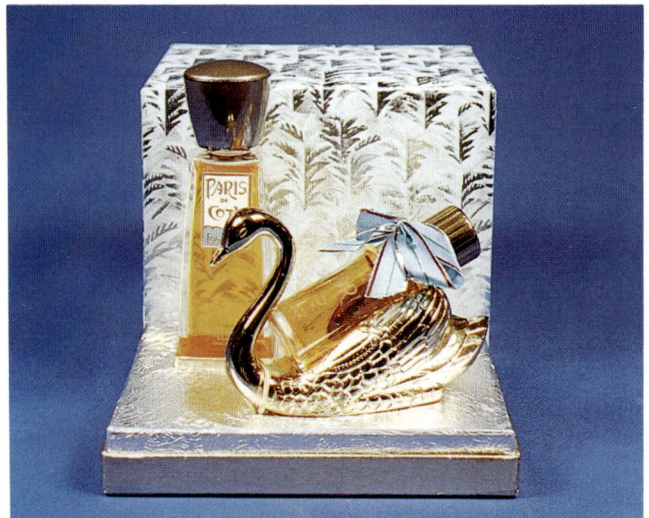

Lot #46. Coty *Paris* set consisting of an *Eau de Toilette* [1 oz.] clear glass bottle and gold cap, 3.9" [9.9 cm], and a clear glass p*arfum*, 2.5" [6.4 cm] with gold cap mounted in a swan; the set is presented in a charming foil box covered with Christmas trees. Est. $75.00-$125.00.

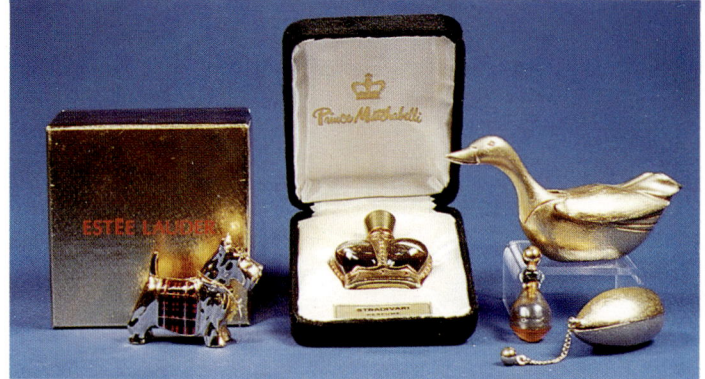

Lot #47. Estée Lauder *Knowing* gold metal solid perfume in the shape of a Scottie, 1.6" [4 cm] tall, with a red plaid enamel coat, unused condition, gold tag label, in its box; Mosell gold metal goose with a gold metal egg inside which holds a clear glass perfume, 1.4" [3.6 cm], Matchabelli *Stradivari* clear glass crown bottle with gold cap, 1.6" [4 cm], full, label on bottom, in its black velvet box. Three items. Est. $150.00-$225.00.

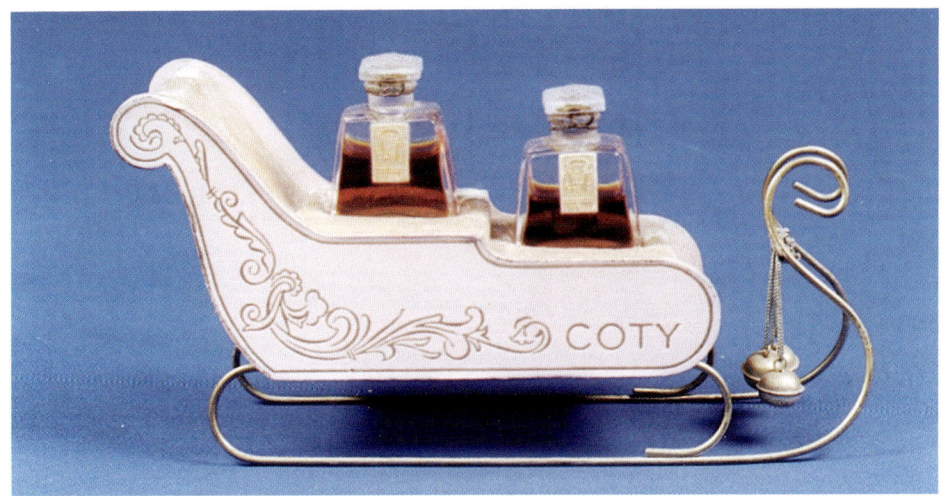

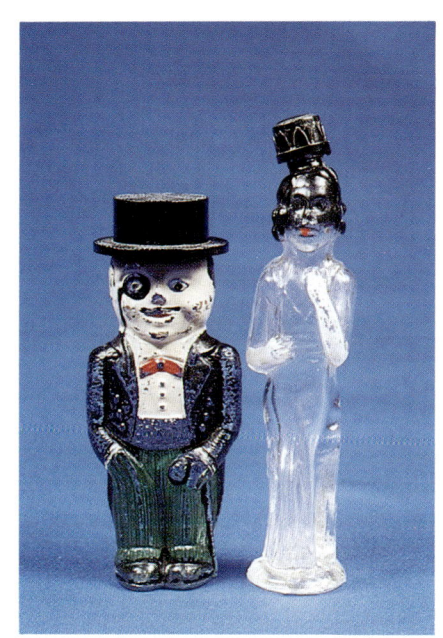

Lot #48. Coty *L'Aimant* ['The Magnet'] pair of clear glass bottles with frosted glass stoppers, bottle height 1.8" [4.6 cm], gold labels on front, with perfume and sealed, stopper with a fishscale motif, on a pink velvet-lined sled with gold bells marked *Coty;* this is a charming old miniature presentation. Est. $250.00-$350.00.

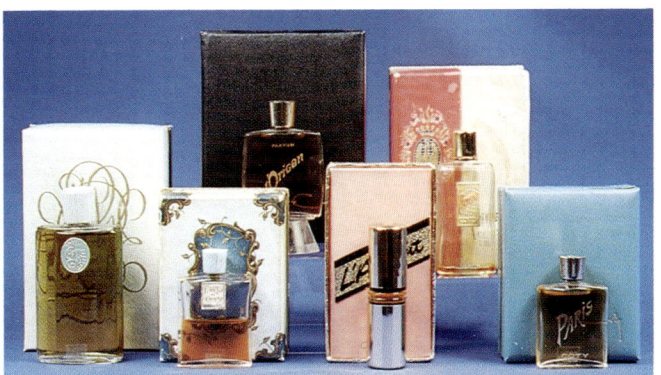

Lot #49. Coty: *L'Aimant* flacon de sac, 2.8" [7 cm], in its peach box; *L'Aimant* glass bottle/gold cap, 3" [7.5 cm], in its box [tear]; *Chypre* clear glass bottle/ blue cap, 3.3" [8.5 cm], in its box; *L'Origan* clear glass mini/gold cap, 2.4" [6 cm]; *Paris* clear glass mini/ gold cap, 2.2" [5.5 cm], in its blue box; *Paris* clear glass mini/blue cap, 2.3" [5.8 cm], in its box. Six boxed items. Est. $150.00-$250.00.

Lot #50. An elegant couple: clear glass bottles with black caps, 4.2" and 3.5" [10.7 and 8.9 cm], molded as a lady in an evening gown and a man with a monocle in a fancy suit, parts enameled in various colors, both empty. Two items. Est. $50.00-$100.00.

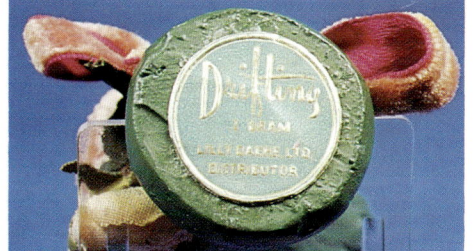

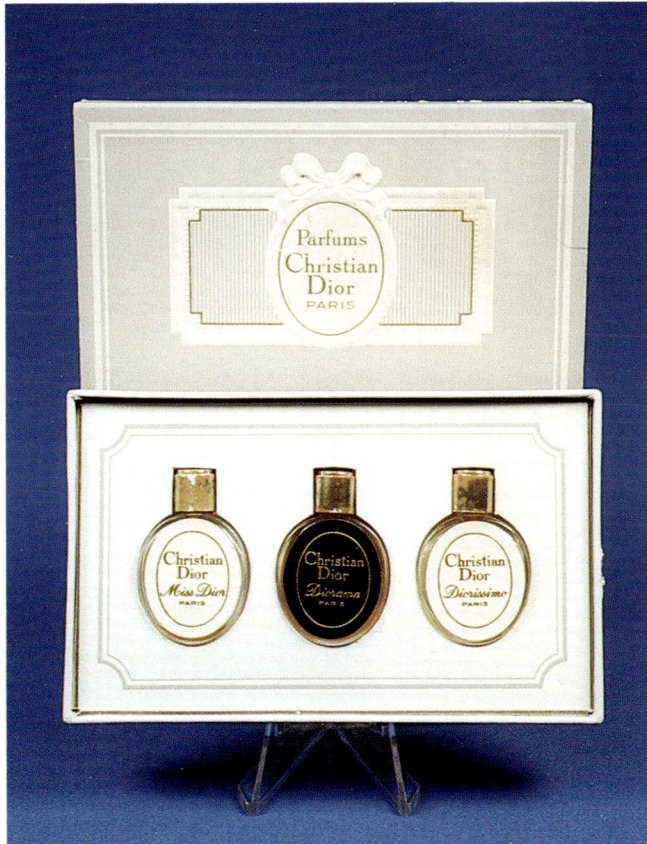

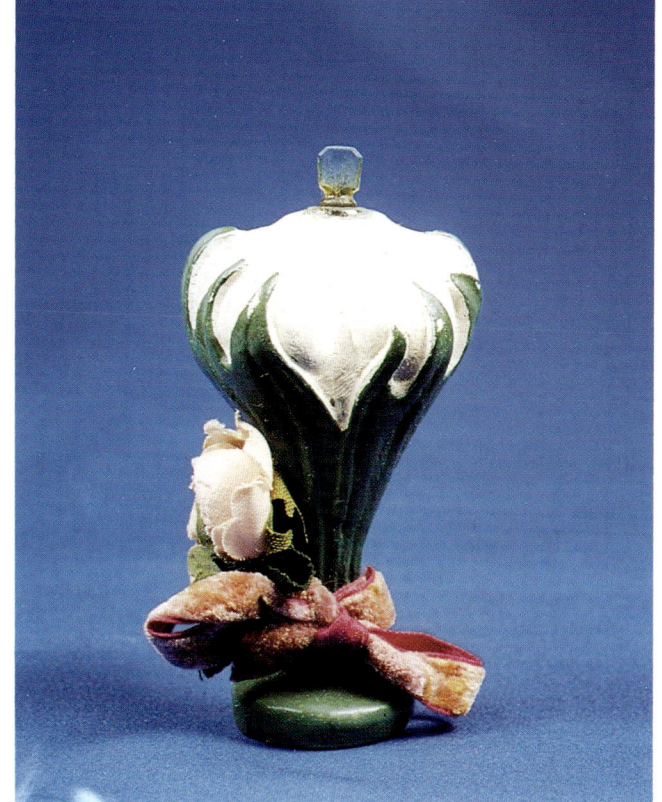

Lot #51. Christian Dior *Diorissimo, Diorama, Miss Dior* set of three glass miniatures with plastic caps, 1.6" [4 cm], each bottle the *galet* or 'cobblestone' shape and molded *France* on back, pretty labels in pink, white, and black, in their grey and white box. Est. $300.00-$400.00.

Lot #52. Lilly Daché *Drifting* glass bottle entirely encased in a composition material shaped as a woman's bust, with plastic stopper, 3.4" [8.6 cm], empty, original ribbon with artificial flowers tied around the bottom, green and gold label on bottom [see photo just above]. Cf. Lefkowith, p. 18, #2; Monsen and Baer, 1996, Lot 72. Est. $600.00-$750.00.

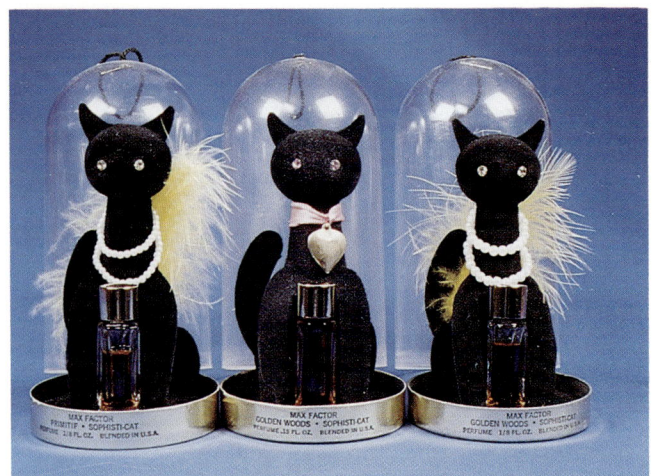

Lot #53. Max Factor *Primitif* and two *Golden Woods Sophisti-Cat* clear glass ribbed bottles with gold caps, 2" [5.1 cm], each held by a black cat [two with pearl necklaces and yellow feathers, one with a heart pendant], each in a plastic dome. Three items. Est. $50.00-$75.00.

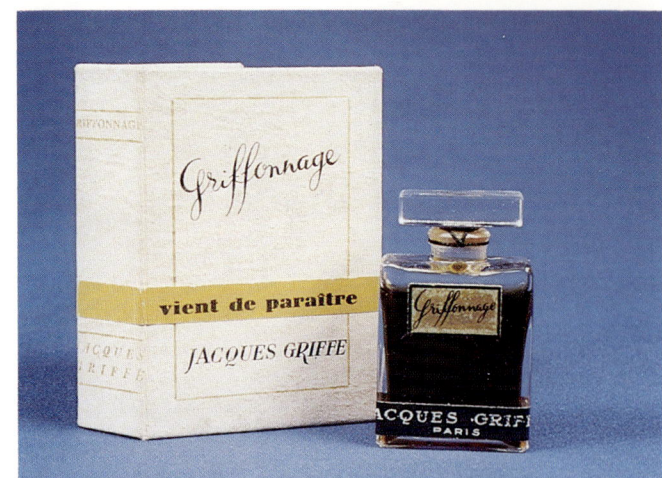

Lot #54. Jacques Griffe *Griffonage* [lit. 'Scribble' but meant as a pun on his name] clear glass bottle and stopper, 1.9" [4.8 cm] of rectangular form, full and sealed, gold and black labels, in its diminutive pink box shaped as a book; the box bears a label stating *Vient de Paraître* ['just issued'], so this is perhaps circa 1949. Est. $100.00-$150.00.

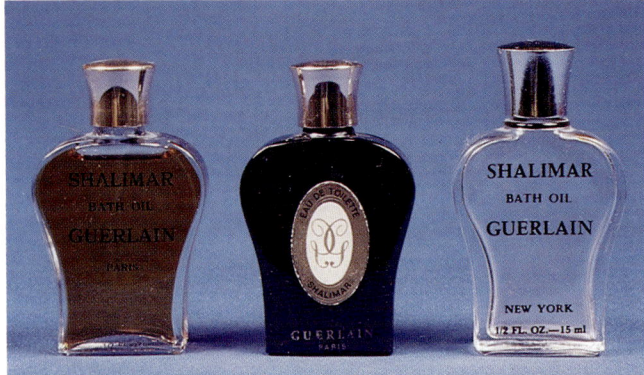

Lot #55. Guerlain *Shalimar eau de toilette* black glass 'lyre' bottle with gold cap, 2.75" [7 cm], empty, gold label on front and *Guerlain* in gold enamel; *Shalimar Bath Oil* identical size clear glass bottle with names in black enamel, full; *Shalimar Bath Oil* clear glass 'lyre' bottle, slightly larger, 3" [7.5 cm], empty, names in black enamel and marked .5 oz/15 ml. Three items. Est. $150.00-$250.00.

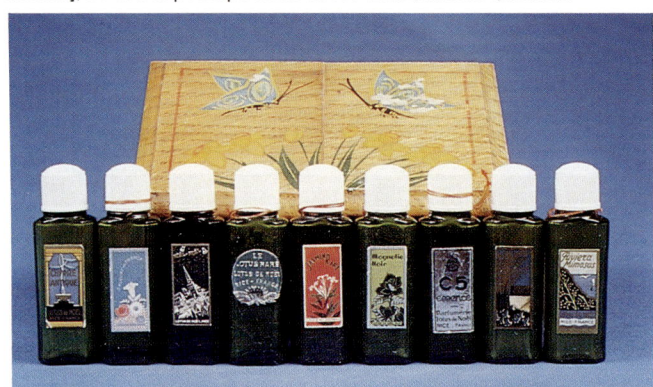

Lot #56. *Lotus de Noël* [Nice] set of 8 green glass bottles and 1 black glass bottle, with white caps: *Cinq Fleurs de France, Chypre Antique, C 5 Essence, Hawaiian Bluebells, Jasmin Rare, Le Lotus Rare, Magnolia Noir, Riviera Mimosas, Noël-Noël* [black]; 2.7" [6.8 cm], empty, with beautiful labels; the set is contained in a unique wood box decorated with daffodils and butterflies. Est. $200.00-$300.00.

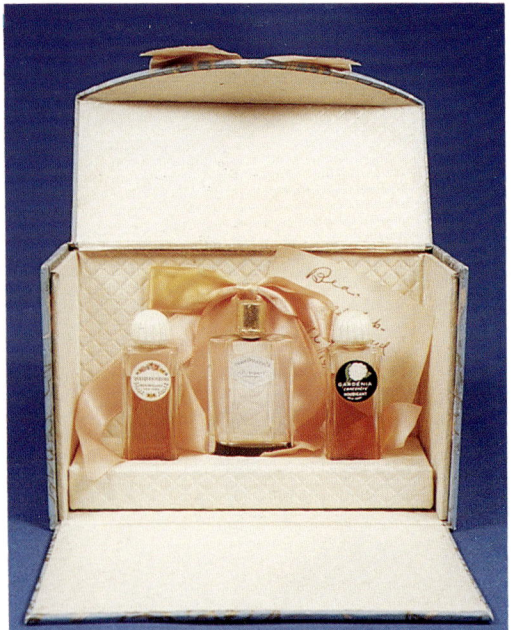

Lot #57. Houbigant set of three miniature glass bottles plastic/metal caps: *Gardenia* and *Quelques Fleurs*, 2.2" [5.6 cm], *Transparence*, 2.3" [5.8 cm], in their drop-front box [top hinge weak]; the box contains an old gift note: "Bea, Dear old Top, Dress up and Smell Good. O. E.". Est. $75.00-$125.00.

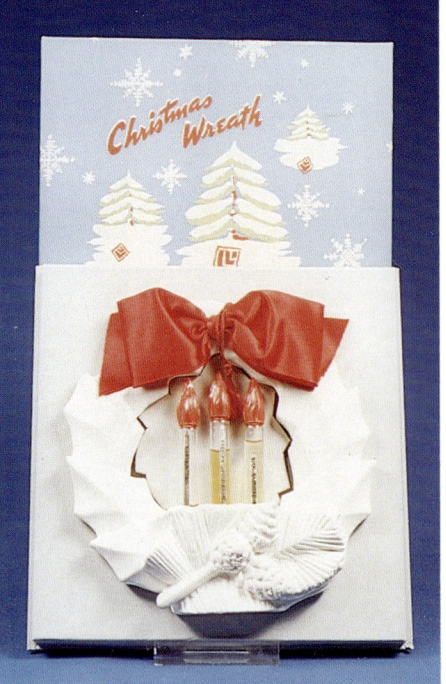

Lot #58. Lucien Lelong *Christmas Wreath - Indiscret, Impromptu, Whisper*, clear glass candle-form bottles with red flame caps, each 2.9" [7.3 cm], with thin gold labels [end of one label torn], mounted in a plaster wreath and in its box and outer box, marked *Christmas, 1945*. Est. $125.00-$175.00.

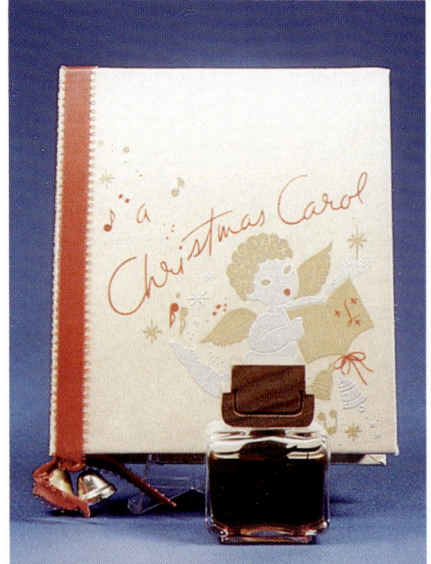

Lot #59. Lenthéric *Tweed* [originally *Risque-Tout* in French] clear glass bottle, inner glass stopper and wood overcap, 2.3" [5.8 cm], unopened, name in black enamel, silver tag label, in a book presentation [and outer box] called *A Christmas Carol* whose frontispiece is a song: "Jingle Bells, Jingle Bells, Jingle all the Way, Oh What Fun it is to give a Lenthéric gift this day!". Est. $175.00-$275.00.

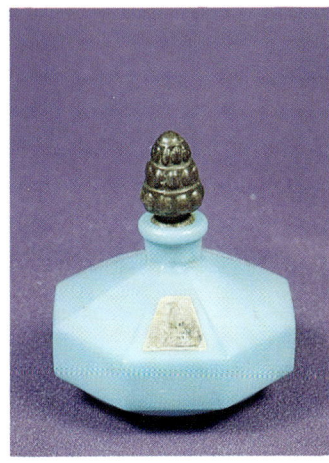
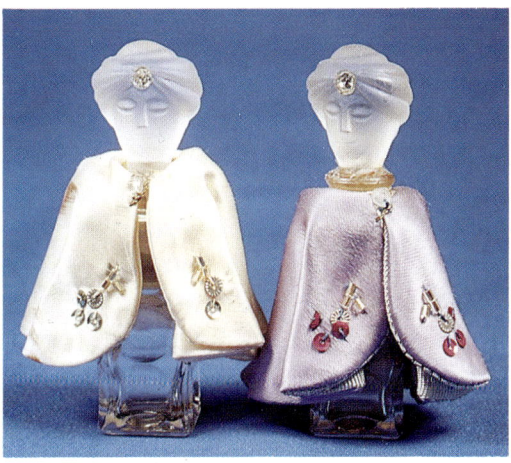
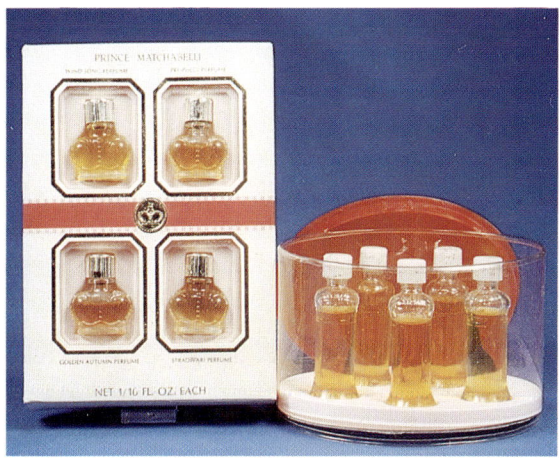

Lot #60. Richard Hudnut *Le Début Bleu* blue glass bottle and stopper, 1.7" [4.4 cm], flat octagonal shape, stopper with silver enamel, silver labels on front and bottom of the bottle, though both are worn [letters faint], empty. Est. $200.00-$300.00.

Lot #61. Marquay *Prince Douka* pair of clear glass bottles with frosted glass stoppers, 3.1" each [7.9 cm], the stoppers molded as the prince's head and each with a rhinestone in the turban, one with a lavendar cape, one with a white cape, empty. Two items. Est. $150.00-$225.00.

Lot #62. Matchabelli *Windsong, Golden Autumn, Prophesy,* and *Strativari* set of four clear glass miniature replicas with gold caps, each 1.4" [3.6 cm], with perfume, gold labels on bottoms, in their gift box with clear windows; *Windsong, Golden Autumn, Prophesy, Beloved,* and *Strativari* set of five clear glass cologne miniatures, 2.6" [6.6 cm], full, labels on bottoms, in a plastic case. Two items, nine minis. Est. $100.00-$175.00.

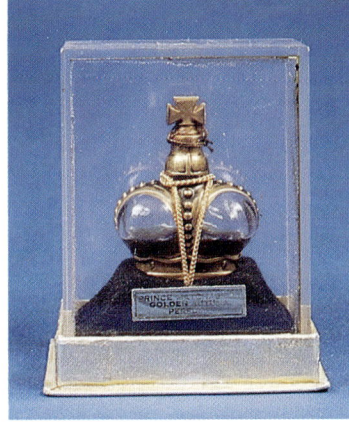
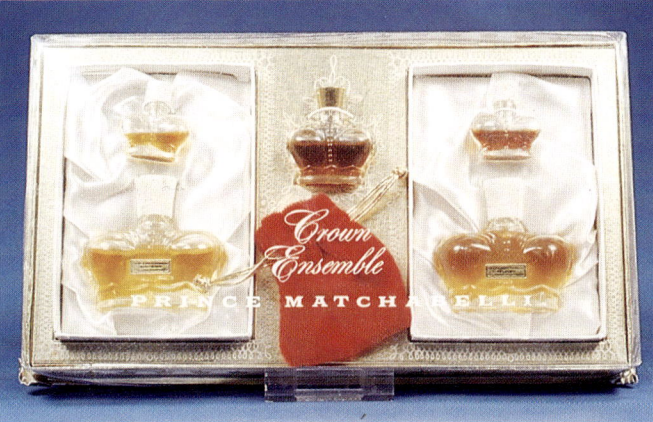
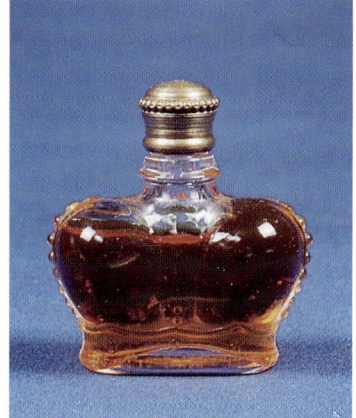

Lot #63. Matchabelli *Golden Autumn* clear glass bottle and stopper in a crown shape, 1.7" [4.3 cm], gold enamel decoration, sealed with some perfume, in a lucite covered box with gold label on side. Est. $75.00-$100.00.

Lot #64. Matchabelli *Crown Ensemble: Beloved* and *Wind Song* clear glass minis with white caps, 1.4" [3.6 cm], unused, gold labels on bottoms, both with a larger size clear glass bottle and white cap, 2.3" [5.8 cm], gold labels on front of each; *Stradivari* clear glass bottle and brass cap, 1.7" [4.3 cm], with perfume, gold label on bottom; all in their presentation box with a celluloid cover. Est. $100.00-$150.00.

Lot #65. Matchabelli *Infanta* rare clear glass miniature bottle and brass metal cap, 1.7" [4.3 cm], crown shape, full, gold label on bottom. Est. $100.00-$150.00.

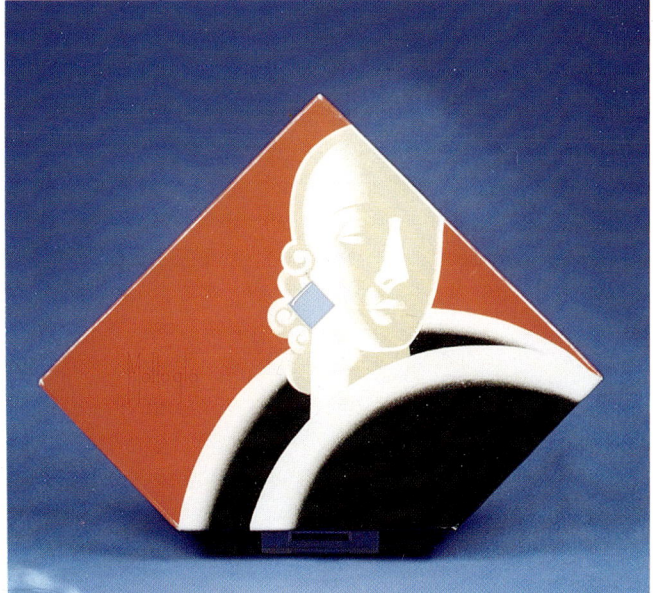
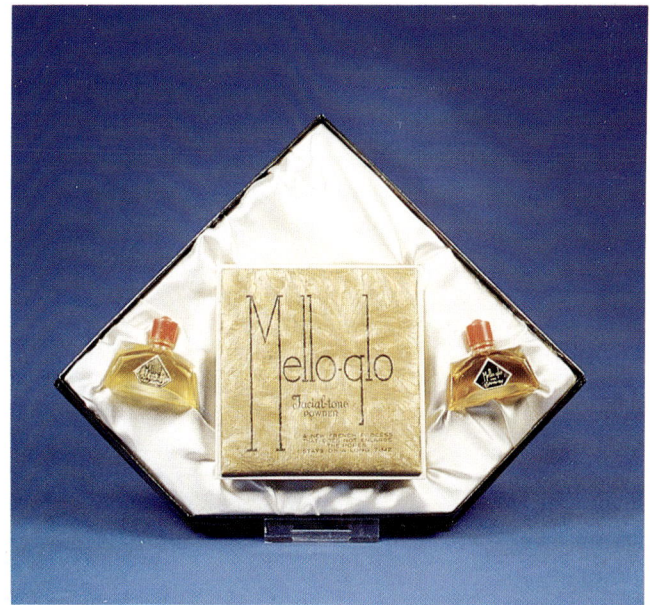

Lot #66. Mello-Glo powder and perfume set: *Daytime* and *Evening* miniature glass bottles with red caps, 1.5" [3.8 cm], gold labels; unopened square powder, in a satin-lined box with a stunning Art Deco graphic in red and black, with outer box. The condition is pristine. Est. $125.00-$175.00.

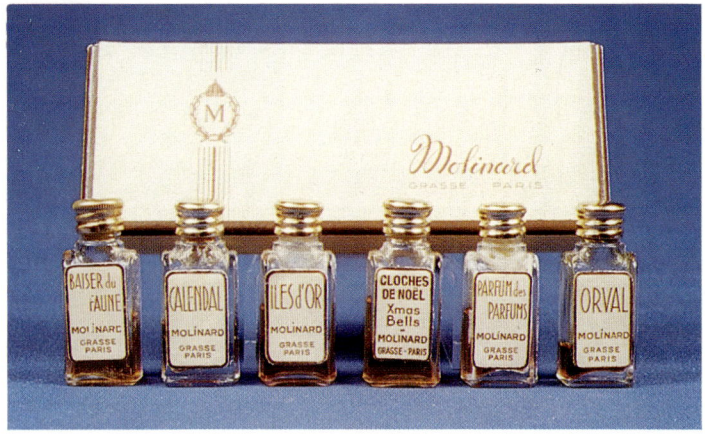

Lot #67. Molinard set of 6: *Baiser du Faune, Calendal, Iles d'Or, Cloches de Noël, Parfum des Parfums, Orval,* each a miniature glass bottle with gold metal cap, 1.5" [3.8 cm], all with intact labels on front, in their box and box cover which are both marked *Compliments of Ralph Wilson*. Est. $100.00-$150.00.

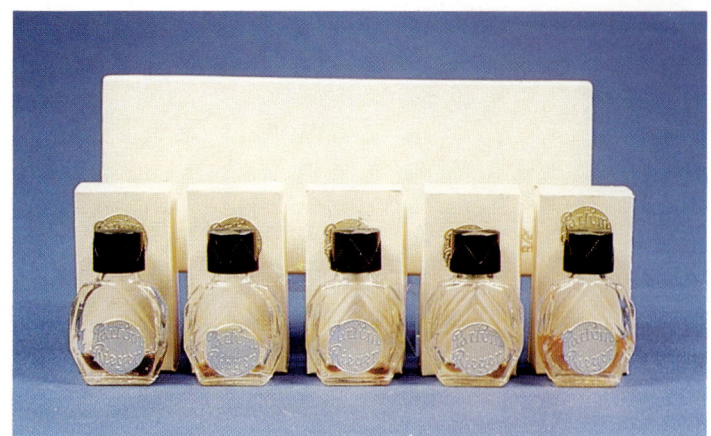

Lot #68. Rieger *Monte Carlo, Lily of the Valley, Mystic Night, Black Velvet, Hollywood Bouquet* set of five miniature bottles with black caps, each 1.9" [4.7 cm], all in unused mint condition but perfume has evaporated, each bottle with gold labels front and back and likewise on its individual box, all in their larger box signed *Rieger Perfumer*. Est. $100.00-$150.00.

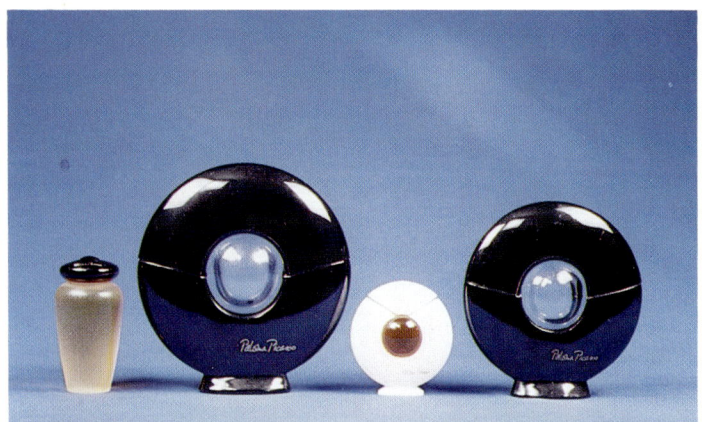

Lot #69. Paloma Picasso group of two clear glass bottles and stoppers encased in a circular black plastic sculpture, 4.5" and 3.8" [11.4 and 9.7 cm], empty, name in gold enamel; miniature replica clear glass bottle similarly encased in white plastic [the white was the original design], 2.3" [5.8 cm], with perfume; miniature bath oil container of plastic with black top, 2.6" [6.6 cm], full. Four items. Est. $100.00-$150.00.

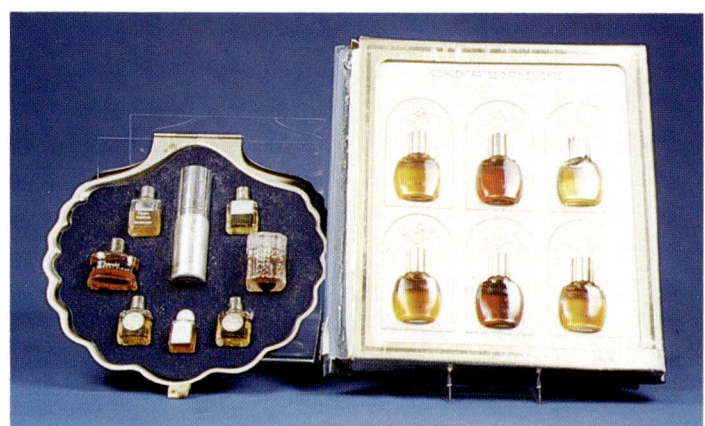

Lot #70. Set of 8 miniatures: Berdoes *Joie,* Smyr, *Tendresse;* Houbigant *Essence Rare, Quelques Fleurs* mini atomizer and a mini bottle with metal cap; Lucien Lelong *Indiscret;* Piguet *Bandit;* all mounted clockform in a metal shell-shaped box; Floris *Florissa, Jasmine, Lily of the Valley, Malmaison, Ormonde, Stephanoitis,* bath essence miniature glass bottles with gold caps, 1.9" [4.8 cm], all mounted in a bookform box, a commemorative presentation for the 250th anniversary of Floris. Two sets of 14 minis. Est. $150.00-$200.00.

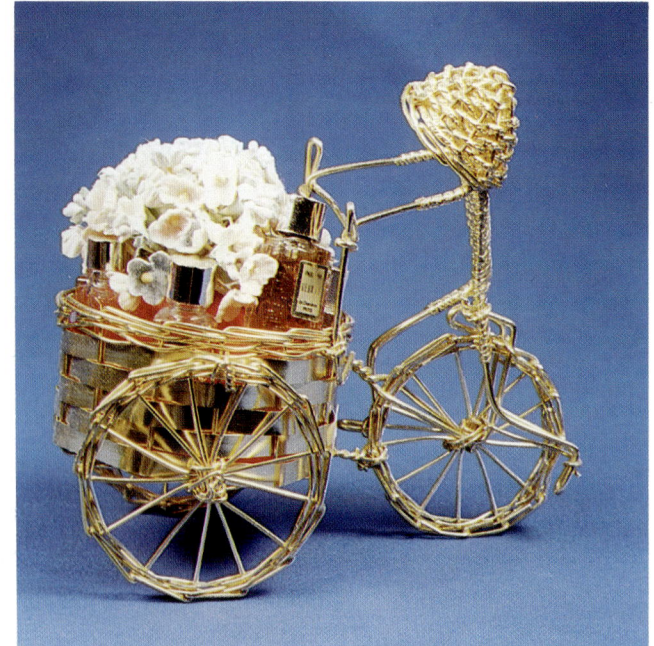

Lot #71. Set of 7 minis: Augier *Garde Moi* ['Keep Me']; Bonnet *Sarine;* Charles V *Versart* and *Parfum Pamyr;* de Charières *Reine de Mai* ['May Queen'], *Bavardage* ['Gossip'], and *Veux-Tu* ['Do You Want'] in a charming wire holder shaped as a flower cart bicycle. Est. $50.00-$75.00.

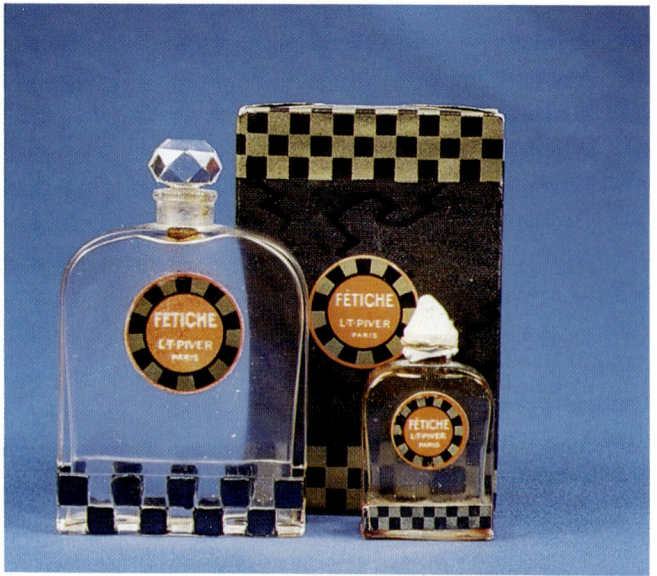

Lot #72. L. T. Piver *Fétiche* ['Fetish'] clear glass bottle and stopper of flask shape, 3.3" [8.4 cm], the base of the bottle enameled with a checkerboard pattern in black, empty, orange label, in its box decorated with conforming motifs; extremely rare replica miniature, 2.1" [5.3 cm], near empty but sealed, orange label and gold and black checkerboard label. Two items. Est. $350.00-$450.00.

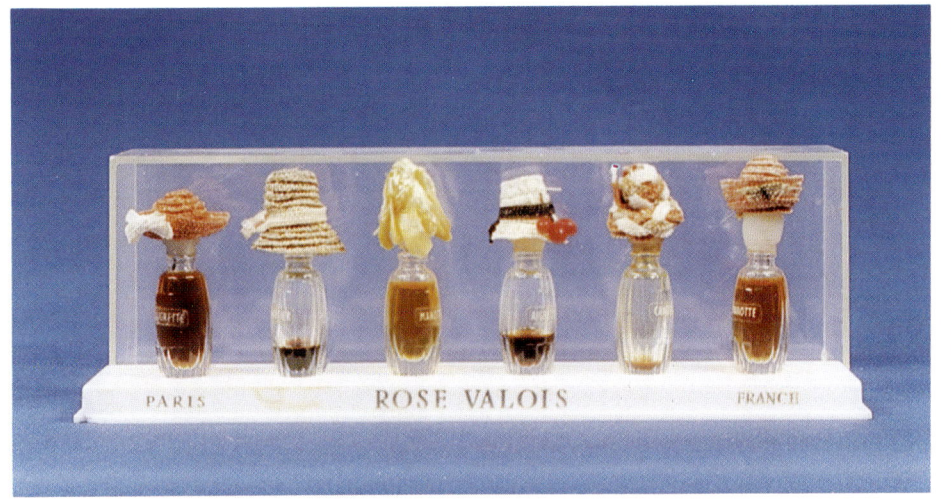

Lot #73. Rose Valois *Aigrette, Canotier, Marotte* [names for hats, such as 'plumed hat,' 'boater,' etc.] unusual set of six clear glass bottles with head-shaped plastic caps and six different hats, 2.4" [6 cm], in a white plastic stand and clear lucite cover [plastic with small chip and lucite with age crack], each with a label and the set with a label underneath. Rose Valois was originally known for haute couture hats; this set is quite rare. Est. $600.00-$750.00.

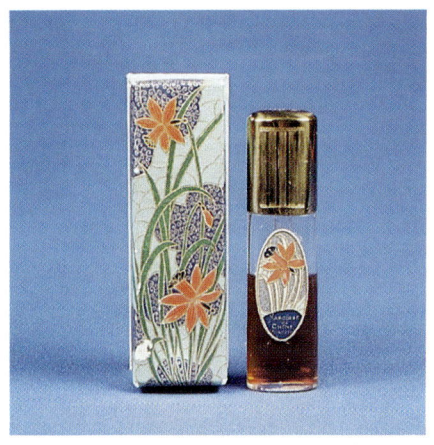

Lot #74. Vivadou *Narcisse de Chine* ['Chinese Narcissus'] clear glass tester bottle and stopper with long dauber and brass overcap, 3.2" [8.1 cm], with perfume and unused, both its label and its box decorated with narcissus in red and gold against a background stylized in the Chinese manner. Est. $50.00-$100.00.

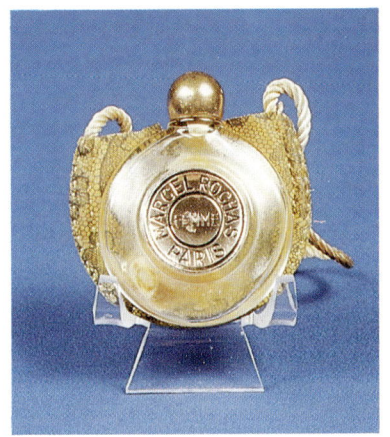

Lot #75. Marcel Rochas *Femme* clear glass round bottle and metal cap, 2.2" [5.6 cm], gold metallic label at center, empty, in its leather pouch with a black lace motif. Est. $75.00-$100.00.

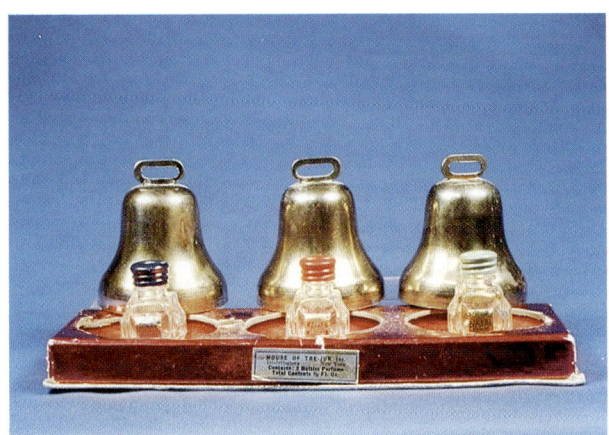

Lot #76. House of Tré-Jur *Apple Blossom, Gardenia, Honeysuckle* set of three clear glass minis with blue, green, and red caps, each 1.4" [3.6 cm], in a Christmas presentation in which they are hidden under brass bells, all empty, gold foil labels. Est. $75.00-$125.00.

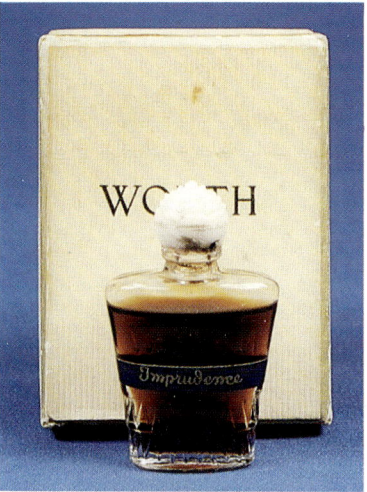

Lot #77. Worth *Imprudence* clear glass bottle with white plastic cap, 2.1" [5.3 cm], the bottle molded with chevrons to replicate the design of the standard bottle, with perfume, blue label, in its cream colored box. Est. $100.00-$150.00.

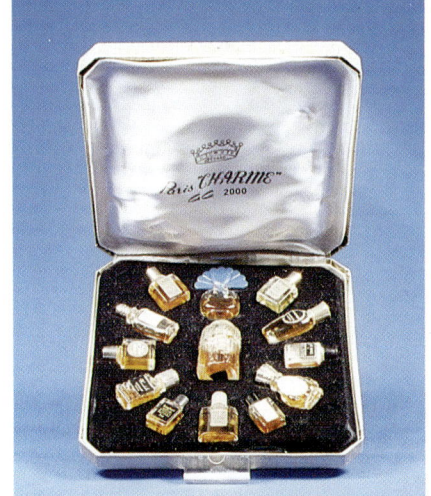

Lot #78. Paris *Charme* set of 13 minis, Balenciaga *Le Dix*; Berdoes *Ambre, Capri, Cordoba, Smyr, Tonka*; Houbigant *Essence Rare*; Marquay *Coup de Feu*; Piguet *Baghari*; Vigny *Heure Intime*; *Parfum Folies Bergere*; Royal Perfumes *C'est*; Weil *Antilope*; all arranged clockform in a gold hinged presentation case. Est. $175.00-$250.00.

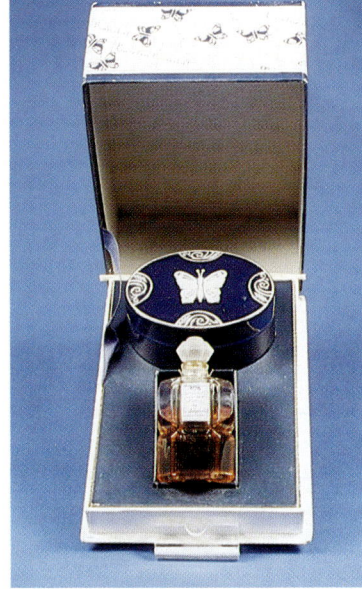

Lot #79. Lucretia Vanderbilt *Concentrated Perfume* clear glass hexagonal bottle and frosted stopper, 2.6" [6.6 cm], silver label; *Face Powder #21* unopened metal powder box; with a pamphlet on beauty, in a lovely box. Est. $125.00-$225.00.

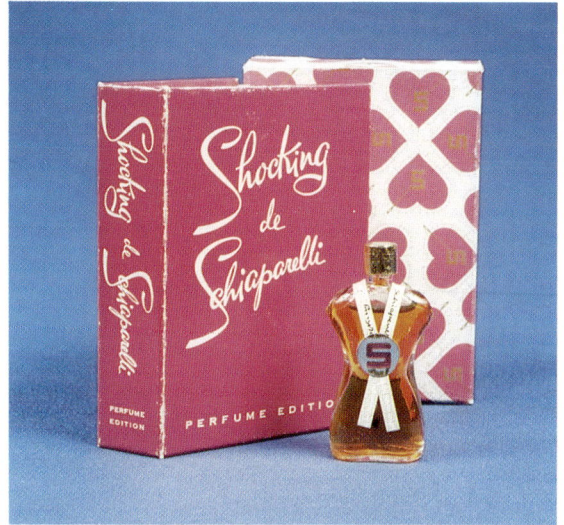

Lot #80. Schiaparelli *Shocking* clear glass bottle with brass cap, 2" [5.1 cm], 1/4 oz., in the dressmaker's dummy shape, full, with tape measure label [small part of label missing on the back only], in a charming book-form presentation marked *Perfume Edition*; with its outer box decorated with hearts. Est. $150.00-$250.00.

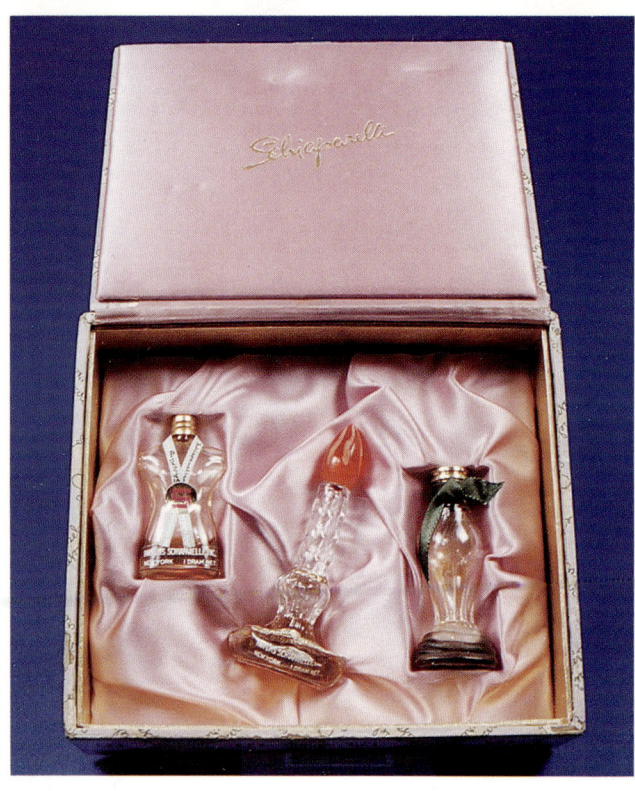

Lot #81. Schiaparelli rare set of three replica miniatures in their box: *Shocking*, clear glass bottle with brass cap, 1.9" [4.9 cm], tape measure label; *Sleeping*, clear glass bottle with red bakelite cap, 3.1" [8 cm], gold label; *Zut*, clear glass bottle with gold cap, 2.3" [5.9 cm], gold labels on cap and bottom; while the top of the box has been taped, it is very unusual to find this set in the box at all; the bottles themselves are in pristine condition. Est. $500.00-$750.00.

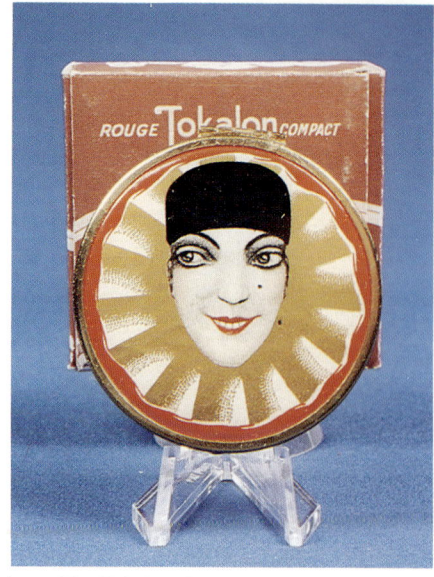

Lot #82. Tokalon *Rouge Oriental* metal compact, 2" [5.1 cm] diameter, the front of the compact beautifully decorated with the face of Pierrot in mulitcolors, mint condition, signed *Tokalon Paris* on the edge, in its box with a Tokalon pamphlet inside. Est. $150.00-$250.00.

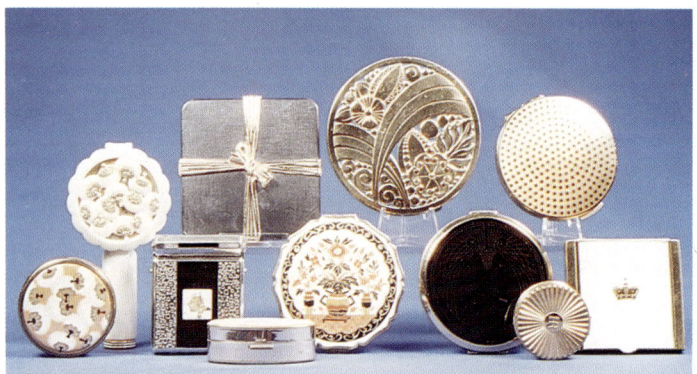
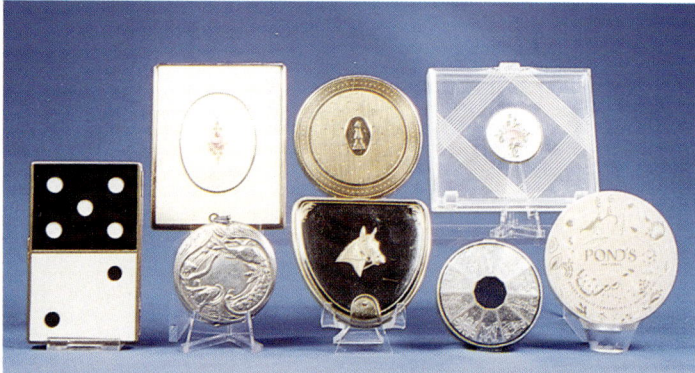

Lot 83. Lot of 19 compacts and related items: Bourjois *Evening in Paris;* Mary Chess; Coro black with horse portrait; Coty, 3 diff., one plastic with lipstick, one brass, one Domino in black and white [inside mirror with chip]; Elgin enamel cigarette case; Max Factor lipstick case; Lancôme black/gold; Prince Matchabelli white/gold; Pond's pink powder box, unused; Rex Fifth Avenue round Art Deco floral design with blue enamel; Helena Rubenstein, 2 diff., one black with gold bow, second round rouge; Stratton, 2 diff, one with an orange, white, and black design of flowers in enamel, second brass with design of stars; Yardley with lipstick; unsigned, Art Nouveau design; lucite case with enamel floral medallion. Total of nineteen items. Est. $190.00-$380.00.

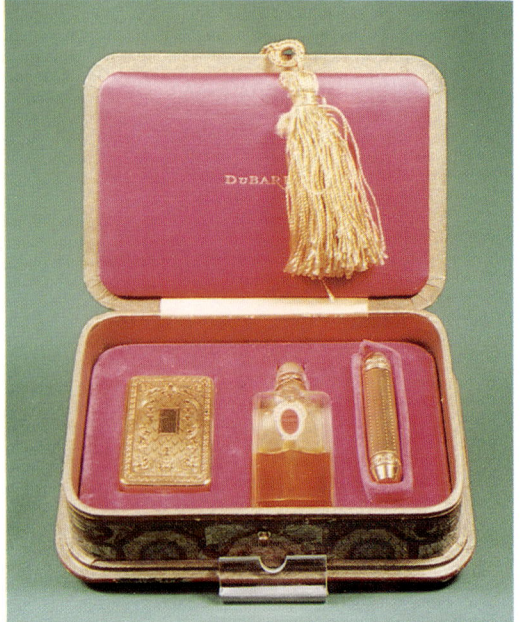

Lot #84. Richard Hudnut *DuBarry* set comprising: clear glass bottle and frosted glass stopper with long dauber, 2.7" [6.9 cm], sealed, label on front; metal lipstick, 2.4" [6.1 cm]; book-shaped compact, 2.1" [5.3 cm], unused, and signed *Richard Hudnut DuBarry;* all in a beautiful case lined with bright pink velvet. Est. $250.00-$350.00.

Lot #85. Richard Hudnut *Deauville* double compact, 2" [5.1 cm] diameter and lipstick, 2.1" [5.3 cm] long, both objects enameled in turquoise, the compact unused and with both rouge and powder, both objects joined together by a chain, in their silk-lined box with velvet cover, marked inside *Deauville*. Est. $150.00-$200.00.

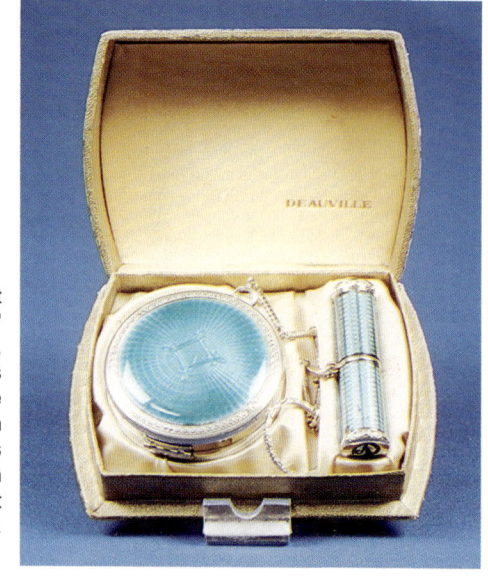

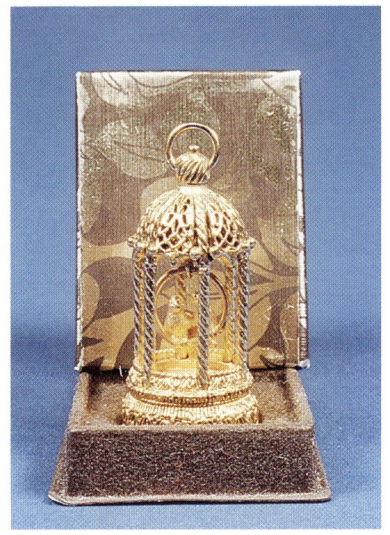

Lot #86. Corday *Fame* lovebirds metal solid perfume container shaped as a cage with two lovebirds, 2.5" [6.4 cm], the bottom part of the cage hinges open for the solid perfume [still present], label on bottom, in its original brown and gold box decorated with foliage. Est. $150.00-$200.00.

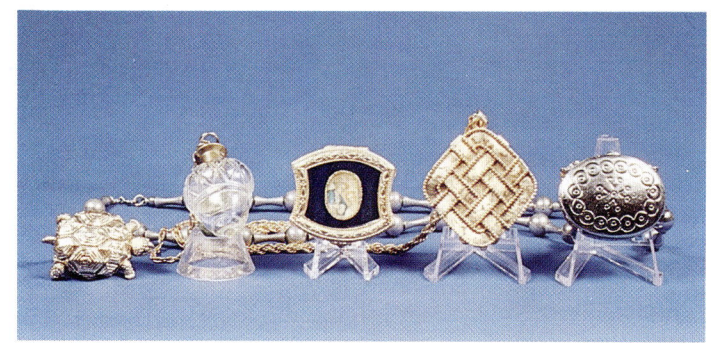

Lot #87. Lauder solid perfume with blue enamel and a tiny cameo of a mother and child, signed *Estée Lauder;* Revlon *Aviance* solid perfume on a long necklace, inside molded *Aviance;* Estée Lauder *Estée* silver metal solid perfume on a long necklace, inside signed *Estée;* Solid perfume pin in the shape of a gold turtle, unsigned; Max Factor *Wild Musk* acorn-shaped clear glass bottle and metal cap on a gold chain necklace. Five items. Est. $125.00-$200.00.

Lot #88. Max Factor *Aquarius Tiny Tusker* creme perfume of gold metal, 1.2" [3.1 cm], the elephant having trappings in the Indian style, red gemstone eyes, on a long gold necklace with its original label, in its original box; *Strawberry Musk* red glass bottle with gold cap, 1.8" [4.6 cm], molded as a strawberry and on a long gold chain, in its original box. Two items. Est. $75.00-$150.00.

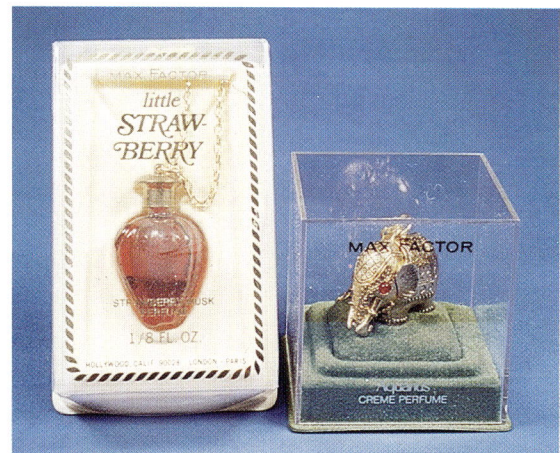

FACTICES
PERFUME LAMPS
FRAGRANCE MEMORABILIA

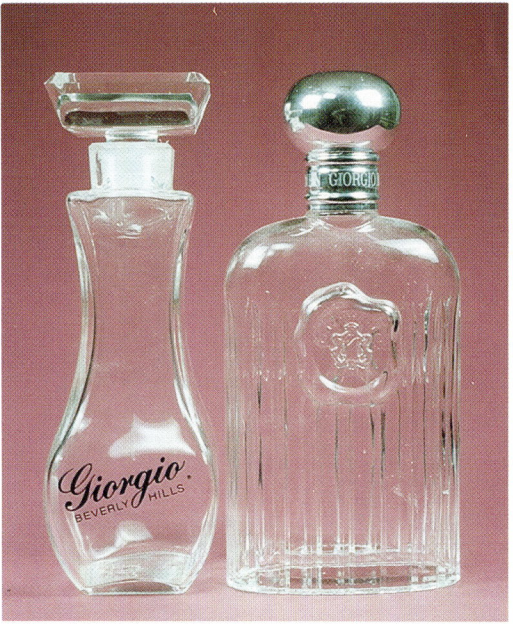

Lot #89. Giorgio *Beverly Hills* clear glass bottle and stopper, 11.8" [30 cm], a combination of curvilinear and rectilinear design, names in black enamel on front, emtpy, signed *Giorgio* on bottom, with emblem, and also *Made in France by Brosse;* Giorgio *Beverly Hills for Men* clear glass bottle of flask shape with silver plastic cap [chips on neck inside], empty, *Giorgio* emblem molded on front in the style of a wax seal, bottom signed *Made in France for Giorgio.* Two items. Est. $300.00-$400.00.

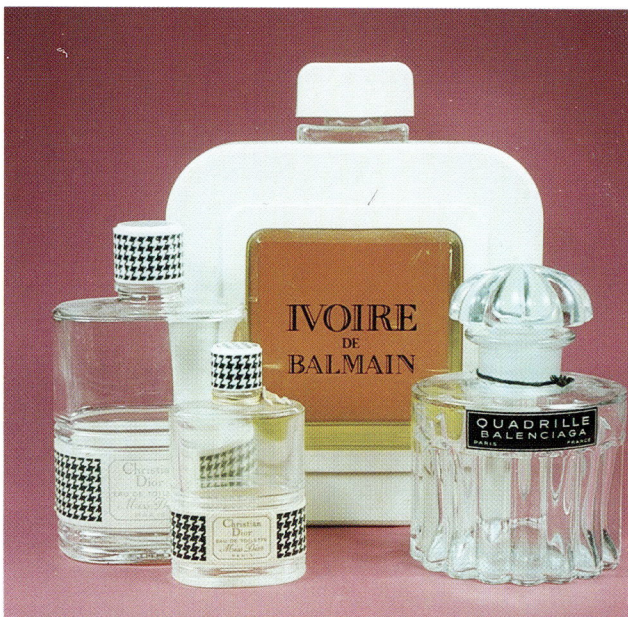

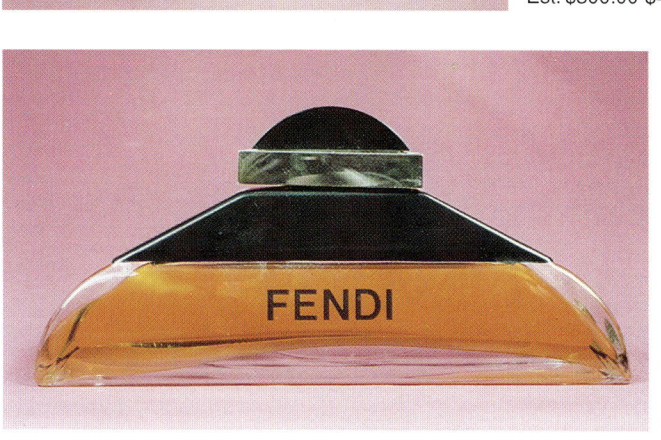

Lot #90. Balmain *Ivoire* plastic replica bottle, 9.5" [24.1 cm], square shaped with rounded corners, names printed on front surface; Christian Dior *Miss Dior Eau de Toilette* pair of clear glass bottles with white caps, 6.5" and 4.5" [16.5 and 11.4 cm], empty, a houndstooth design on labels and caps, bottoms signed *CD* in the mold; Balenciaga *Quadrille* clear glass bottle and stopper, 5.9" [15 cm], designed with scallops around bottle and stopper, empty, black label, bottom signed *Balenciaga* in the mold. Four items. Est. $250.00-$350.00.

Lot #91. Fendi elongated modernistic clear glass perfume factice with black cap and plastic overcap, 11.3" long [28.7 cm] and 5.3" tall [13.4 cm], name in black enamel on front, full. Est. $200.00-$300.00.

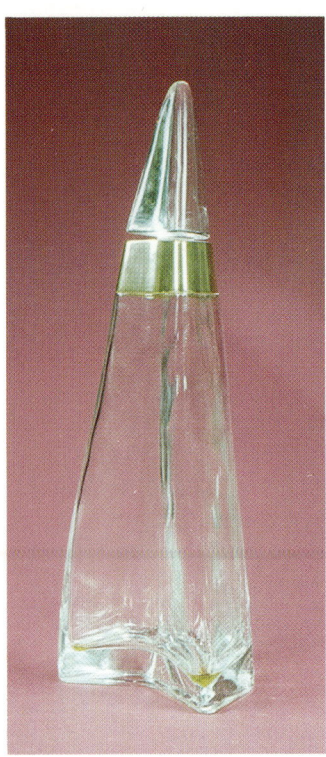

Lot #92. Halston *Night* clear glass bottle and stopper with plastic tip, 14" [35.6 cm], shaped as an icicle, gold plastic neck, empty, bottom with names in black enamel and signed *Halston Fragrances*. Est. $175.00-$275.00.

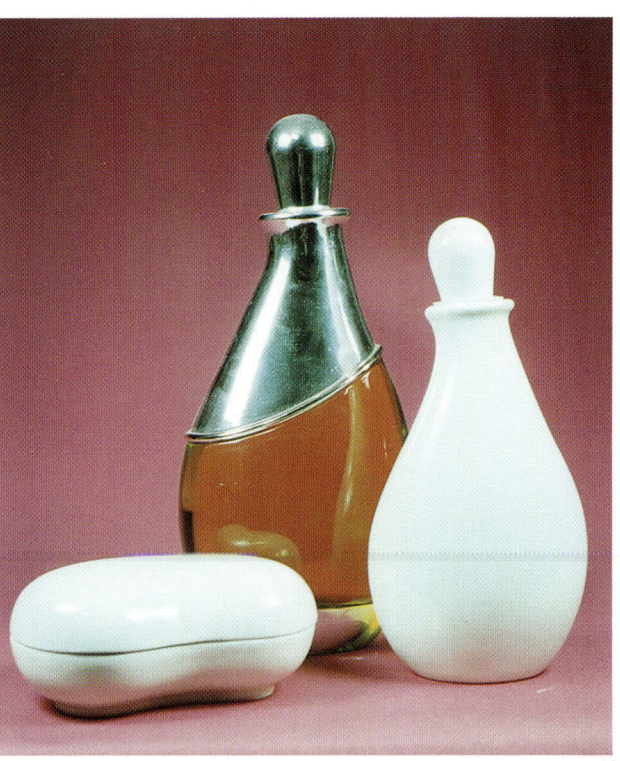

Lot #93. Halston *Couture* clear glass bottle with silver stopper, 12" [30 cm], full, bottom with label marked *factice;* porcelain bottle and stopper, 9.5" [24 cm] of identical design, bottom signed *Halston;* porcelain box and cover, 6" long and 2.2" tall [15.2 and 5.5 cm], bottom signed *Halston;* these three items all designed by Elsa Peretti. Three items. Est. $250.00-$350.00.

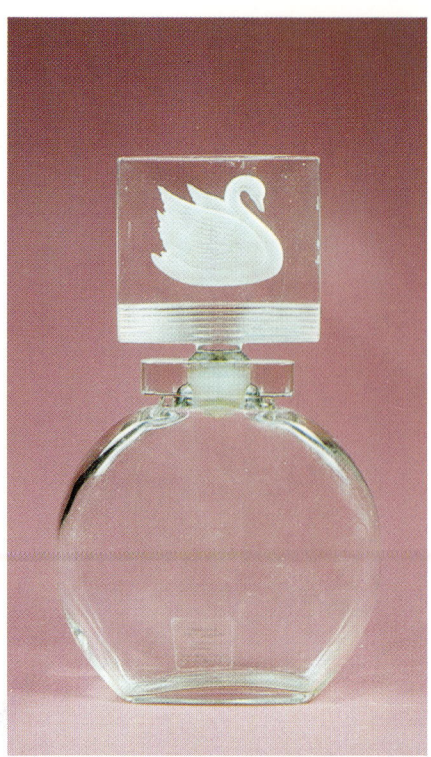

Lot #94. Gloria Vanderbilt *Vanderbilt* clear glass bottle and stopper with plastic tip, 9.9" [25 cm], the bottle of flattened round shape with a rectangular neck, the stopper intaglio cut and frosted with a swan, label on back, empty. Est. $175.00-$250.00.

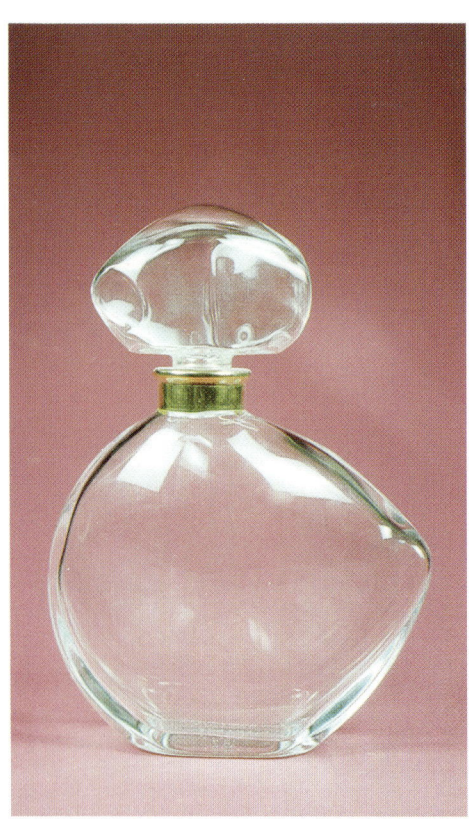

Lot #95. Jaclyn Smith *California* clear glass bottle and stopper, 10.4" [26.4 cm], an abstract design of softly curving lines not dissimilar from the movements of the wind, gold neck, empty, bottom marked *Made in France*. Est. $150.00-$250.00.

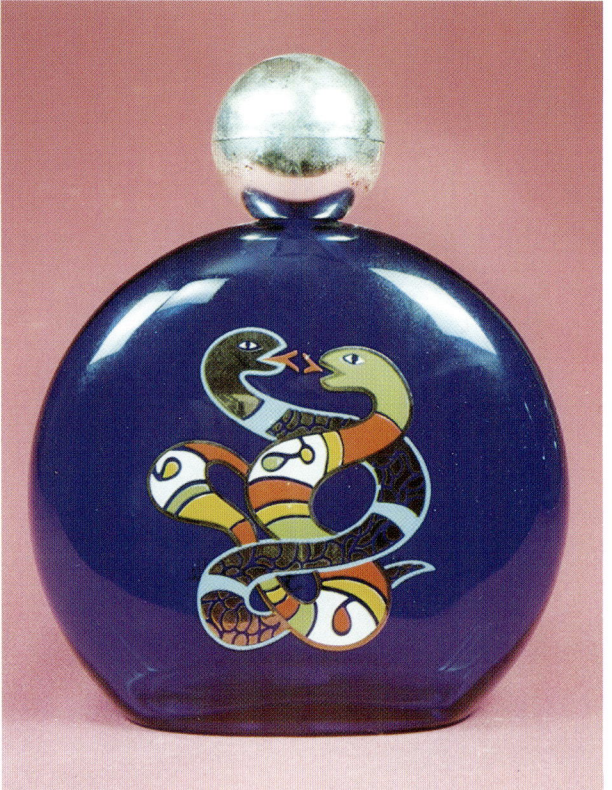

Lot #96. Niki de Saint Phalle rarely seen blue glass bottle and silver plastic stopper, 8.4" [21.3 cm], of flattened round shape, the front enameled in bright colors with intertwined snakes, empty, bottom with *Dummy* label, back of bottle signed *Niki de Saint Phalle* in gold enamel. Est. $200.00-$300.00.

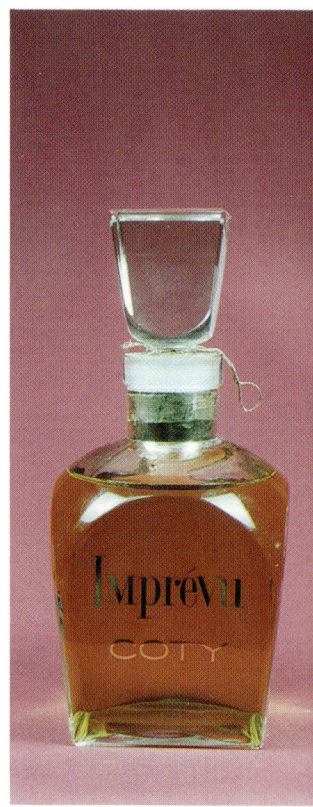

Lot #97. Coty *Imprévu* ['Unforesee clear glass bottle and stopper w plastic tip, 9.5" [24.1 cm], the fou sided bottle enameled with the nam in gold, full, bottom marked *Dumm* Est. $150.00-$250.00.

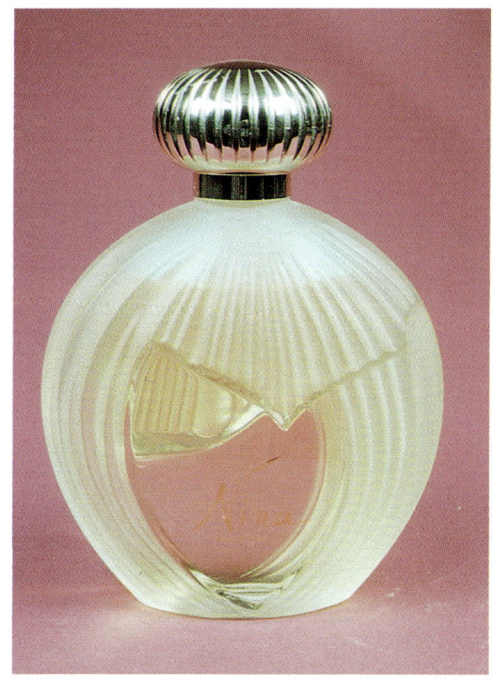

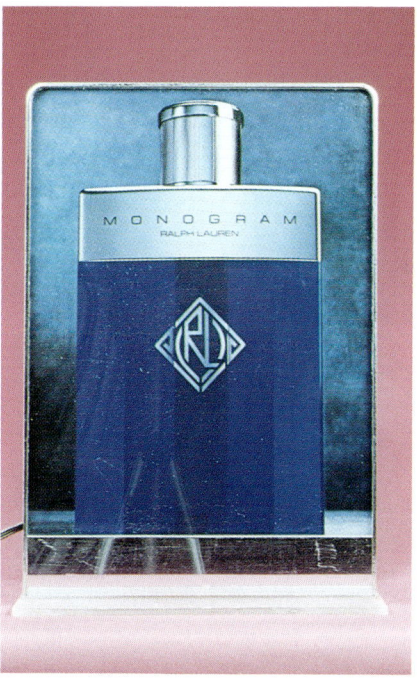

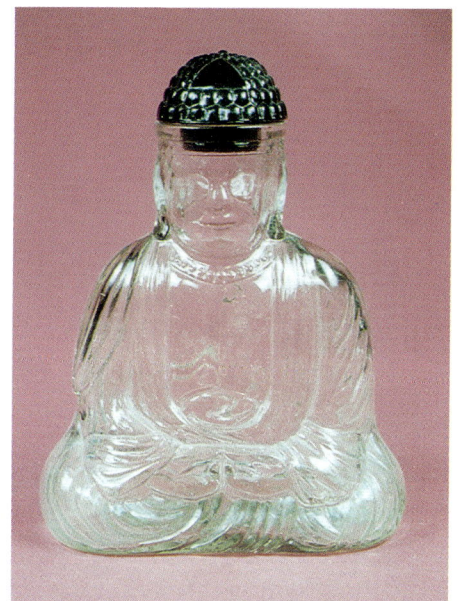

Lot #98. Nina Ricci *Nina* clear and frosted glass bottle with silver plastic cap, 7.2" [18.3 cm], the round form draped with satin folds of material as in a jabot, a heart-shaped window of clear glass with the name in gold enamel, bottom marked *factice* and signed *Lalique* in the mold, designed by Marie-Claude Lalique. Utt #NR-116. Est. $300.00-$400.00.

Lot #99. Ralph Lauren *Monogram* unusual electric display lighting fixture, 16" tall and 11" wide [40.6 x 28 cm], with a picture of the blue glass bottle covering most of the surface; this is an unusual and attractive item to light up a perfume collection. Est. $100.00-$200.00.

Lot #100. Vantine's early clear glass bottle and amber glass stopper, 6.5" [16.5 cm], in the shape of an oriental figure in the lotus position, with the folds of his robe open at the chest, empty, bottom signed *Vantine's* in the mold. Est. $250.00-$350.00.

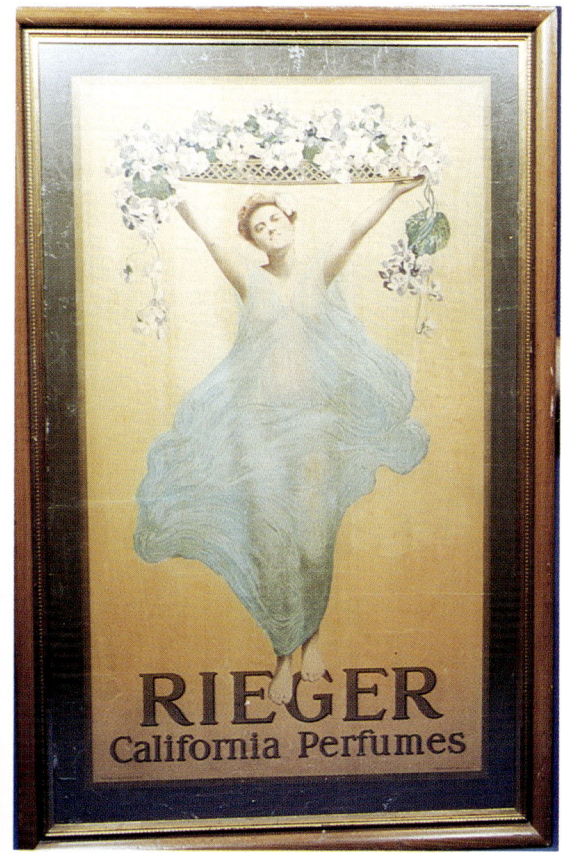

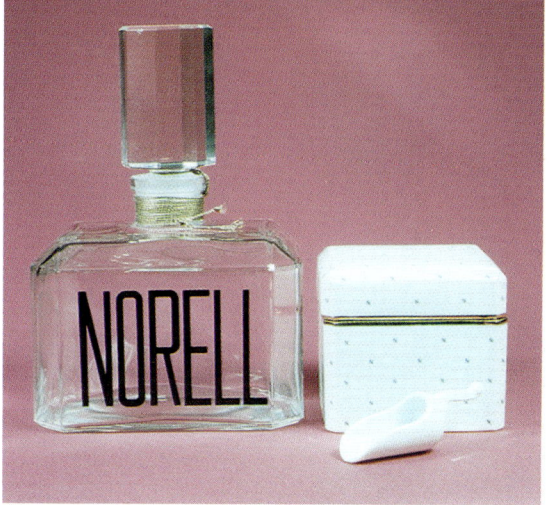

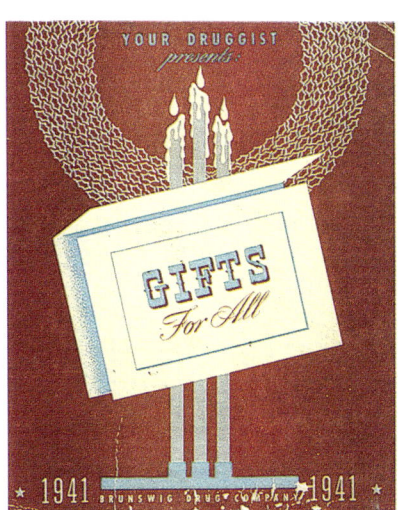

Lot #101. Norell *Norell* clear glass bottle and stopper with plastic tip, 8.2" [20.8 cm] with faceted columnar stopper, name in black enamel on front, empty; porcelain powder box and cover in a design matching the bottle, with a porcelain scoop, edges of the box enameled in gold and the initial *N* enameled in a symmetrical pattern covering the entire surface, bottom signed *Norell* and *Made Expressly for Norell in Seto City Japan*. Two items. Est. $200.00-$300.00.

Lot #102. Early publicity poster for Rieger California Perfumes, depicting, in the Art Nouveau style, a woman in a diaphanous green robe holding aloft an overflowing basket of flowers mounted in a wood frame, artist signed *Urquhart Wilcox* at bottom, printed by Mutual Lithography Co, San Francisco; some wear and creasing to the poster, total framed dimensions 27.3" x 41.8" [69.3 cm x 106 cm]. Est. $300.00-$400.00.

Lot #103. Brunswig Drug Company 1941 catalogue, a spiral bound book, mostly in color, with gift items of all kinds [cameras, pens, etc.] as well as fragrances: 2 pages each on Williams, Karoff, Nassour, Pinaud, Stuart, Vigny, Charbert, Ciro, Lanvin, Gabilla, Wembdon; 3-4 pages each on Babs, Olde New England, Cardinal, Houbigant, Roger & Gallet, Wrisley, as well as extensive coverage of Coty [16 p]; Bourjois [12p]; H. H. Ayer [10 p]; Hudnut [10 p]. Overall very good condition but with slight water damage at the very bottom on some pages. Est. $200.00-$300.00.

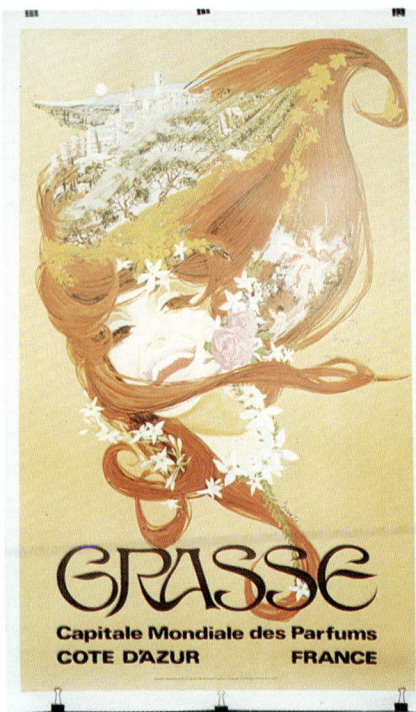
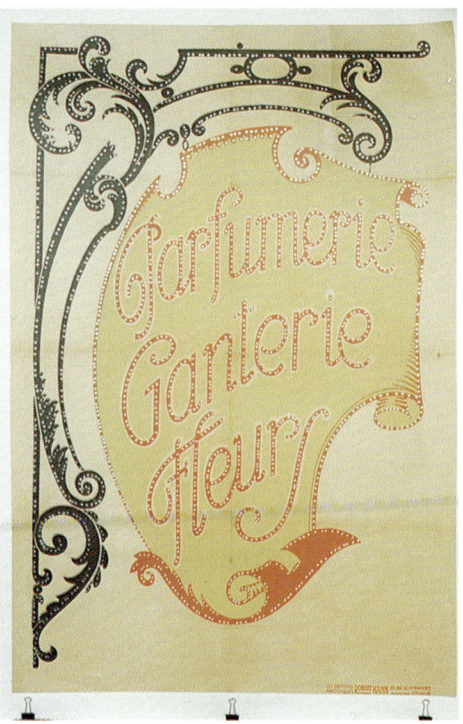
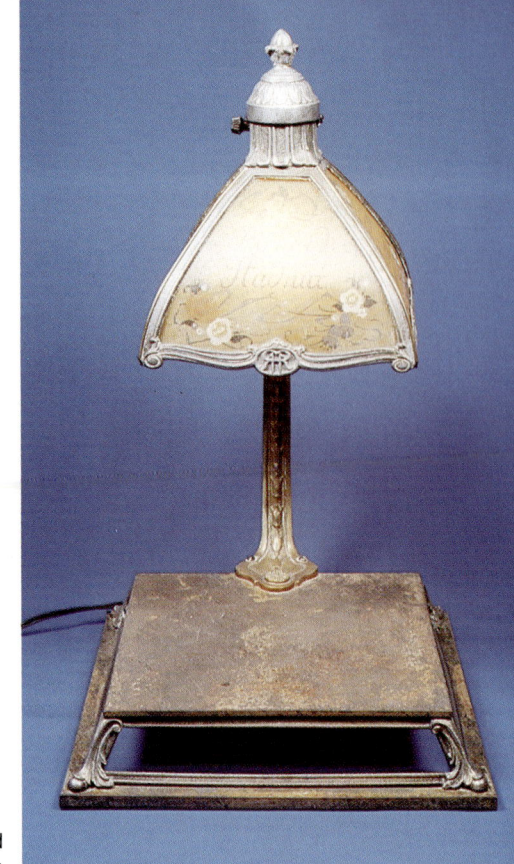

Lot #104. Lot of two perfume related posters: *Grasse Capitale Mondiale des Parfums* ['World Capital of Perfumes'], 37" x 22.5" [94 x 57 cm], produced by the Grasse Syndicat d'Initiative; *Parfumerie Ganterie Fleur*, 38" x 26" [96.5 x 66 cm]; both posters are canvas-backed and in excellent condition. Two posters. Est. $250.00-$350.00.

Lot #105. Richard Hudnut metal lamp with reverse painted glass shade, 20" [50.8 cm], the metal base with a large square platform for the display of perfumes [it may originally have had glass panels around the base; the metal parts to hold glass accompany it], the metal frame for the shade molded with the *Hudnut* logo, each panel of the shade with the words *Richard Hudnut* and decorated with various flowers. Est. $500.00-$750.00.

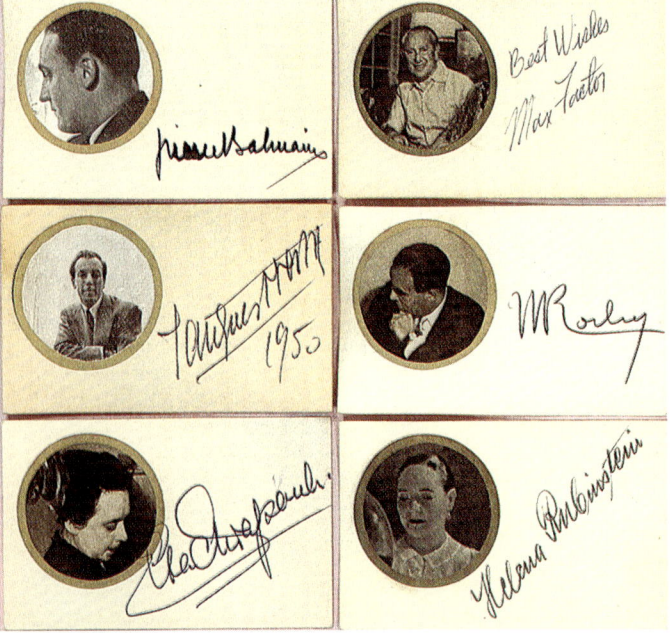

Lot #106. A collection of six autographs: *Pierre Balmain, Max Factor, Jacques Fath, Marcel Rochas, Helena Rubenstein, Elsa Schiaparelli*; each autograph is on an identical card, 2.7" x 4.5" [7 cm x 11.4 cm] on which the collector has placed a picture of each designer. Est. $600.00-$750.00.

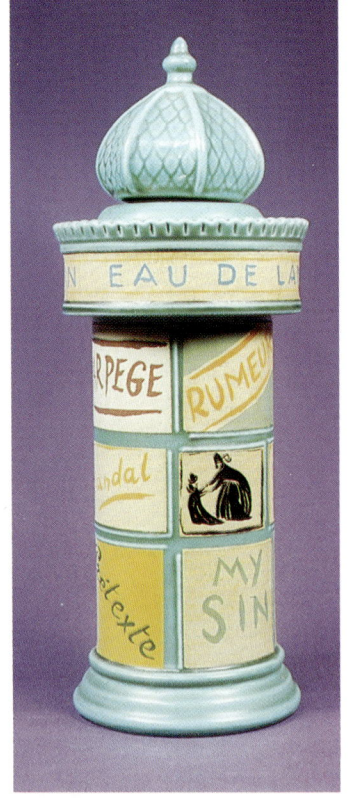
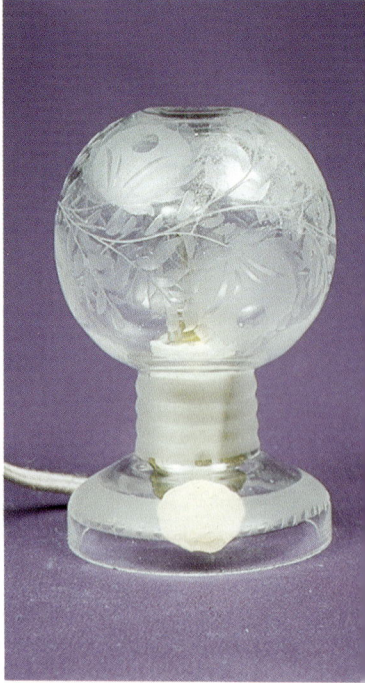

Lot #107. Lanvin ceramic publicity bottle, 10.5" [26.7 cm], shaped as a Parisian kiosk in green, with the names of important Lanvin fragrances mounted in découpage around the sides; the top is removable and has a small bruise; the bottom is molded *Executé à Paris pour Lanvin Parfums par Franor-Royale*. Est. $300.00-$400.00.

Lot #108. Clear crystal perfume lamp in a ball shape, 4.1" [10.4 cm], wheel-cut with a design of flowers and leaves, original electrical apparatus intact, I.Rice paper label and acid-stamped *Czechoslovakia*. Est. $200.00-$250.00.

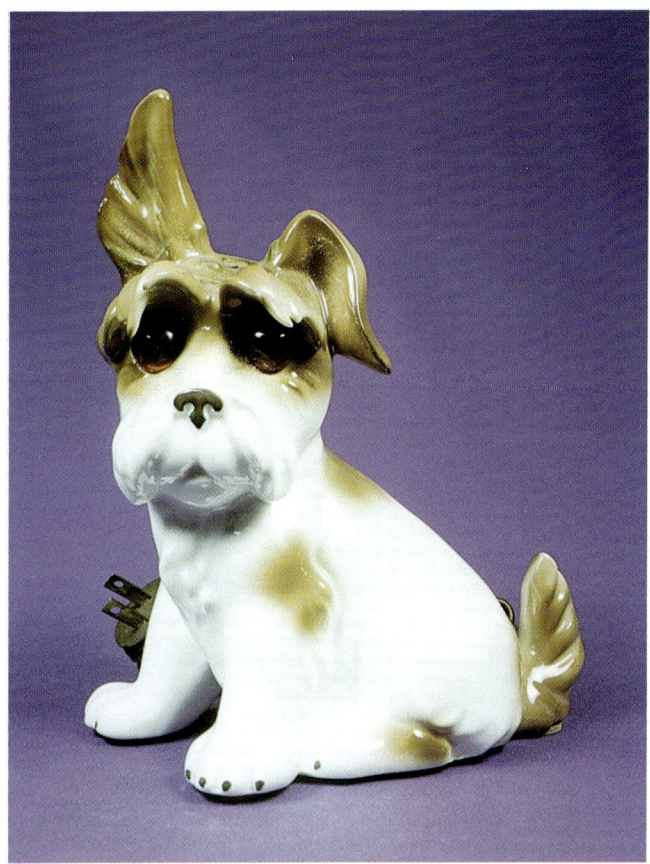

Lot #109. German porcelain figural perfume lamp, 7.9" [20 cm], in the shape of an adorable terrier puppy with one ear cocked up, a well in head for the perfume, unsigned, original electrical wiring. Est. $450.00-$550.00.

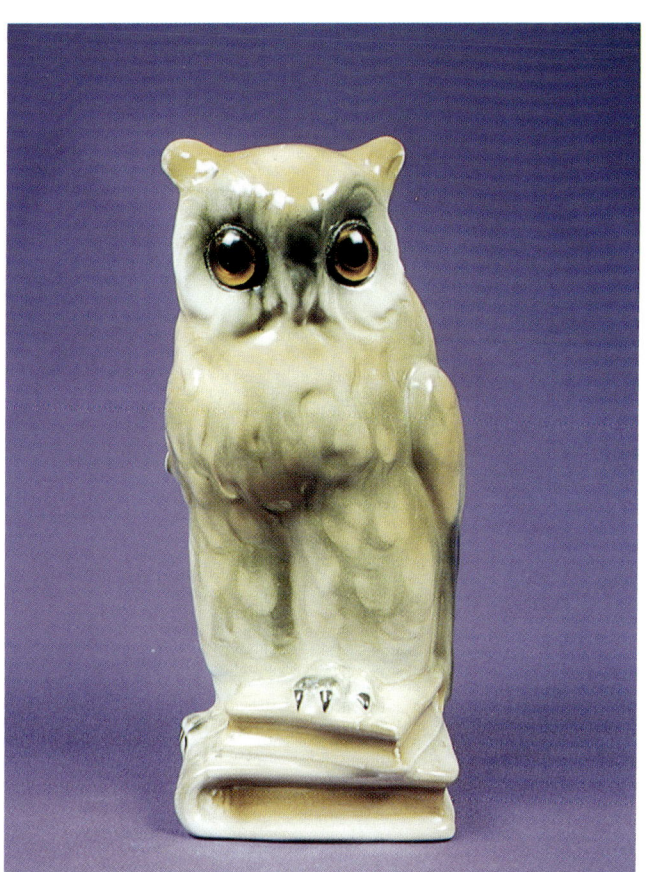

Lot #110. German porcelain perfume lamp in the shape of an owl, 7.5" [19 cm], the owl perched upon two books, realistically painted in brown tones, amber eyes, a well in the side for perfume, totally unwired, German factory emblem inside. Est. $200.00-$300.00.

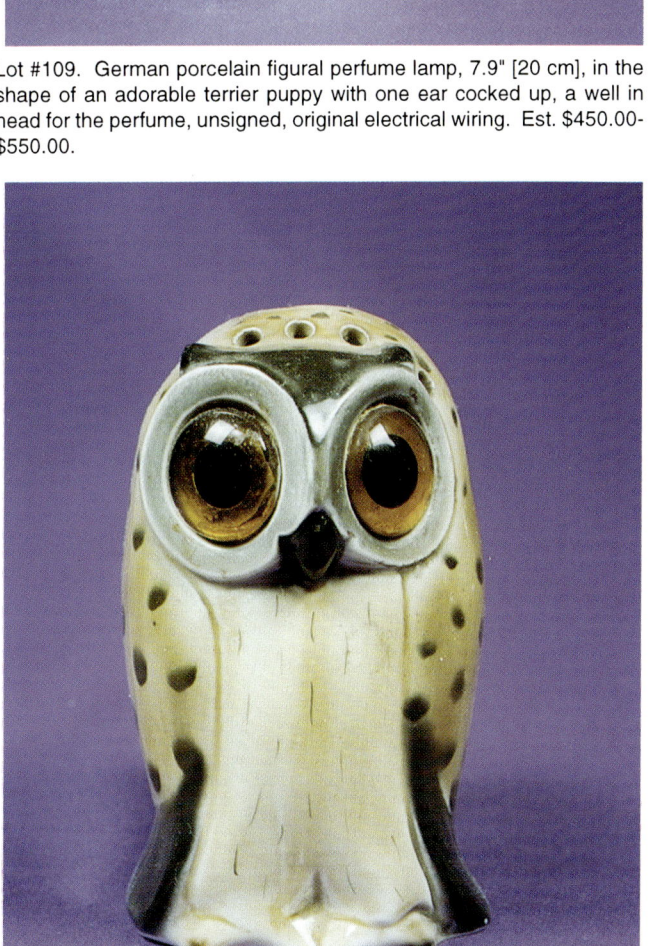

Lot #111. Goebel porcelain perfume lamp in the shape of an owl stylized in the Art Deco manner, 5" [12.7 cm], a well on top for perfume, painted in gray and brown with huge amber eyes, electrified, stamped *Germany* and signed with the logo for *W. Goebel*. Est. $400.00-$500.00.

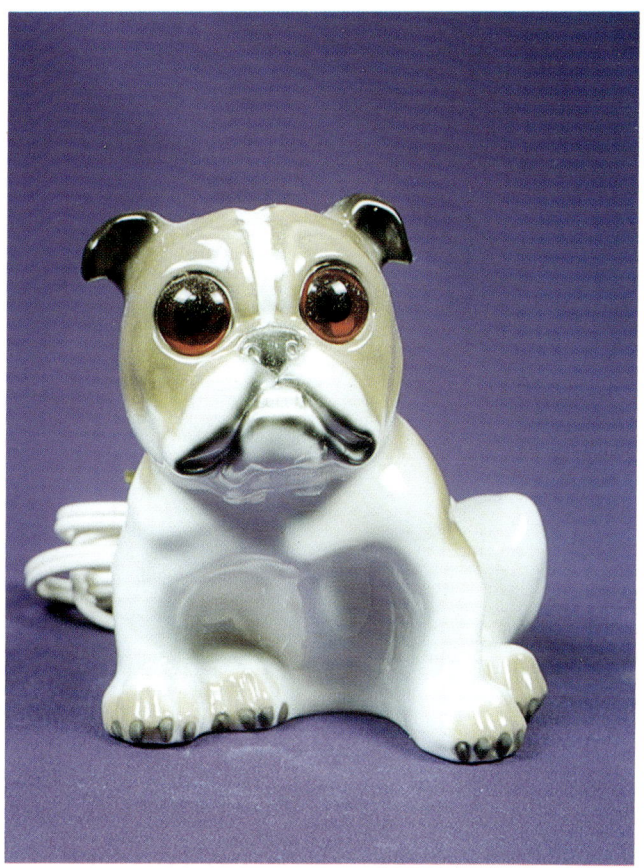

Lot #112. Goebel porcelain perfume lamp in the shape of a French bulldog, 4.6" [11.7 cm], the dog with a well in the back for perfume, large red eyes, rewired for working condition, signed underneath with Goebel Crown and *WG* in ink and in the mold, model *#EF 256*. Est. $450.00-$550.00.

CROWN TOP - PORCELAIN - DECORATIVE BOTTLES

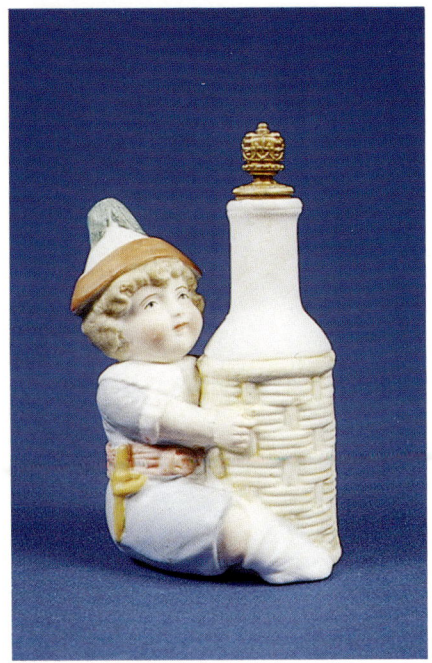

Lot #113. Bisque ceramic figural bottle and metal crown stopper, 3.5" [8.9 cm], shaped as a baby holding a giant bottle in a wicker holder, beautifully painted in multicolors, probably of German or English manufacture. Est. $150.00-$200.00.

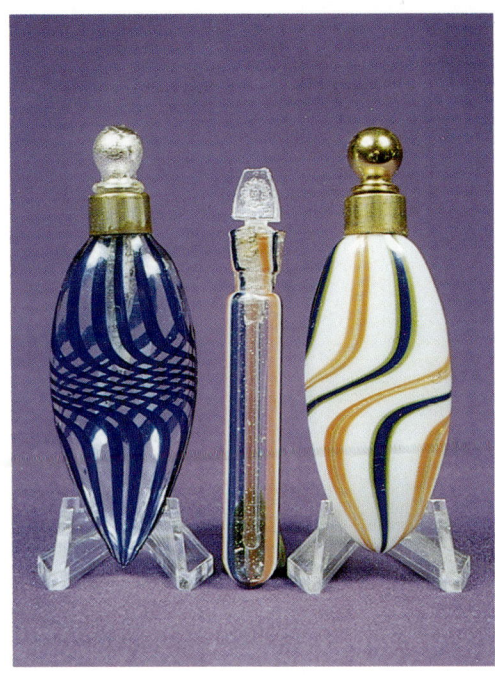

Lot #114. Blown glass perfume vial with gold mercury glass dauber, 2.8" [7 cm] the white glass with swirls of blue, orange, green, and gold; tiny glass vial with clear glass stopper and dauber, 2.8" [7 cm], clear glass with blue, white, and orange; blown glass perfume vial with silver mercury glass dauber, 3" [7.6 cm], blue swirls in the clear glass. Three items. Est. $150.00-$200.00.

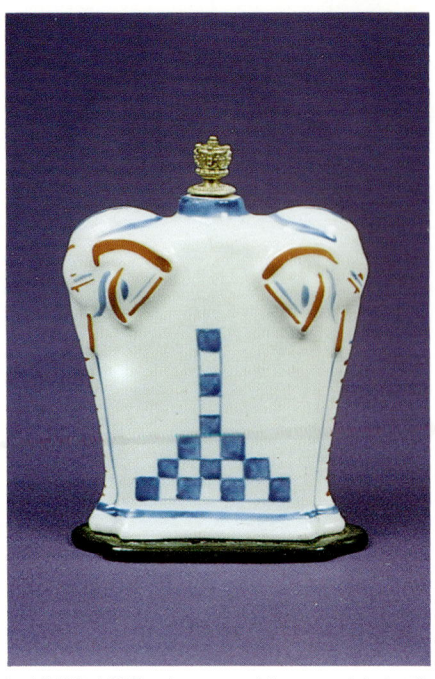

Lot #115. HD Boulogne sur Mer porcelain bottle with metal crown stopper, molded with two stylized elephant heads on the sides of the bottle and painted in red and blue, artist-signed *Liane*, bottom stamped with anchor mark in blue, on its wooden plinth. Est. $175.00-$250.00.

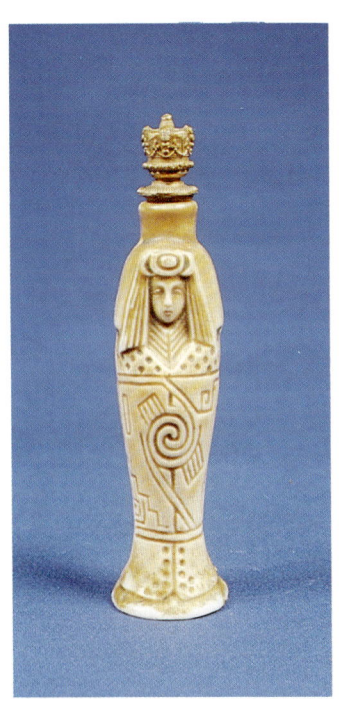

Lot #116. Ceramic bottle and gold metal crown stopper, 3.4" [8.6 cm], shaped as an Egyptian mummy with a brown glaze, mold *#14690* on back, of German manufacture. Est. $100.00-$150.00.

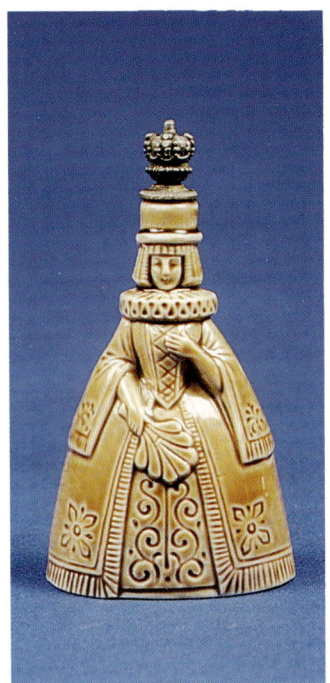

Lot #117. Ceramic bottle and metal crown stopper in the shape of an Elizabethan lady, 3.4" [8.6 cm], brown glaze, of German manufacture. Est. $100.00-$150.00.

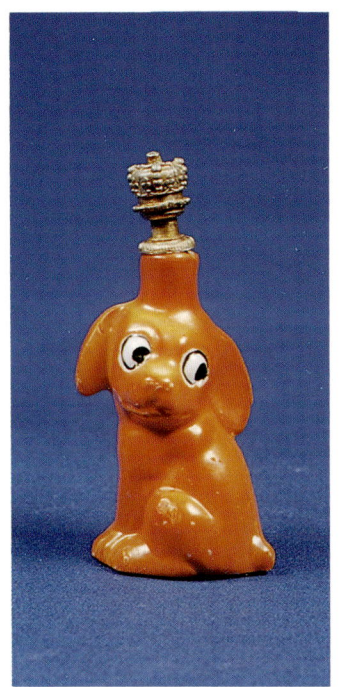

Lot #118. Ceramic figural bottle and metal crown stopper, 2.5" [6.4 cm], shaped as a dog with goolie eyes painted in orange enamel, signed *Germany #3756* on back of bottle. Est. $75.00-$125.00.

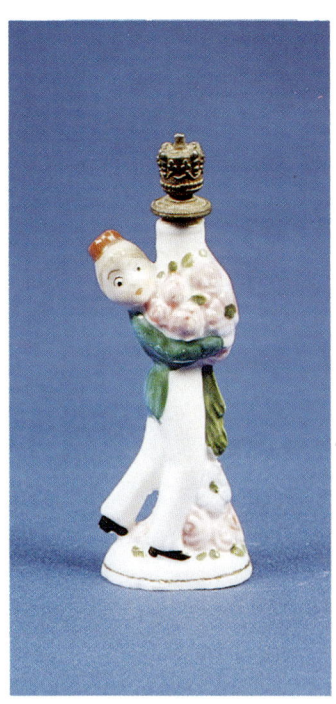

Lot #119. Ceramic figural bottle and metal crown stopper, 3.2" [8.1 cm], shaped as a surprised bellboy carrying a bouquet of flowers, signed *Germany* in the mold on the back. Est. $125.00-$175.00.

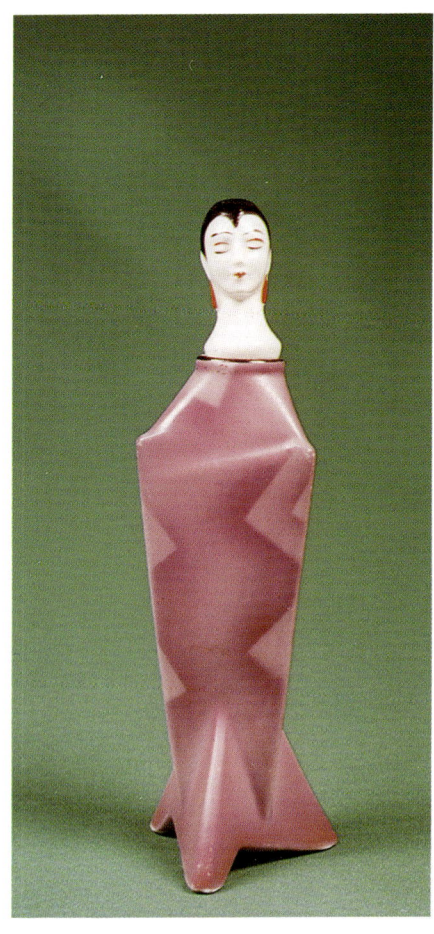

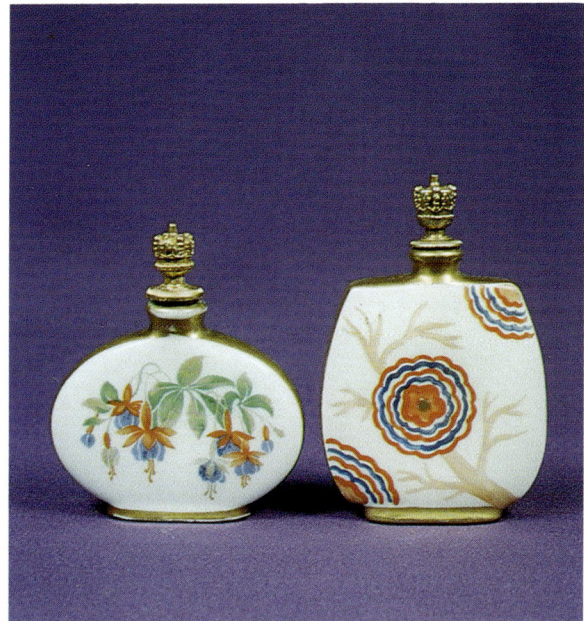

Lot #121. Pair of porcelain bottles with metal crown stoppers, 2.5" and 2.9" [6.4 and 7.4 cm], the taller painted with an abstract Art Deco floral motif, the smaller enameled with fuschias, sides enameled in gold, unsigned but of German manufacture. Two items. Est. $150.00-$200.00.

Lot #120. Figural porcelain bottle and stopper, 6" [15.2 cm], the bottle an angular Art Deco form and painted in violet with zigzag motifs, the stopper shaped as a woman's head, long glass dauber, bottom signed *Germany*. Est. $175.00-$250.00.

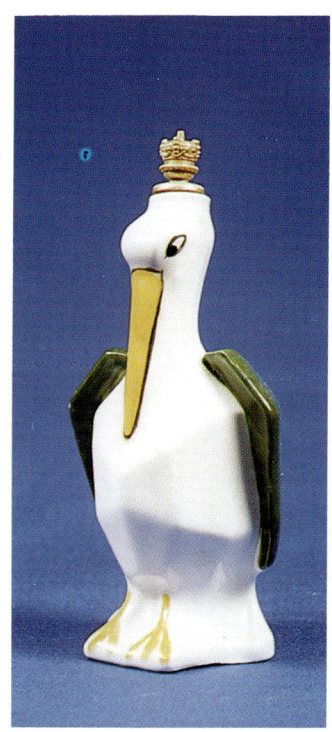

Lot #122. Garnier porcelain figural bottle in the shape of a stylized pelican, parts painted green and yellow, gold metal crown stopper, originally for liquor, bottom signed *Garnier France*. Est. $100.00-$150.00.

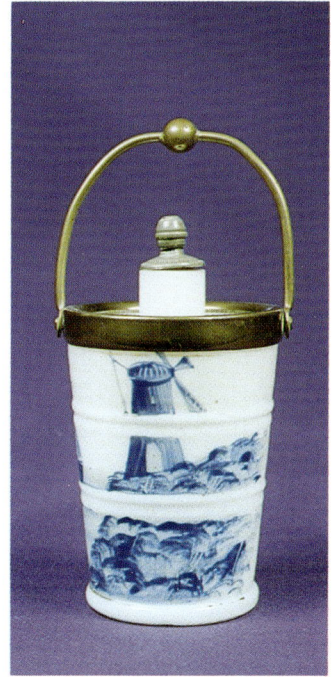

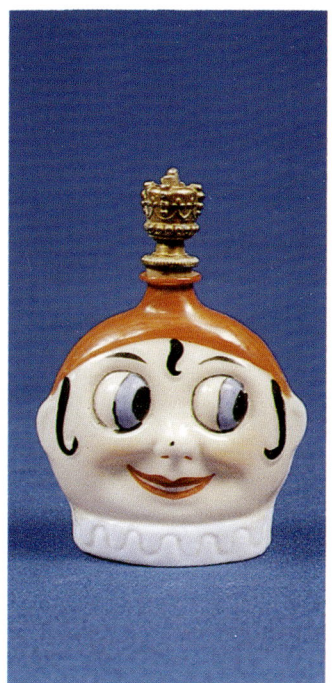

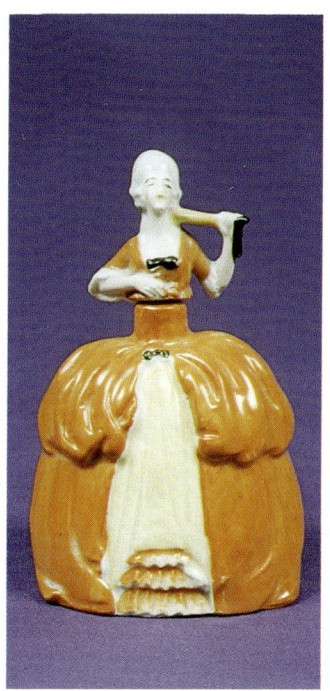

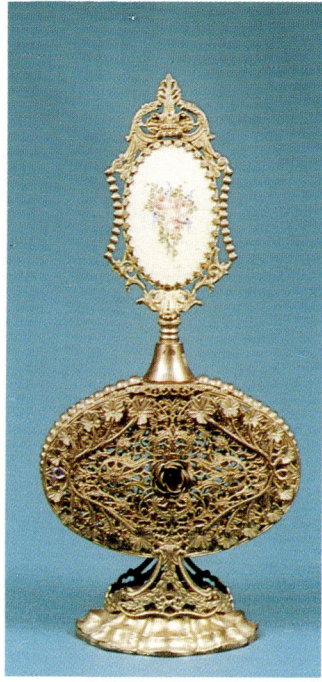

Lot #123. Unusual opaque white glass bottle and metal crown stopper in the shape of a milk pail, 3.9" [10 cm] to top of crown, the top of the pail fitted with a brass rim and handle, painted with a Windmill and shoreline with a boat in blue, probably of Dutch manufacture. Est. $150.00-$200.00.

Lot #124. White glass perfume bottle and crown stopper in the form of a smiling, googlie-eyed Pierrot, beautifully enameled in red, blue, black, 2.4" [6 cm], bottom stamped *Germany*. Est. $100.00-$175.00.

Lot #125. German porcelain figural bottle and stopper, 4.6" [11.7 cm], shaped as an 18th century lady in a ballgown holding a fan near her face, painted realistically in flesh tones with the gown in deep orange and yellow, unsigned. Est. $125.00-$175.00.

Lot #126. Clear glass perfume bottle contained in an elaborate gold metal reliquary type holder, 8.7" [22.1 cm], the filagree metalwork embellished with roses and leaves, the stopper with a long glass dauber and white enamel medallion with roses. Est. $100.00-$150.00.

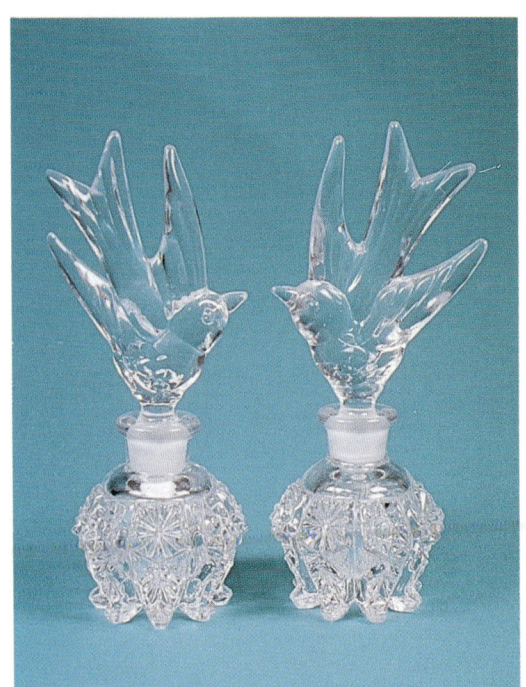

Lot #127. Pair of pressed glass bottles with stoppers molded as birds in flight, 7" [17.8 cm], the bottles molded with facets to resemble cut glass. Two items. Est. $75.00-$100.00.

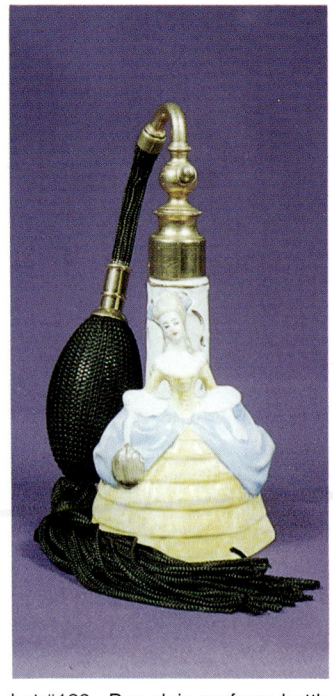

Lot #128. Porcelain perfume bottle with metal atomizer top, 5.7" [14.5 cm] to top of atomizer, in the form of an 18th century courtesan in a yellow gown, porcelain of German manufacture [small flat chip on bottom of bottle], atomizer marked *France*, new ball and tassel. Est. $100.00-$150.00.

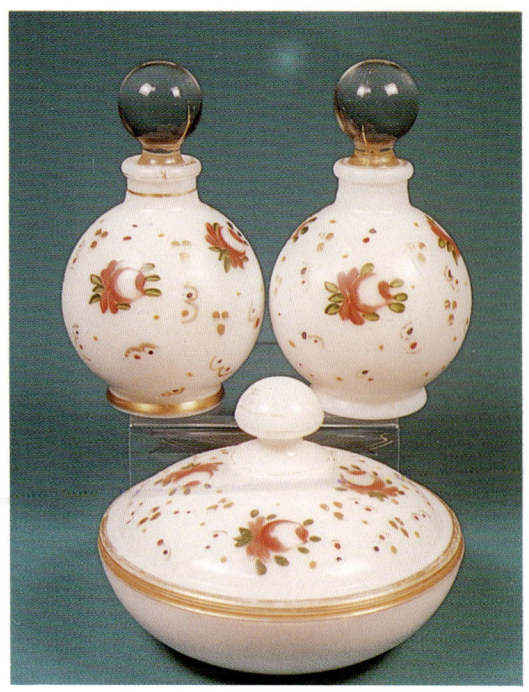

Lot #129. Early twentieth century dresser set of three items: pair of opaque white glass bottles with clear ball stoppers, 5" [12.7 cm], decorated with handpainted roses in red and green and with gold dots; opaque white powder box and cover, 3.5" [8.9 cm], conforming decor, unsigned. Three items. Est. $100.00-$200.00.

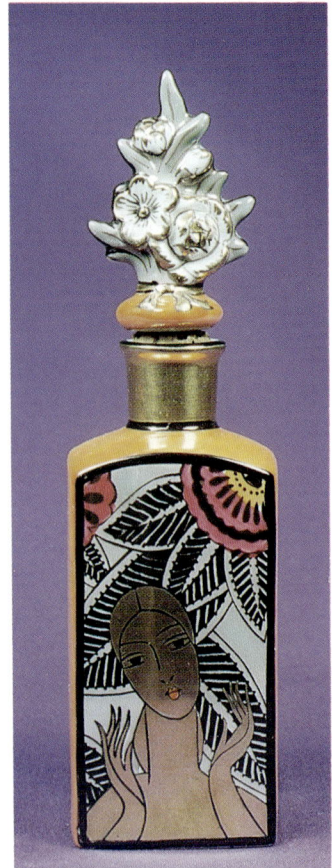

Lot #130. Noritake porcelain cologne bottle and cork-lined stopper with porcelain dauber, 6.5" [16.5 cm], beautifully decorated with the figure of a woman in gold surrounded by large blossoms in the Art Deco style, all against a background of aqua and orange, signed *Noritake* in red on the bottom. Est. $250.00-$300.00.

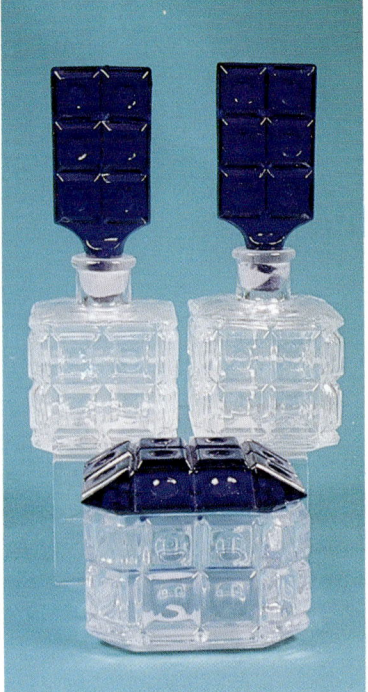

Lot #131. American pressed glass dresser set of 3 items: pair of clear glass perfumes with cobalt glass stoppers, 5.7" [14.5 cm], molded with a square thumbprint design; glass powder box and cover, 2.5" [6.4 cm], of conforming design; all unsigned. Three items. Est. $75.00-$125.00.

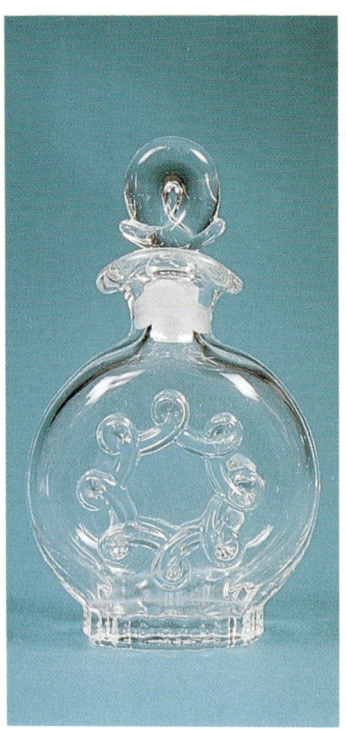

Lot #132. Heisey *Lariat* clear glass perfume bottle and stopper, 5.7" [14.5 cm], the round bottle molded on both sides with a design of rope loops, unusual curved and elongated lip to the bottle, unsigned. Est. $75.00-$125.00.

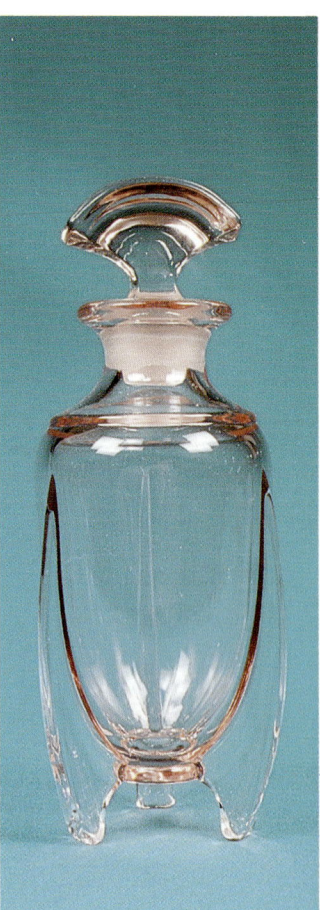

Lot #133. American depression era pink glass perfume bottle and stopper, 6.2" [15.6 cm], the bottle molded with three wing-like feet and having a very futuristic appearance. Est. $100.00-$150.00.

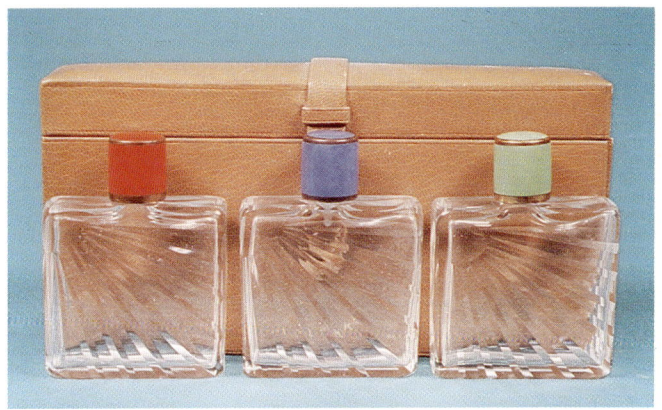

Lot #134. Art Deco set of three clear crystal bottles with inner stoppers and metal overcaps, each 3.3" [8.4 cm], each bottle cut with facets in a sunray motif, the caps enameled red, green, and blue, in their satin-lined leather case signed *J. E. Caldwell Co. Philadelphia*. The sunray motif was one of the most recurrent decorative themes in the Art Deco era. Est. $100.00-$175.00.

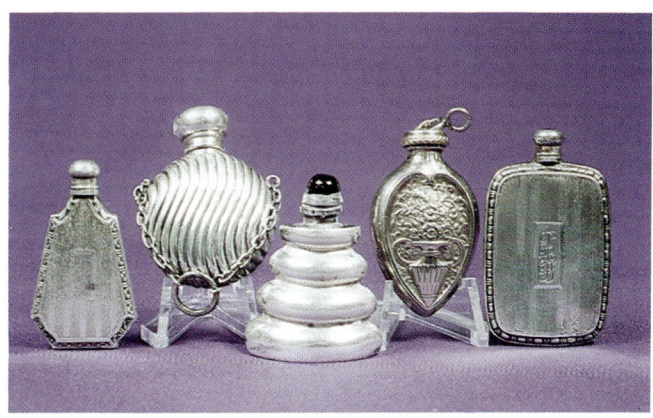

Lot #135. Lot of 5 miniature metal flasks: silver flask in a stepped pyramid design, stopper with purple stone, 1.5" [3.8 cm], bottom marked *Sterling Mexico*; round metal bottle molded with curved lines, 1.6" [4.1 cm], with loop and chains at sides; heart-shaped flask molded with an urn of flowers on both sides, 1.6" [4.1 cm], loop on stopper; triangular shaped flask, 1.7" [4.3 cm], marked *Sterling*; silver flask with initials, 1.9" [4.8 cm], marked *Sterling*. Five items. Est. $150.00-$250.00.

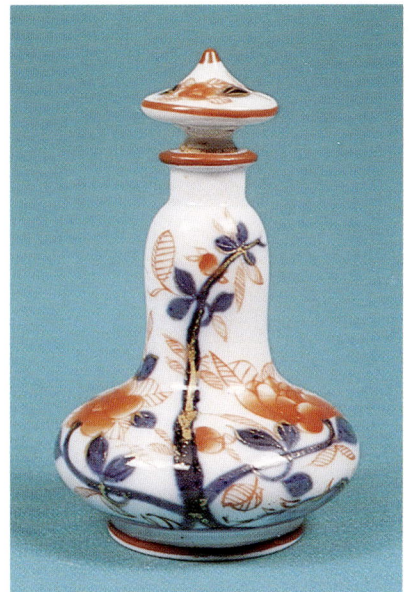

Lot #136. Imari Japanese porcelain scent bottle and stopper, 4.2" [10.7 cm], the bell-shaped bottle decorated in the signature colors of deep navy blue and orange, with gold highlights, bottom signed underglaze with blue square. Est. $200.00-$250.00.

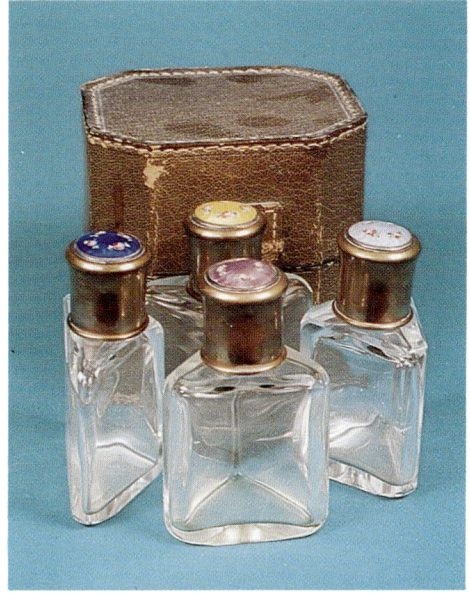

Lot #137. Set of four clear glass bottles with inner glass stoppers and enameled metal overcaps, each 3.2" [8.1 cm], the bottles of triangular shape, the caps beautifully enameled with flowers in light blue, deep blue, violet, and yellow, in their leather carrying case. Est. $125.00-$175.00.

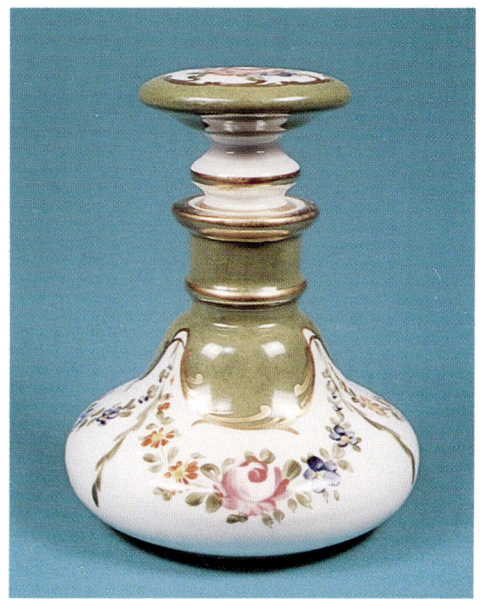

Lot #138. Sèvres type large porcelain cologne bottle, 5.5" [14 cm], of bell shape beautifully decorated with garlands of flowers in multicolor against a white and green background embellished with flourishes of gold, bottom signed *France* and with a Sèvres type mark underglaze in blue. Est. $100.00-$200.00.

ATOMIZERS & DEVILBISS

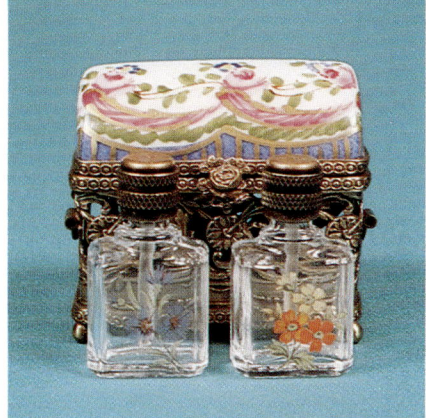

Lot #139. Limoges porcelain metal box for two miniature glass perfume bottles with metal caps, bottle height 1.4" [3.6 cm], the box and the bottles gaily painted with flowers in pink, green, blue, and gold, signed underglaze *Limoges France* in blue. Est. $75.00-$125.00.

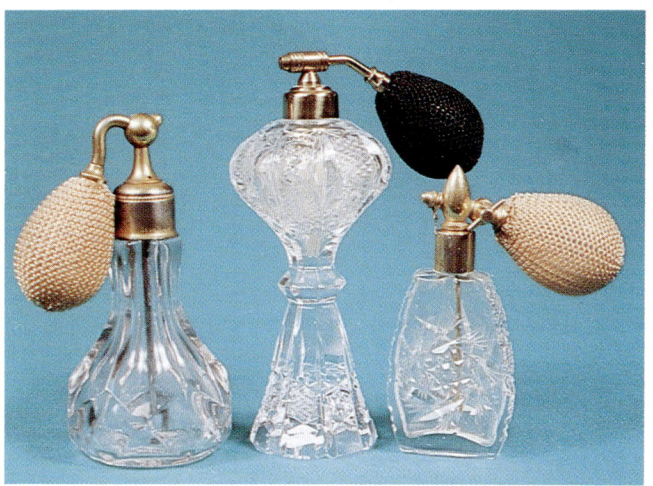

Lot #140. DeVilbiss clear glass bottle with metal atomizer, 4.3" [10.9 cm], small chip on side of bottle, replaced ball, collar signed *DeVilbiss*; pressed clear glass bottle of tower form with metal atomizer, 5.1" [13 cm], new ball, unsigned; thin clear glass bottle with atomizer attachment, 3.7" [9.4 cm], new ball, bottle with an elaborate star design, unsigned. Est. $150.00-$225.00.

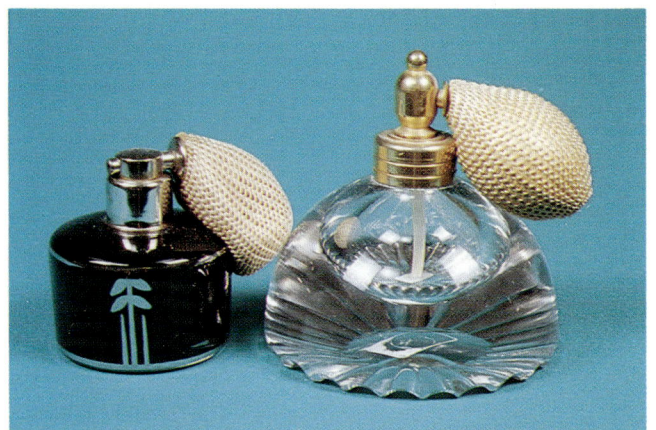
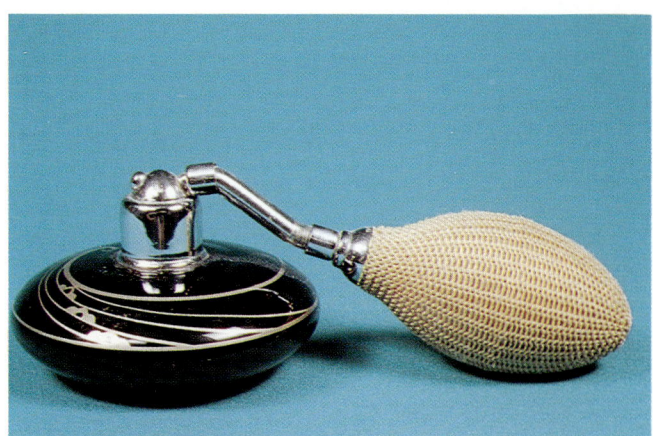

Lot #141. Small glass perfume bottle with chrome atomizer, 2.3" [5.8 cm], internally decorated with black enamel, silver enamel on the outside, original ball; heavy hemispherical perfume bottle of paperweight glass with gold metal atomizer, 3.3" [8.4 cm], the bottom molded with scallops; both bottles unsigned. Two items. Est. $100.00-$150.00.

Lot #142. DeVilbiss black glass bottle and silver atomizer attachment, 1.7" [4.3 cm], the bottle shaped as a round disc and decorated with silver swirls, with original atomizer stamped *DeVilbiss* and with DeVilbiss label on bottom. Est. $150.00-$250.00.

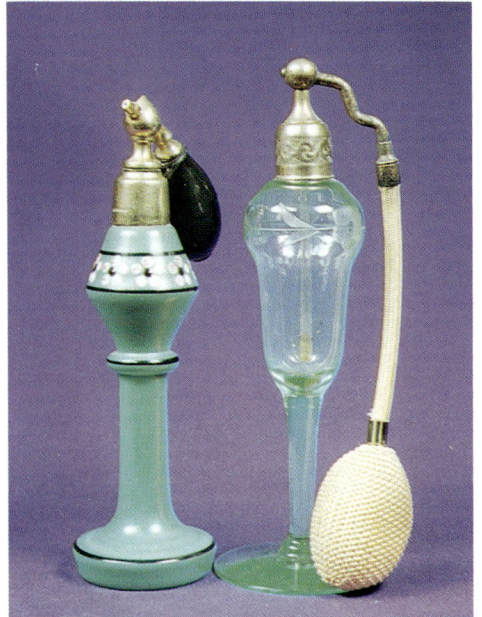
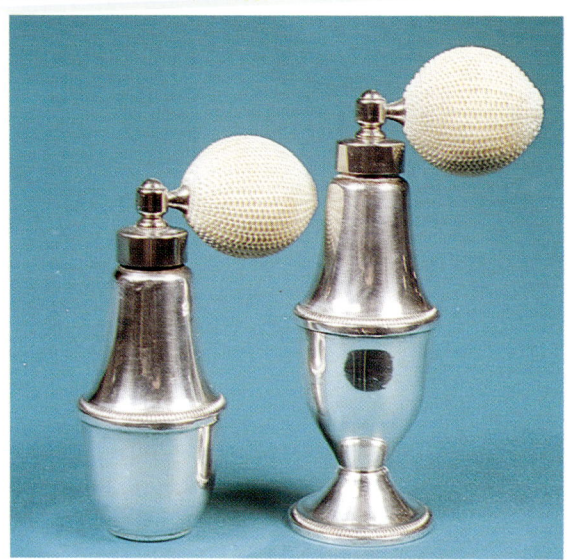

Lot #143. Translucent green glass bottle and metal atomizer attachment, 6.5" [16.5 cm], the bottle wheel-cut with flowers and leaves, unsigned, but of American manufacture; clear glass bottle and metal atomizer attachment, 6.2" [15.7 cm], totally enameled in green with white flowers, metal signed *Czechoslovakia*. Two items. Est. $150.00-$225.00.

Lot #144. Pair of sterling silver-clad glass bottles with atomizer attachments, 4" and 5" [10.1 and 12.7 cm], each of baluster shape, the taller with a pedestal base, both signed *Duchin Creation* and stamped *Sterling* on the bottom. Est. $100.00-$175.00.

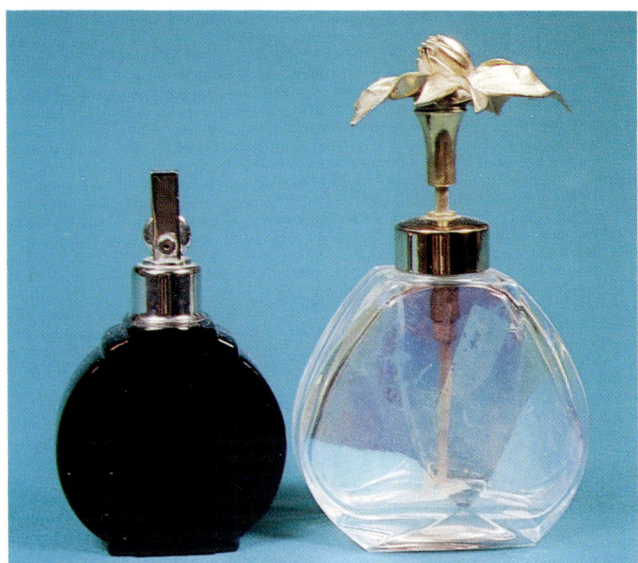
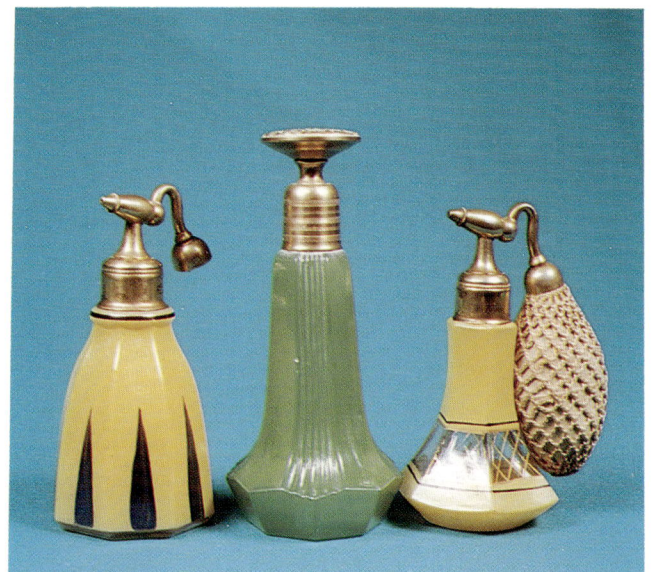

Lot #145. DeVilbiss clear glass bottle with gold atomizer attachment, 5" [12.7 cm], the bottle designed with broad facets and the glass with a slight irridescence, the atomizer shaped as a flower with leaves, signed with a DeVilbiss paper label model #750-53; DeVilbiss black glass bottle with silver metal atomizer attachment, 3.7" [9.4 cm], of circular form with a sculpted vertical panel, ball lacking, bottom signed *DeVilbiss* in acid. Two items. Est. $100.00-$200.00.

Lot #146. DeVilbiss clear glass hexagonal atomizer bottle, 4.1" [10.4 cm], enameled in yellow and black with a clear window all around, original ball, unsigned; DeVilbiss clear glass octagonal atomizer bottle, 4.2" [10.6 cm], enameled in yellow and black, ball lacking, signed *DeVilbiss* on hardware and with paper label; clear glass bottle with metal neck and metal stopper embossed with flowers and with glass dauber, 5" [12.7 cm], enameled in green, unsigned. Three items. Est. $200.00-$300.00.

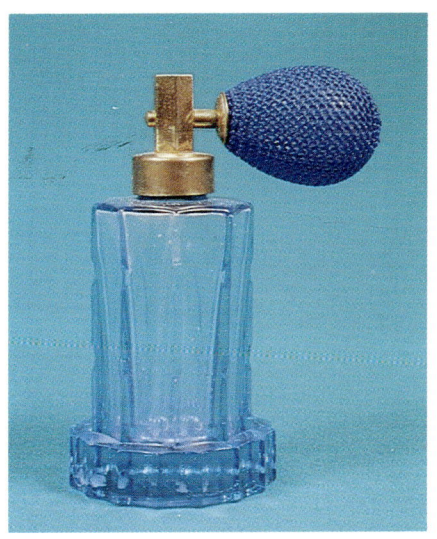

Lot #147. Pretty bright blue glass perfume bottle with metal atomizer, 4" [10.2 cm], nine-sided with a scalloped pedestal base, gold paper label marked *Holmspray*, bottle marked in the mold *USA*. Est. $75.00-$100.00.

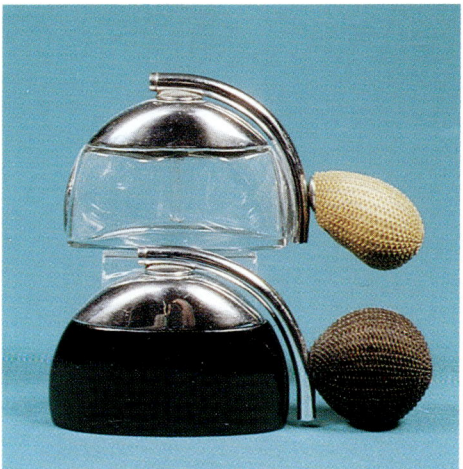

Lot #148. DeVilbiss pair of Art Deco atomizers in the streamline style, each 2.3" [5.8 cm], one of black glass, one clear, both with chrome atomizers and original balls; the clear glass one is unsigned, the other has a partial DeVilbiss label. Two items. Est. $200.00-$300.00.

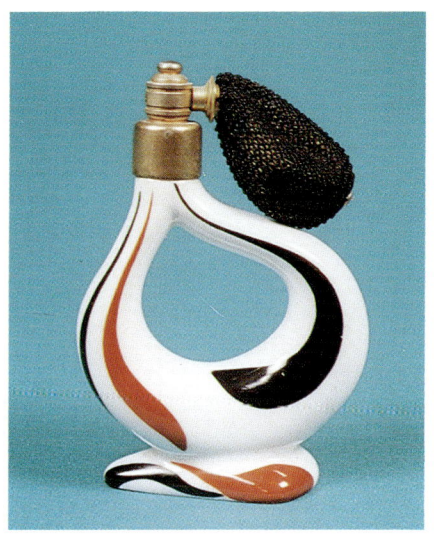

Lot #149. Limoges porcelain atomizer bottle, 4" [10.2 cm], of abstract modern design decorated with swirls of black and deep orange, hardened atomizer ball, bottom and also the side signed *Limoges France*. Est. $125.00-$175.00.

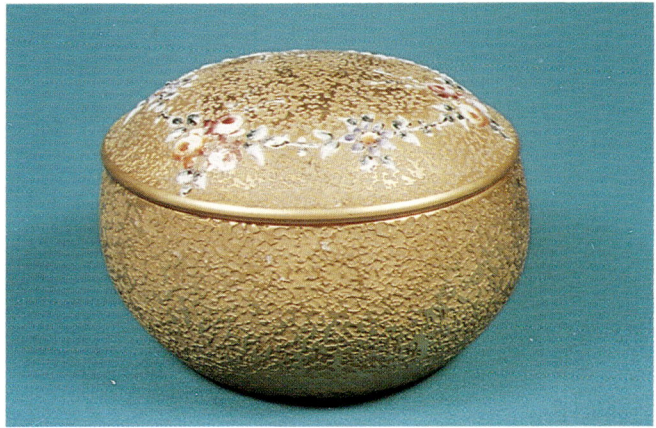
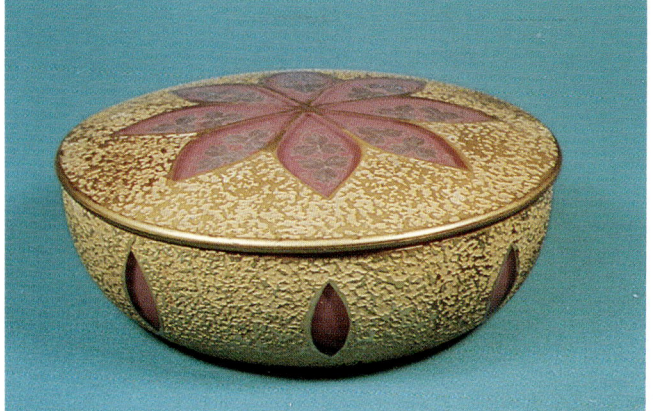

Lot #150. Pair of DeVilbiss glass powder boxes: acid-etched box in a variegated pattern, diameter 4.5" [11.4 cm], the whole surface enameled in gold and decorated with multicolor flowers, unsigned; acid-etched box, diameter 5.7" [14.5 cm], the inner surface of the lid wheel-cut with ivy leaves and enameled in violet, the exterior surface enameled in gold with a flower shape on the cover and with petal-shaped windows around the sides of the box, bottom with DeVilbiss paper label. Two items. Est. $300.00-$450.00.

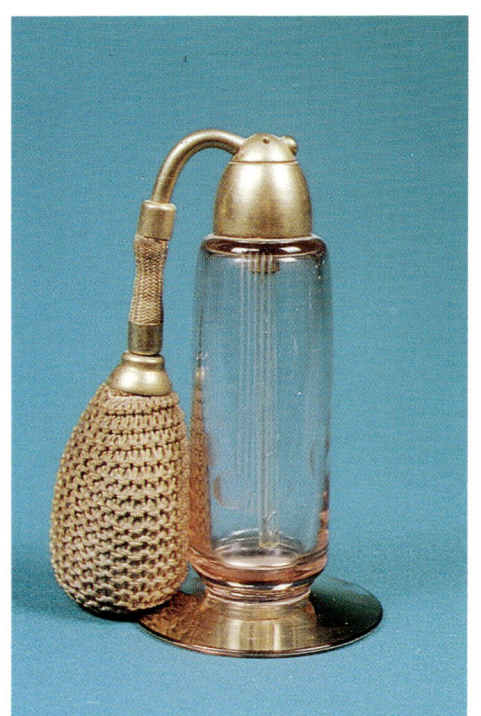

Lot #151. DeVilbiss pink glass atomizer bottle and gold metal atomizer attachment, 3.8" [9.7 cm], the bottle wheel-cut with an Art Deco design of lines and circles and having a pedestal base enameled in gold, with its original atomizer parts signed *DeVilbiss*. Est. $150.00-$250.00.

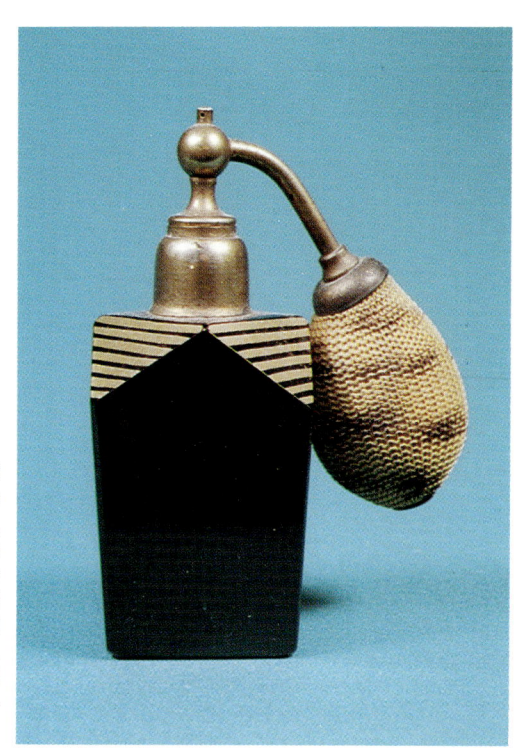

Lot #152. Black glass Art Deco perfume bottle with metal atomizer attachment, 3.7" [9.4 cm], the square shape faceted at the shoulder and decorated with gold bands, metal attachment signed *Fizz Btle. S. D. G. France*; it retains the original atomizer ball. Est. $100.00-$175.00.

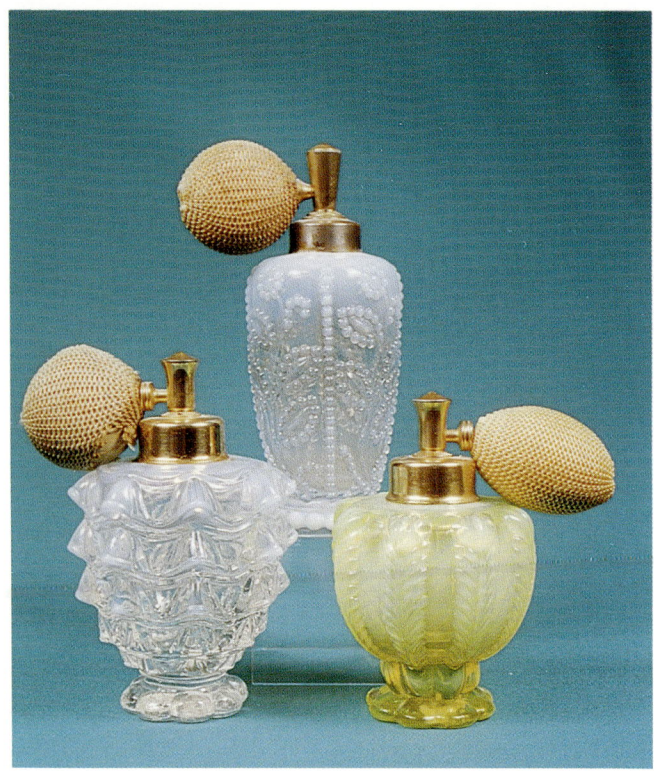

Lot #153. Lot of 3 atomizers: DeVilbiss clear and semi-opalescent glass bottle, 4.4" [11.3 cm], molded with tiers of ruffles, original ball, by Fenton Glass; clear and white opalescent glass bottle with metal atomizer, 4.9" [12.5 cm], molded with a beaded design of leaves, original ball; citrine yellow and semi-opalescent bottle, 3.9" [10 cm], molded with a leaf design; all three unsigned. Three items. Est. $175.00-$250.00.

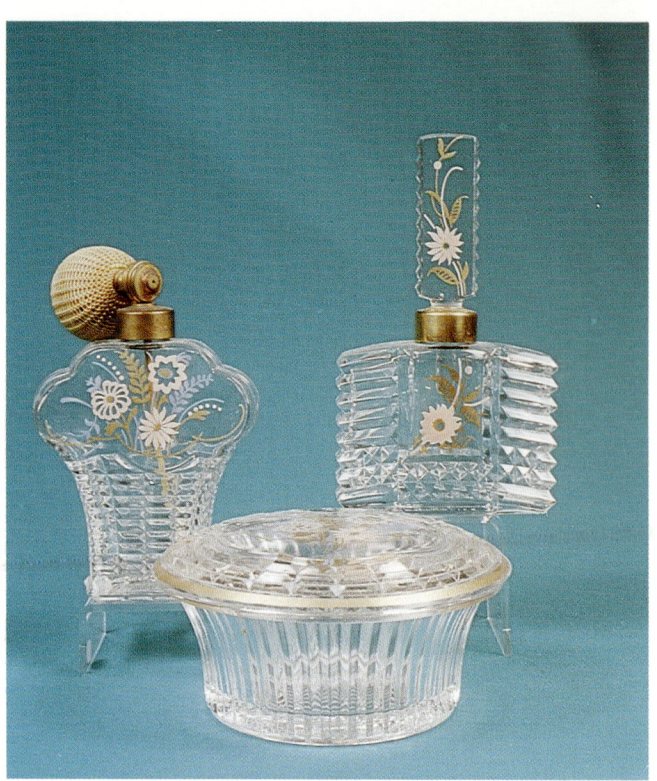

Lot #154. Devilbiss set of three DeVilbiss clear glass items: perfume atomizer shaped as a flower basket with original ball, 4.7" [12 cm], molded *DeVilbiss* on bottom; dropper bottle with a metal collar 5.3" [13.5 cm], molded *DeVilbiss* on bottom; powder box and cover, 2.2" by 4.5" [5.6 by 11.4 cm]; all three items with a design of blue, pink, and gold flowers. Three items. Est. $150.00-$225.00.

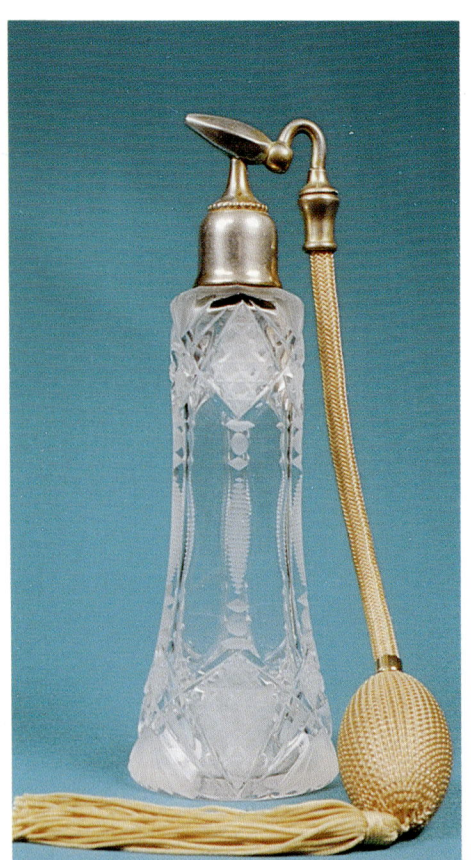

Lot #155. Cut crystal perfume bottle with atomizer attachment, 8" [20.3 cm], cut with geometric facets which have then been frosted in parts to enhance the design, replaced ball and tassel, unsigned. Est. $150.00-$250.00.

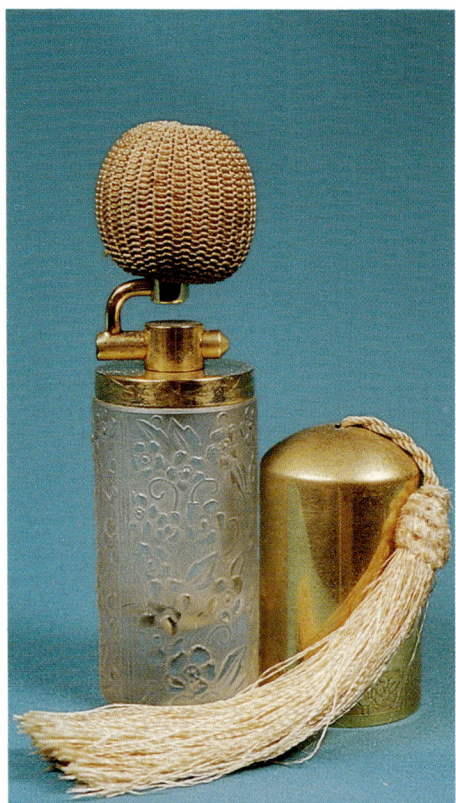

Lot #156. DeVilbiss frosted glass atomizer bottle with gold metal overcap, 5.2" [13.2 cm], the cylindrical bottle molded with a design of forget-me-nots, the overcap with its original tassel also molded with a border of the same flowers, functioning original atomizer, bottom with a silver DeVilbiss label and acid-etched *DeVilbiss USA*. Est. $200.00-$300.00.

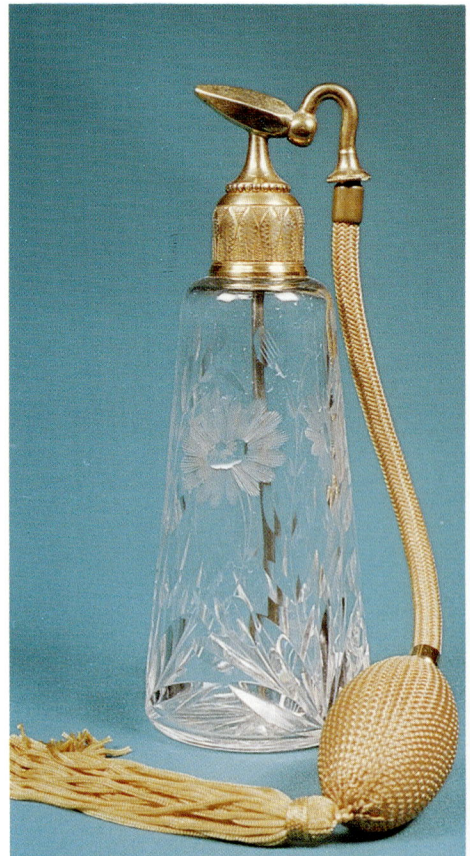

Lot #157. Wheel-cut clear crystal bottle with gold metal atomizer attachment, 7.2" [18.3 cm], beautifully designed with flowers and leaves, bottom cut with a starburst, replaced ball and tassel, unsigned. Est. $150.00-$250.00.

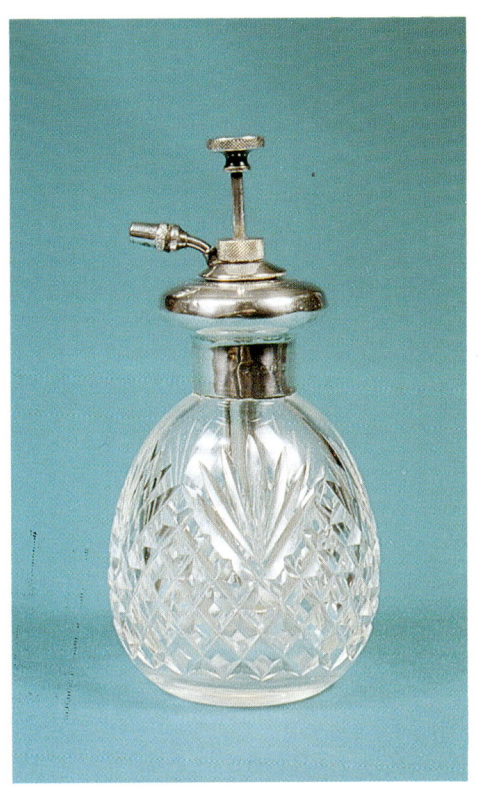

Lot #158. English clear crystal bottle with sterling silver atomizer top, 6" [15.2 cm], the ovoid bottle cut with diamond-shaped facets, the elaborate pump atomizer fixture in excellent condition and stamped with Sterling silver hallmarks for Birmingham, England, 1924, by Elkington Mason & Co. Est. $125.00-$175.00.

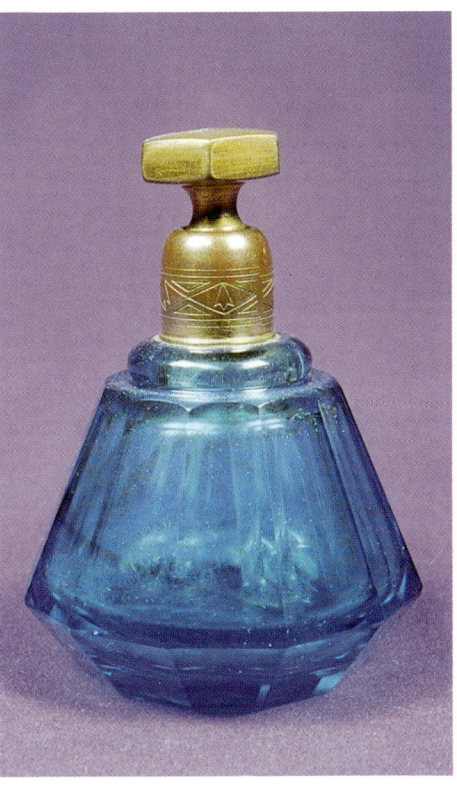

Lot #159. Volupté royal blue crystal bottle and metal dropper, 3.5" [9 cm], the bottle designed with twelve rectangular facets, metal stopper with glass dauber, stopper signed *Volupté*. Est. $150.00-$200.00.

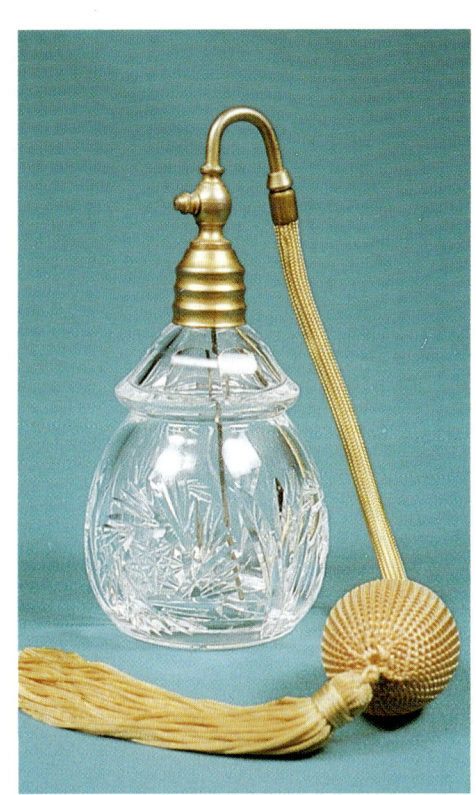

Lot #160. American brilliant period cut glass bottle with metal atomizer top, 5.8" [14.8 cm], the bottle cut with a swirl and star motif, the bottom also cut with a star, new ball and tassel, unsigned. Est. $150.00-$250.00.

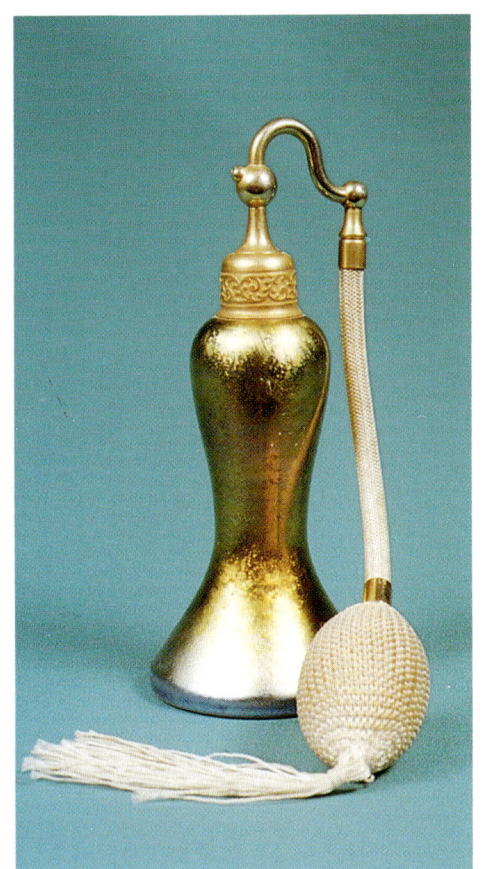

Lot #161. DeVilbiss Steuben gold Aurene glass atomizer bottle, 6" [15.2 cm], of baluster form with a wide base, brilliant gold color shading to blue and violet at the base, replaced ball and tassel but with original atomizer hardware, unsigned. Est. $400.00-$550.00.

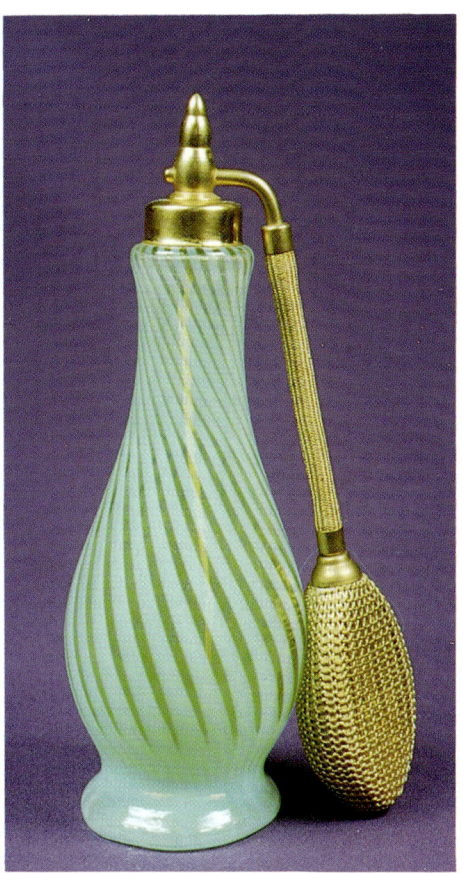

Lot #162. DeVilbiss translucent light green glass bottle with white swirls and gold-plated metal atomizer attachment, 6.9" [17.5 cm], of baluster shape with a round pedestal base, original hardware and ball, bottom with DeVilbiss label CS-200-3, bottom signed in acid *DeVilbiss*. Est. $275.00-$375.00.

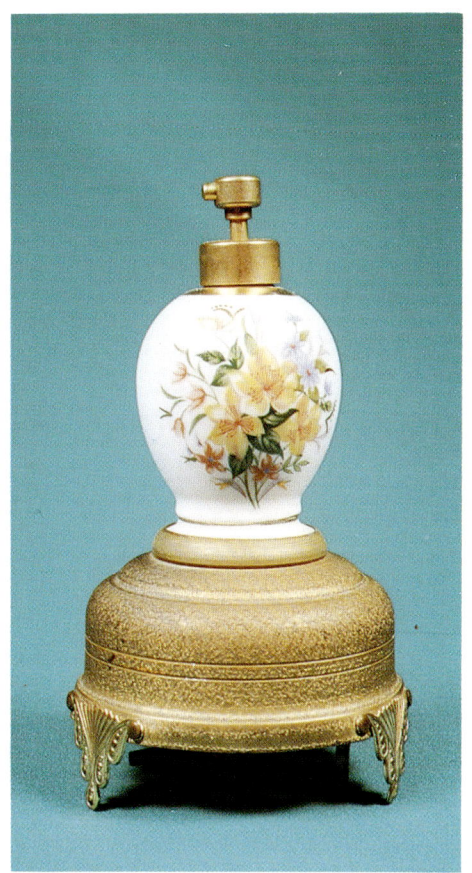

Lot #163. Porcelain perfume bottle with gold metal pump atomizer mounted on a music box, 5.5" [14 cm], the bottle painted front and back with a colorful bouquet of flowers, the music box plays when the bottle is picked up. Est. $75.00-$125.00.

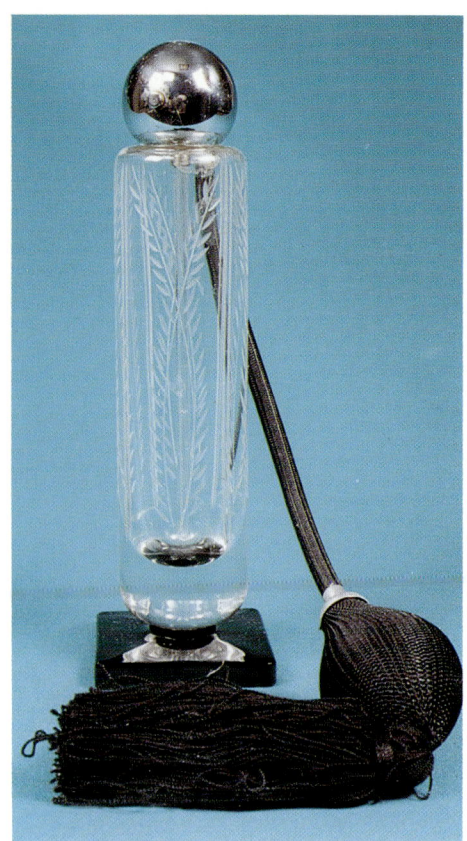

Lot #164. Statuesque DeVilbiss Art Deco atomizer of clear and black glass with chrome atomizer and black ball and tassel, 8" [20.3 cm], the cylindrical bottle wheel-cut with leaves, signed on bottom with a DeVilbiss black paper label. Est. $400.00-$500.00.

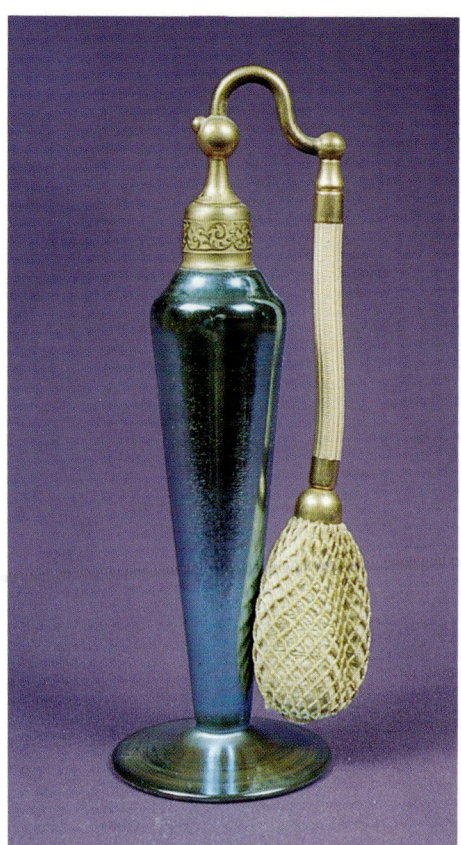

Lot #165. DeVilbiss Steuben blue Aurene perfume bottle and gold metal atomizer hardware, 7.2" [18.3 cm], the glass characterized by exceptionally rich silvery blue iridescence with some gold highlights, original ball, unsigned. Est. $600.00-$750.00.

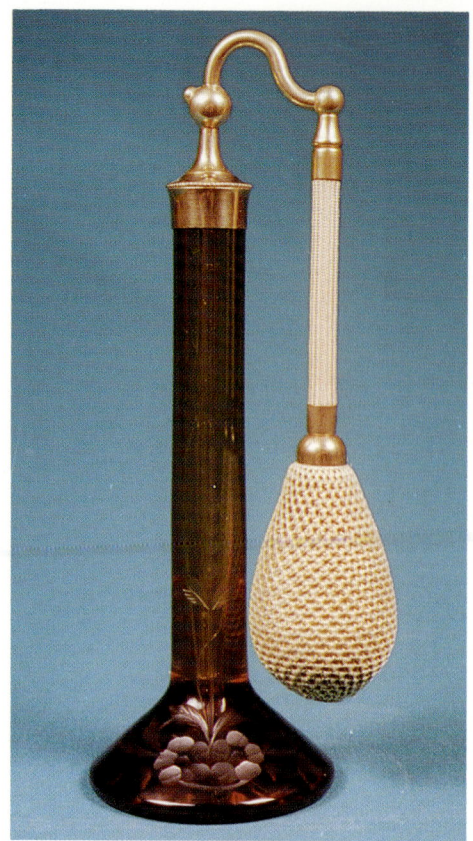

Lot #166. DeVilbiss amber glass bottle with metal atomizer, 7.5" [19 cm], of trumpet form wheel cut with a design of flowers and leaves, original atomizer ball, glass by Steuben, bottom signed *DeVilbiss* in gold. Cf. Sloan, p. 52. Est. $350.00-$450.00.

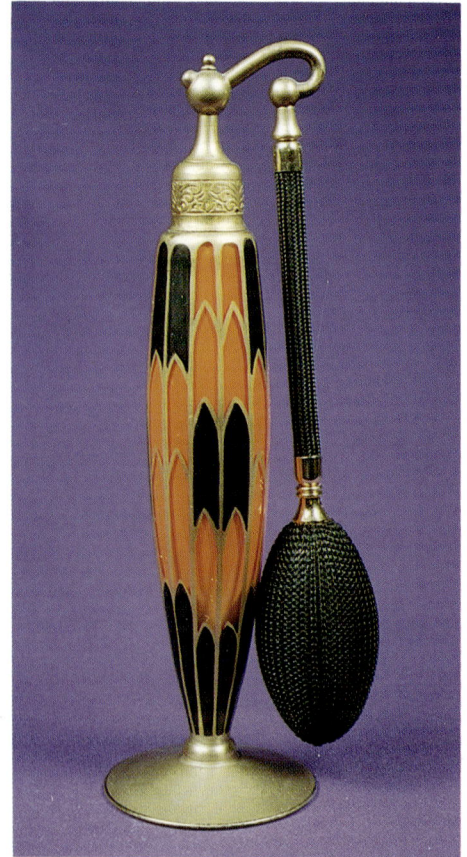

Lot #167. DeVilbiss clear glass perfume bottle and metal atomizer, 7.4" [18.8 cm], of slender shape internally decorated in orange, the exterior elaborately hand-enameled with abstract motifs in black and gold, new ball and tassel, bottom signed *DeVilbiss* in gold. Est. $500.00-$600.00.

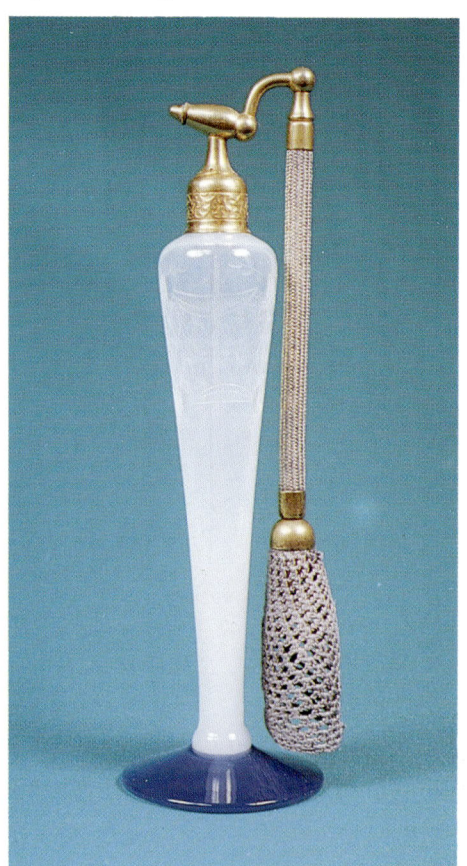

Lot #168. DeVilbiss blue and opalescent white glass perfume bottle with a metal atomizer, 8" [20.4 cm], the opalescent bottle wheel-cut with a trellis and scroll design, original blue crocheted bag [ball lacking], unsigned, possibly by Fry Glass. No. G2 in the DeVilbiss catalogue. Est. $600.00-$750.00.

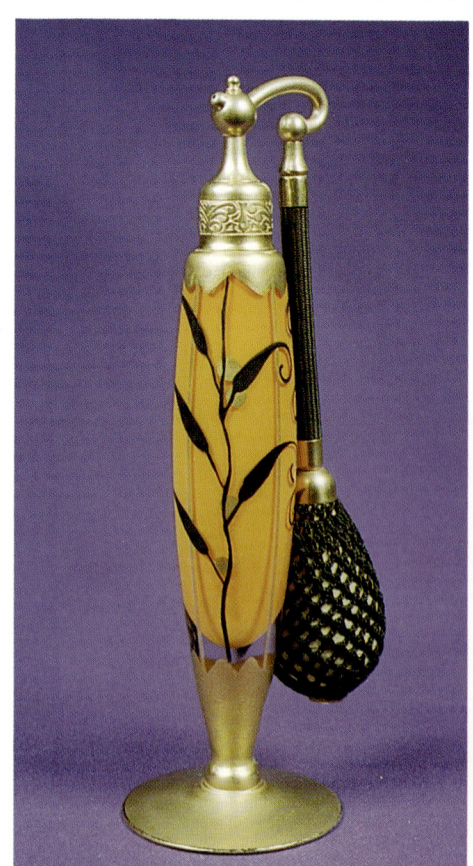

Lot #169. DeVilbiss glass bottle with metal atomizer, 7.3" [18.5 cm], the bottle internally enameled in orange, and decorated on the outside with an abstract leaf design in black and gold, some regilding at base, original ball and crocheted net, signed on bottom *DeVilbiss* in gold. Est. $300.00-$400.00.

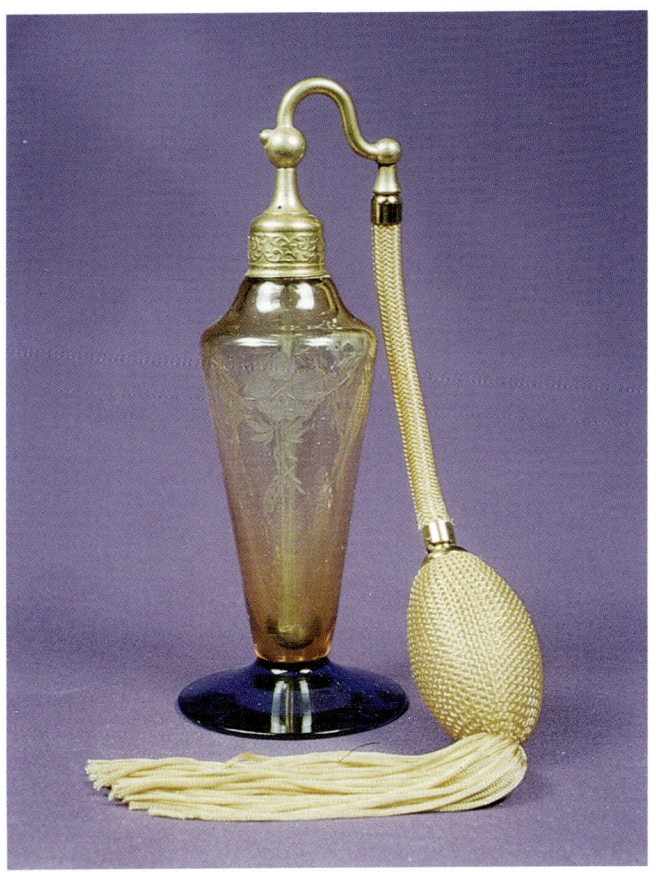

Lot #170. DeVilbiss translucent amber and blue glass atomizer bottle with gold metal atomizer attachment, 6.6" [16.8 cm], the bottle of baluster form with wheel-cut flowers and leaves, long glass siphon, new atomizer ball and tassel, the glass probably by Steuben, unsigned. No. L7 in the DeVilbiss catalogue. Est. $400.00-$500.00.

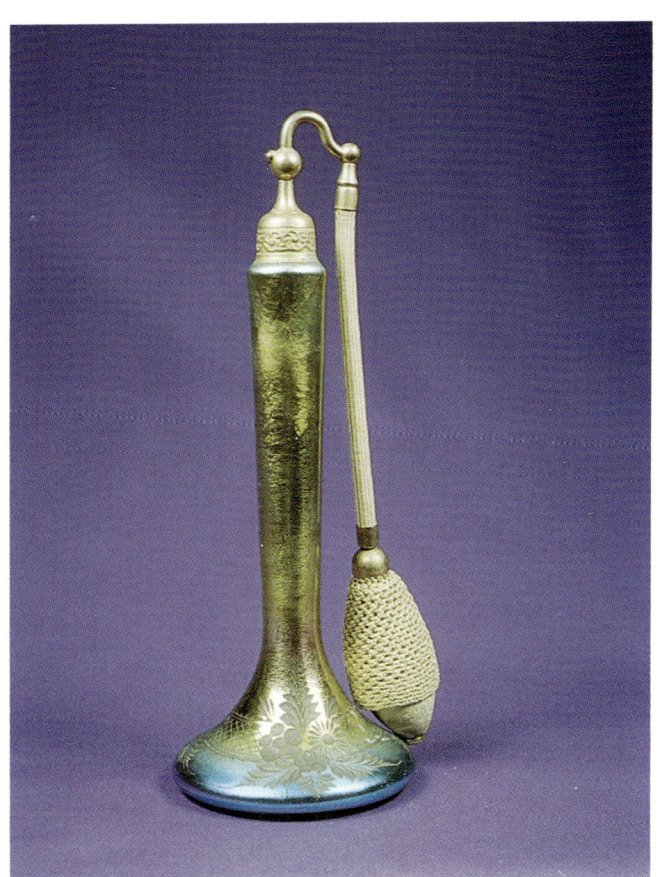

Lot #171. DeVilbiss Steuben gold and blue Aurene perfume bottle and gold metal atomizer hardware, 9" [22.9 cm], the glass shades from gold at the top to iridescent blue at the bottom, wheel-cut with flowers and a trellis, original ball, unsigned. Est. $1,200.00-$1,500.00.

NINETEENTH AND EARLY TWENTIETH CENTURY DECORATIVE BOTTLES

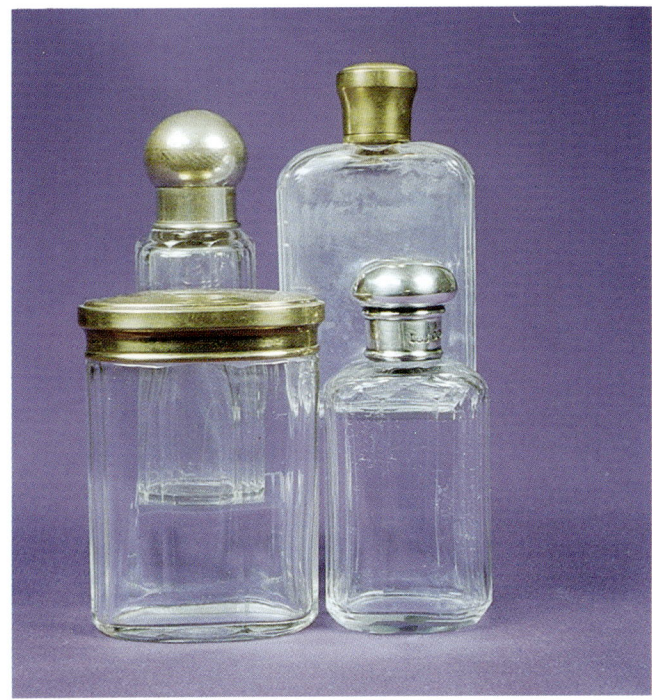

Lot #172. Lot of 4 clear crystal and glass dresser bottles: crystal bottle with sterling silver cap engraved with initials, 3.8" [9.6 cm], long vertical facets, the cap with hallmarks for sterling silver Sheffield, England, 1894; three glass bottles with brass caps [one with dent and an inner glass stopper], various heights from 4.3" to 3.4" [10.9 to 8.6 cm]. Four items. Est. $125.00-$175.00.

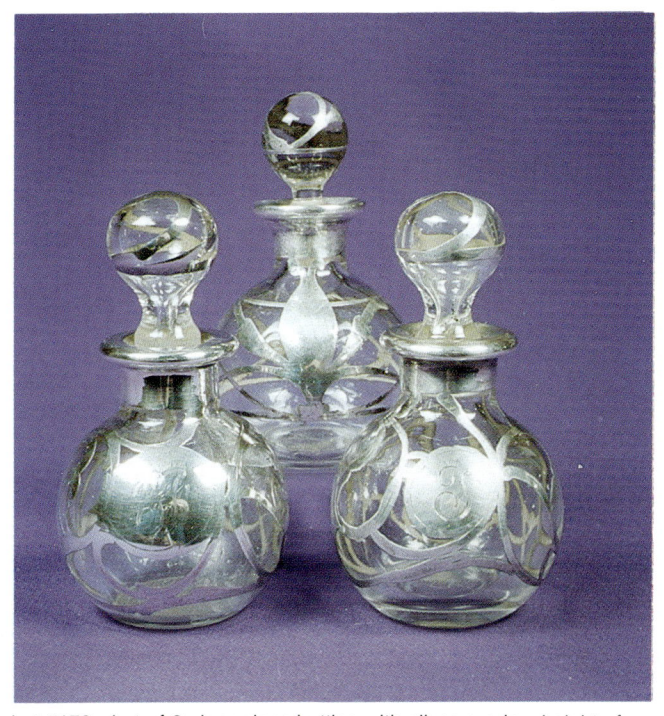

Lot #173. Lot of 3 clear glass bottles with silver overlay, heights from 3.7" [9.4 cm] to 3.5" [8.9 cm], silver deposit in a scrollwork design on all sides of the bottles and on the stoppers, two inscribed with initials. Three bottles. Est. $200.00-$300.00.

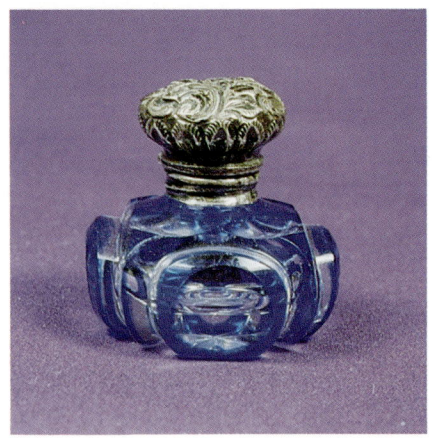

Lot #174. Blue cut back to clear crystal bottle with silver repoussé cap, 1.5" [3.8 cm], shaped with four sides, the hinged cap covers a perforated silver liner, probably for smelling salts or to be used as a vinaigrette. Est. $100.00-$125.00.

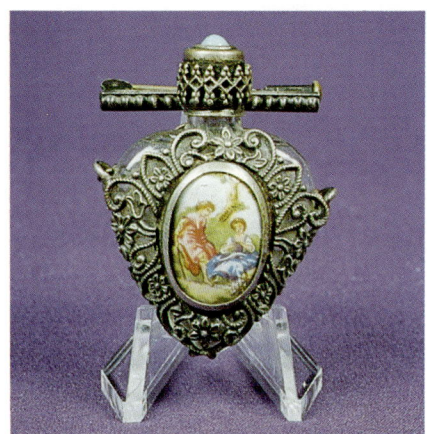

Lot #175. Heart-shaped clear glass bottle with metal cap encased in metal and mounted on a metal bar pin, the stopper with a glass dauber and a turquoise stone, the front of the bottle holding a porcelain medallion of an couple in a pastoral setting. Est. $100.00-$150.00.

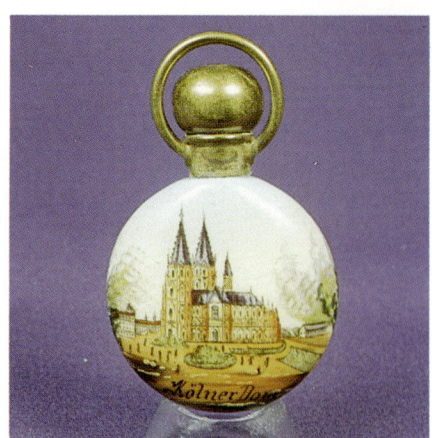

Lot #176. Porcelain scent bottle with brass cap and loop, 2.6" [6.6 cm] to top of loop, of flat round shape, beautifully hand-painted with a portrait of the Cathedral of Cologne, marked *Kölner Dom*, the reverse side painted with plants. Est. $150.00-$200.00.

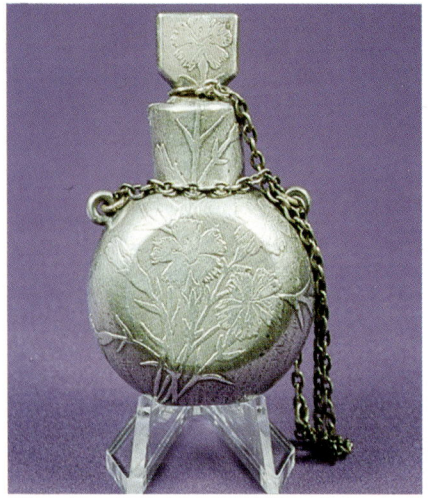

Lot #177. Early glass bottle and stopper encased in silver metal, 2.4" [6.1 cm], the metallic coat beautifully embossed with a design of pinks on both bottle and stopper, metal chains unite the stopper and bottle and allow it to be suspended from a chatelaine. Est. $125.00-$175.00.

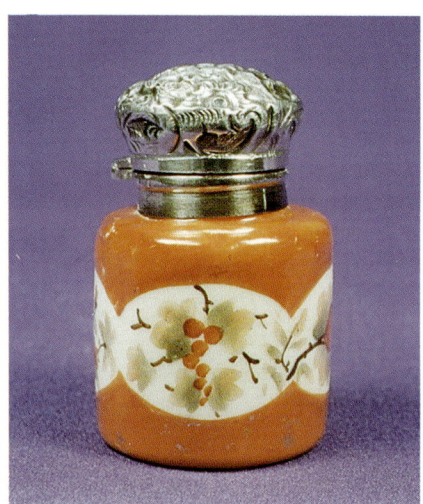

Lot #178. Diminutive porcelain scent bottle, inner glass stopper, and silver metal overcap, 1.7" [4.3 cm], painted in deep orange with a design of a bird and branches of leaves, cap heavily embossed with flowers. Est. $125.00-$175.00.

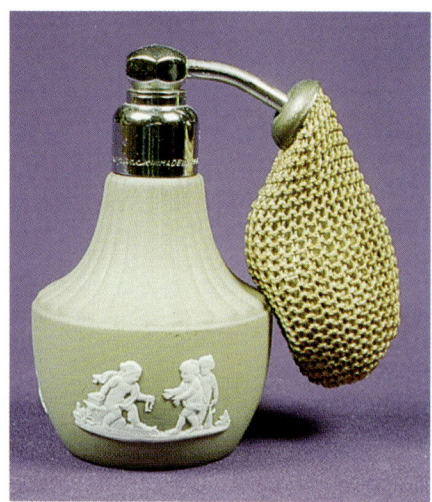

Lot #179. Wedgewood bisque porcelain perfume bottle and atomizer top, 3.3" [8.4 cm], decorated with white cameos of three different scenes of cupids, metal atomizer top with original [hardened] ball and signed *Marcel Frank*, bottom signed *Wedgewood England*. Est. $150.00-$200.00.

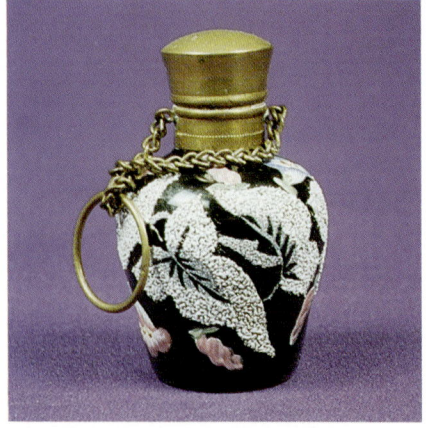

Lot #180. Black glass bottle, black glass inner stopper, and brass metal overcap, 2.2" [5.6 cm], the bottle enameled with white leaves whose thick enamel has a beaded effect, with red and blue flowers. Est. $150.00-$250.00.

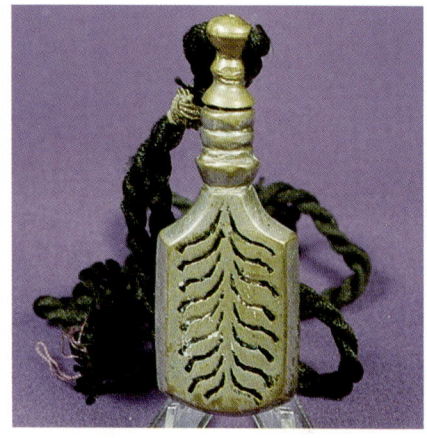

Lot #181. Unusual and very old metal bottle and stopper, 2.6" [6.6 cm], both sides of the bottle carved with a leaf-like motif, the stopper attached with a long black cord, country of origin unidentified. Est. $75.00-$125.00.

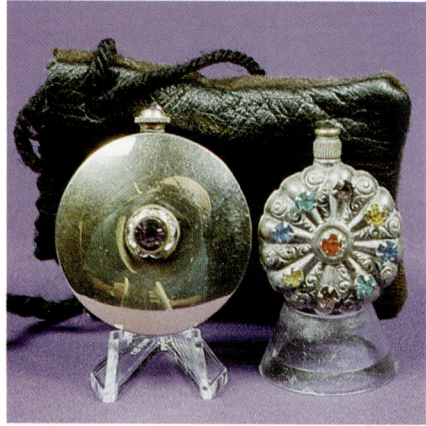

Lot #182. Pair of two different metal perfume purse flacons: round flat gold metal flask with violet stones on front and on cap, 2" [5.1 cm]; silver round metal flask, 1.6" [4.1 cm], festooned with multicolored stones and mounted as a brooch with a pin attachment. Two items, both in pouches. Est. $75.00-$125.00.

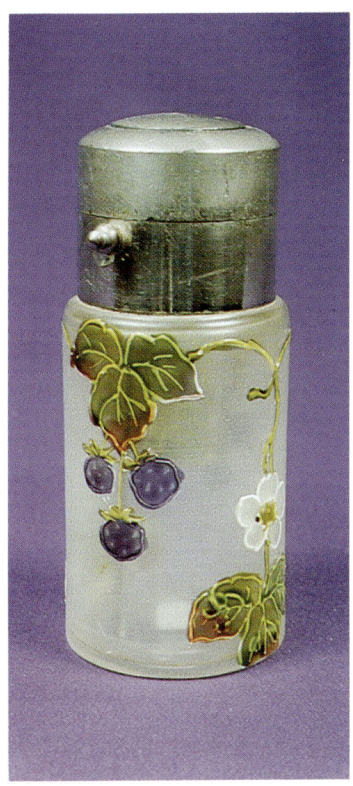

Lot #183. Frosted glass atomizer with a metal pump top, 4.3" [11 cm], enameled with a design of blackberries and flowers, functioning atomizer, unsigned. Est. $125.00-$175.00.

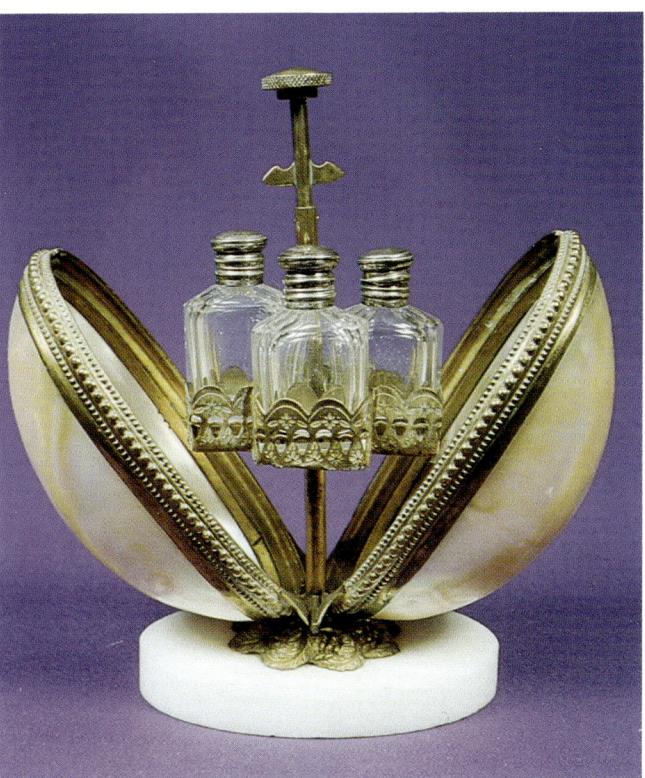

Lot #184. Unusual holder for miniature glass scent bottles created by two shells with a metal frame and mounted on a polished white stone base, 5.7" [14.5 cm] to top, containing three small crystal bottles [fourth one lacking], each 1.8" [4.6 cm], with silver caps [continental hallmarks], beautiful iridescence to the pearl-like shell. Est. $350.00-$450.00.

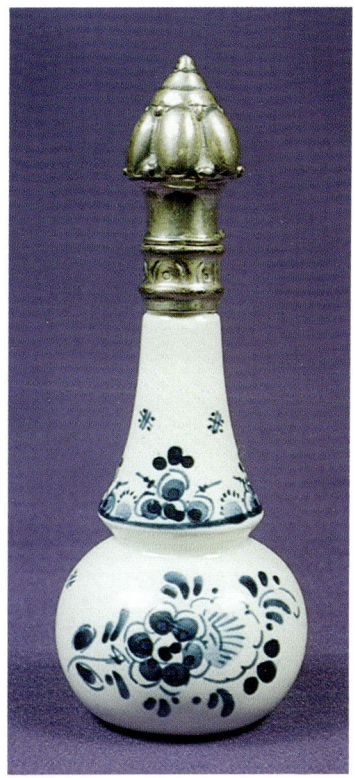

Lot #185. Delft ceramic bottle, inner stopper and sterling silver overcap, 4.2" [10.6 cm], navy blue flowers and leaves, indistinct hallmark on cap, signed *Delft Holland*. Est. $150.00-$200.00.

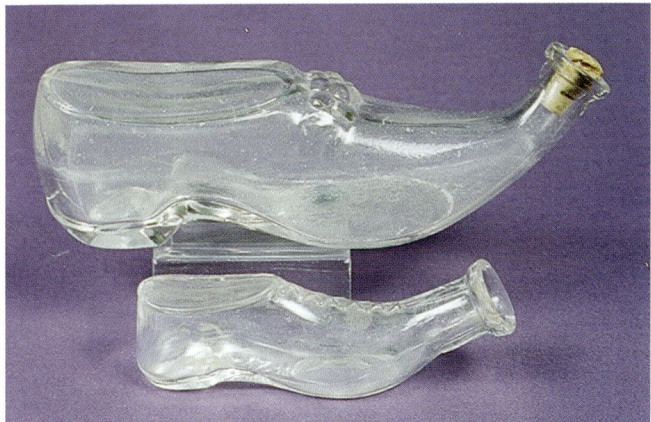

Lot #186. Two early pressed glass bottles in the shape of shoes, probably originally for commercial perfume: one 3.7" [9.4 cm], molded *R* and *M* on bottom; one 6" [15.2 cm], molded *B 18,* both empty. Two items. Est. $75.00-$125.00.

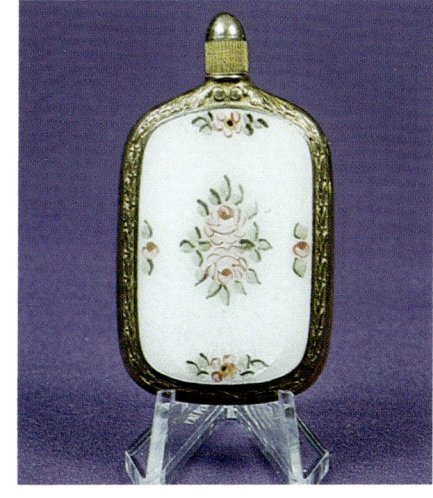

Lot #187. Metal purse flacon and cap, 2.3" [5.7 cm], covered in white enamel on both sides, the front also enameled with red roses and leaves, stopper with metal dauber. Est. $125.00-$175.00.

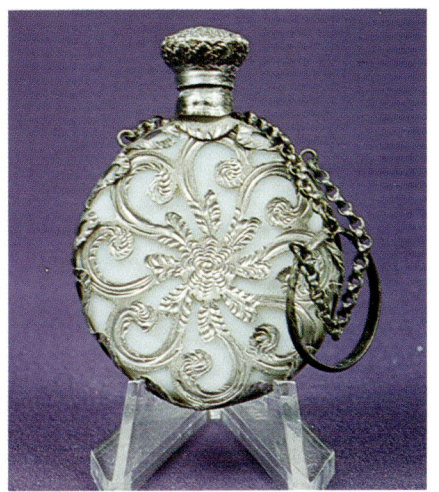

Lot #188. White glass scent bottle, tiny glass inner stopper, and metal cap, 1.8" [4.6 cm], the flat circular bottle entirely covered on both sides with an intricate design of scrolls in metal, with chain attachment and loop. Est. $125.00-$175.00.

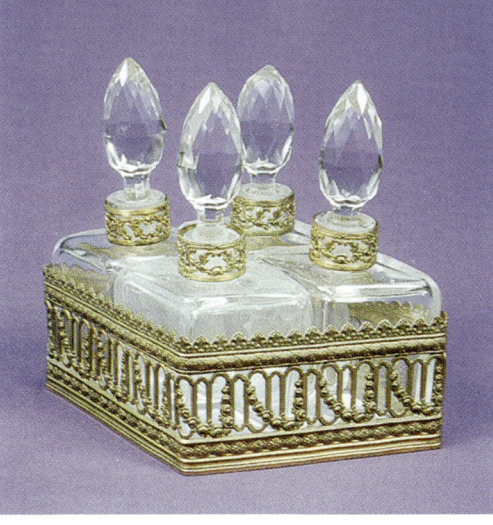

Lot #189. French crystal dresser set of four diamond shaped bottles, each 4.7" [11.9 cm], highly faceted teardrop stoppers, the neck of each bottle with a gold metal collar, all unsigned, in their gold metal holder festooned with garlands of flowers, metal holder signed *France* in a circle and in an oval. Est. $400.00-$500.00.

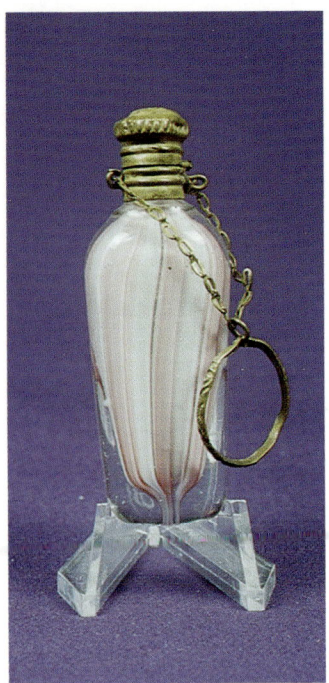

Lot #190. Scent bottle of pink and white glass cased in clear glass, 2.2" [5.6 cm], the neck affixed with a metal cap and chain attached to a ring. Est. $100.00-$150.00.

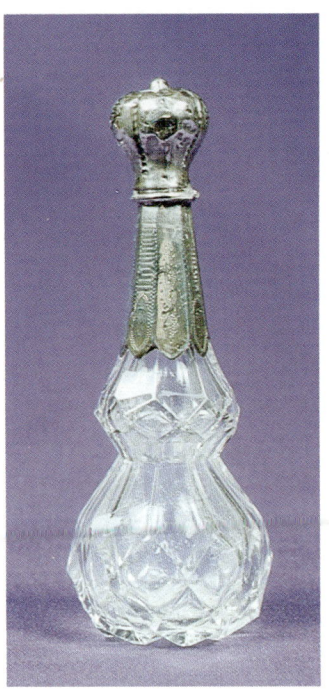

Lot #191. Clear crystal bottle with silver neck and cap, 4.4" [11.1 cm], an interesting and unusual shape, inner stopper lacking and with small hole in the silver, neck stamped with the Dutch hallmark for 833 silver. Est. $100.00-$200.00.

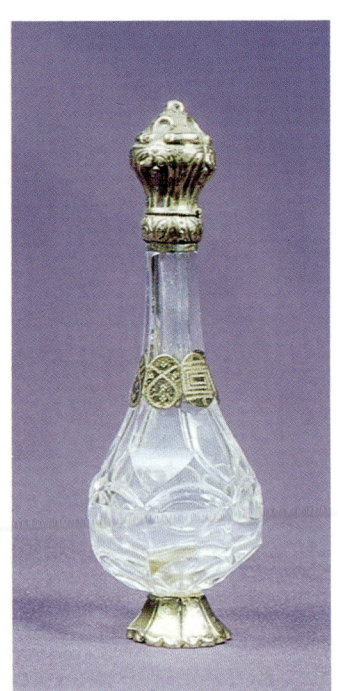

Lot #192. Clear crystal bottle with silver neck and cap, 5" [12.7 cm], standing on a silver pedestal and with a decorative silver band around the middle, inner stopper lacking, the metal parts bearing a gold tint, middle band stamped with the Dutch hallmark for 833 silver. Est. $200.00-$300.00.

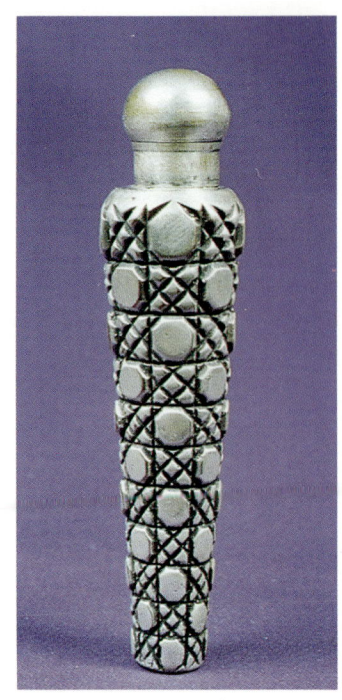

Lot #193. Unusual clear glass bottle totally clad in sterling silver over copper, 5" [12.7 cm], the metal designed with a geometric motif in high relief, screw on cap of silver, shoulder of bottle stamped *Sterling*. Est. $150.00-$200.00.

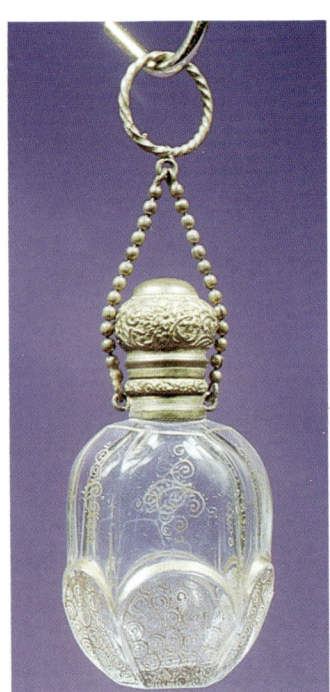

Lot #194. Clear crystal chatelaine-type scent bottle with brass fitting and cap with a loop and chain, 2.9" [7.4 cm] to top of cap, petal-like facets at the base decorated with hand-enameled gold swirls [with gentle wear], inner stopper lacking. Est. $200.00-$300.00.

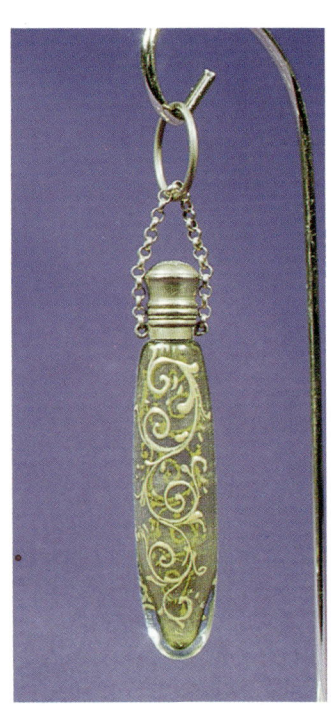

Lot #195. Light olive green glass perfume bottle with tiny inner glass stopper and metal overcap with a chain and loop, height to top of cap 3.3" [8.4 cm], both sides of the bottle intricately enameled with fanciful scrolls in gold and yellow. Est. $125.00-$175.00.

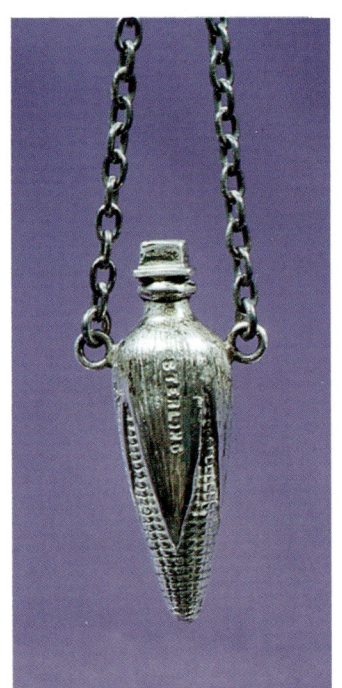

Lot #196. Sterling silver perfume flask and stopper in the shape of an ear of corn, 1.6" [4 cm], with loops on two sides and a chain with a loop, stamped *Sterling* on both sides. Est. $125.00-$175.00.

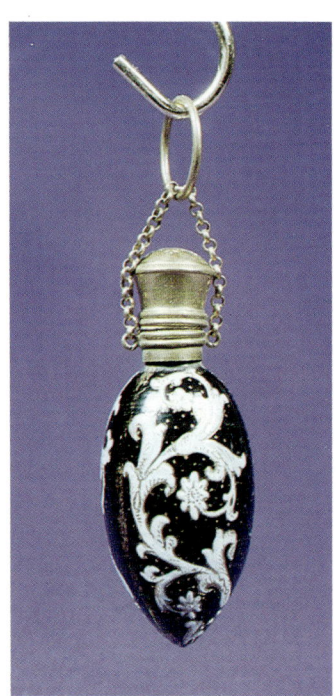

Lot #197. Dark blue glass bottle, clear glass inner stopper, and brass neck and cap with a chain attachment and loop, 3.1" [7.9 cm], the bottle of ovoid form decorated with leaves and scrolls of white and gold enamel. Est. $150.00-$250.00.

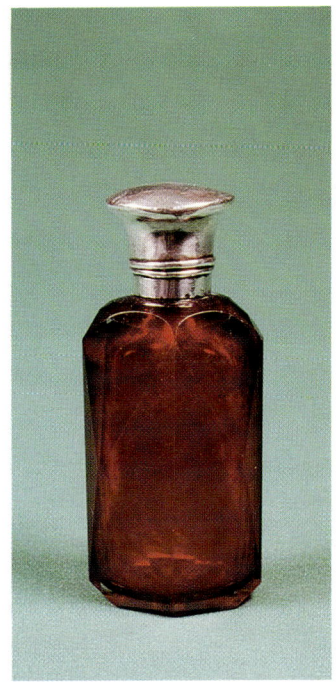

Lot #198. Red crystal perfume bottle with clear glass inner stopper and silver cap, 3.6" [9.1 cm], the bottle designed with large diamond-shaped facets, gently worn, unsigned. Est. $175.00-$250.00.

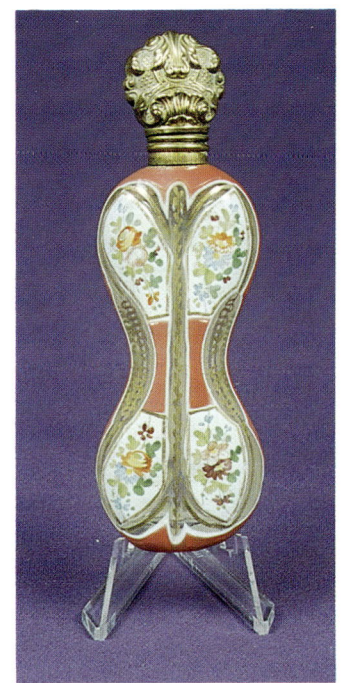

Lot #199. Pink over white cut back to clear crystal scent bottle with glass stopper and brass cap, 4.5" [11.4 cm], of hour-glass shape flattened on two sides, highly decorated on both sides with multicolor flowers and gold enamel. Est. $250.00-$350.00.

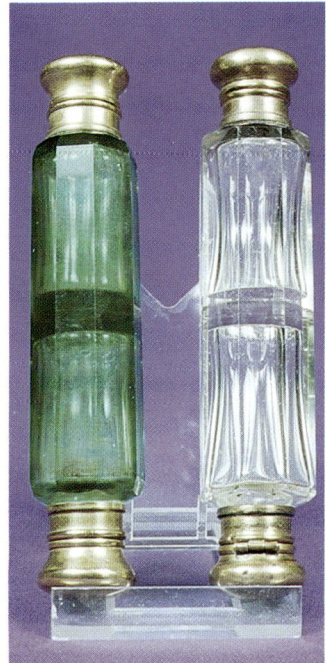

Lot #200. Green crystal double-ended flacon with metal hinged lids, 5.1" [12.9 cm], the bottle with nine sides and two separate perfume wells; similar clear crystal double-ended flacon, 5.3" [13.5 cm], inner stoppers lacking to both; possibly of English manufacture. Two items. Est. $150.00-$250.00.

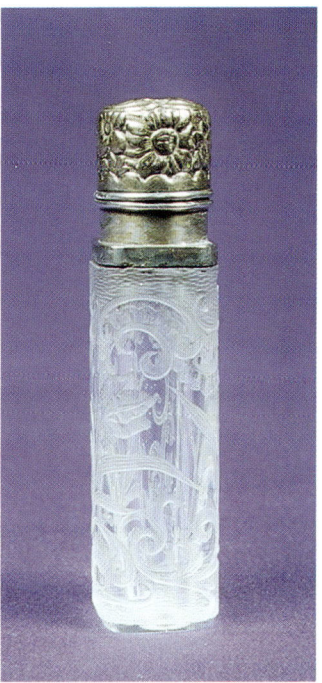

Lot #201. Cut crystal perfume flacon with sterling silver neck and cap, 3.4" [8.6 cm], the bottle wheel-cut with irises and scrolls, the hinged cap molded with flowers, inner stopper lacking, neck stamped *Sterling* and with hallmarks for Birmingham, England, 1830. Est. $200.00-$275.00.

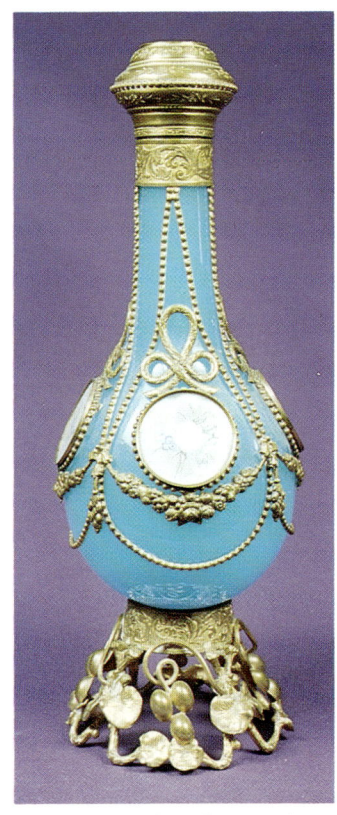

Lot #202. Blue 'Bristol' glass cologne bottle with a clear glass inner stopper, gold metal base and elaborate fittings, 9.6" [24.4 cm], decorated with paintings of flowers mounted under circular glass medallions around the bottle and on the cap; this bottle is of very large size and brilliant color. Est. $500.00-$600.00.

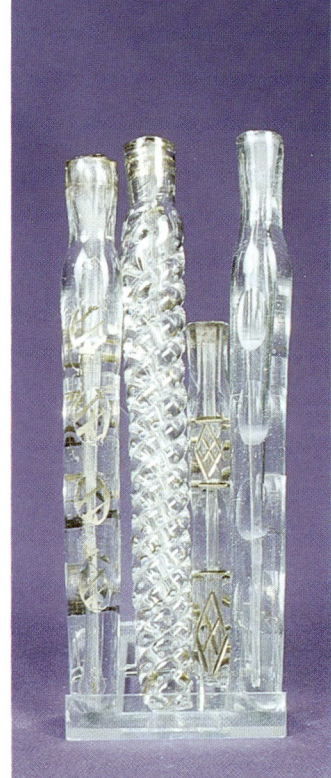

Lot #203. Lot of four different 19th century 'lavender' or 'attar of roses' bottles, heights from 4" to 6.2" [10 to 15.7 cm], the tallest in a swirl design with blue enamel dots, the others cut with scalloped facets and decorated with gold enamel, without stoppers, as is typical. Four items. Est. $100.00-$200.00.

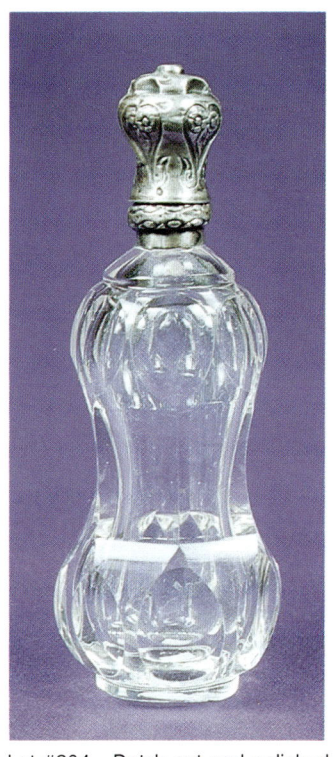

Lot #204. Dutch cut and polished crystal bottle sterling silver fitted cap, 5" [12.7 cm], the silver cap and neck hammered with flowers and decorative motifs, no inner stopper, Dutch hallmark for 833/1000 silver, signed with the maker's mark of Johannes van Vliet who worked from 1884-1914. Est. $125.00-$175.00.

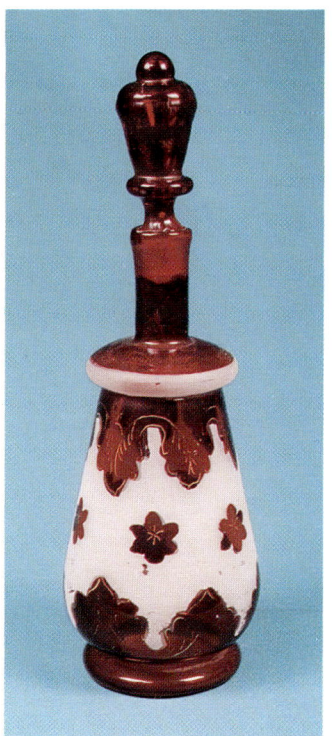

Lot #205. Victorian clear and frosted cologne decanter, 9.5" [24.1 cm], the bottle and stopper flashed with ruby red color in a design of scrolls and flowers and parts also frosted, possibly of American manufacture. Est. $100.00-$175.00.

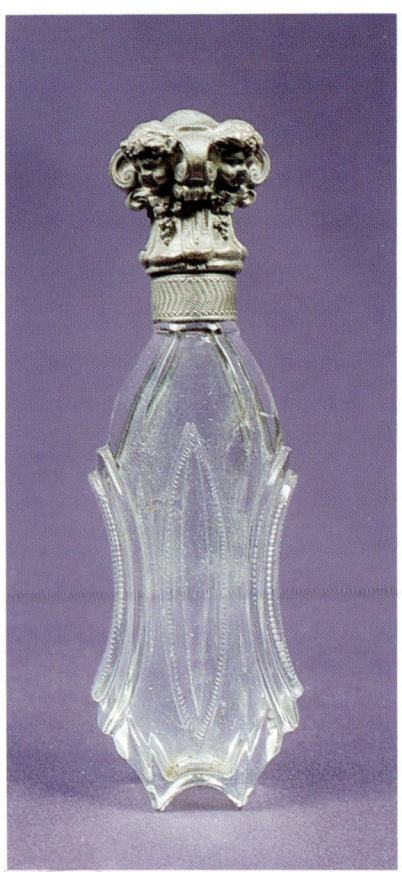 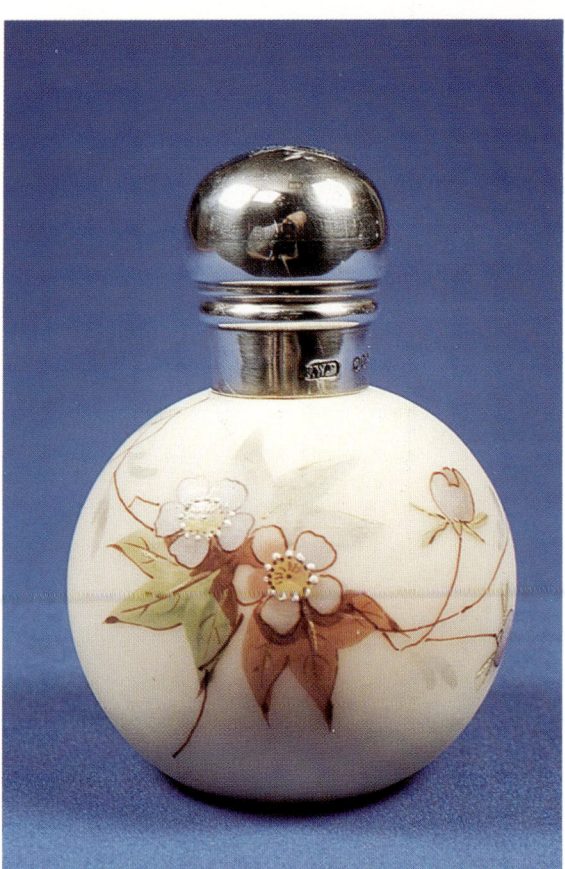 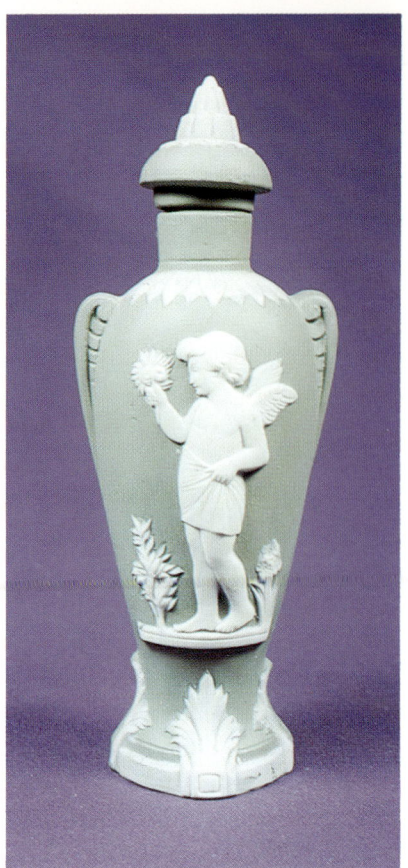

Lot #206. Russian clear crystal and silver fitted perfume flask, 4.6" [11.7 cm], the crystal cut with oval facets, the silver cap beautifully designed with heads of Cupid on four sides, the neck and the cap impressed with hallmarks for .875 silver and St. Petersburg, Russia, circa 1896. Est. $250.00-$350.00.

Lot #207. Webb Burmese scent botttle with glass inner stopper and sterling silver overcap, 3.5" [8.9 cm], the glass shading from yellow at the base to light peach at the top, enameled with flowers and leaves, silver cap stamped with English hallmarks for London, 1886. Est. $450.00-$600.00.

Lot #208. Green jasperware bottle and stopper with long glass dauber, 6.1" [15.5 cm], shaped as a miniature covered vase, beautifully molded with a wingèd cupid standing and admiring a bouquet of flowers, unsigned, possibly of German or English manufacture. Est. $300.00-$400.00.

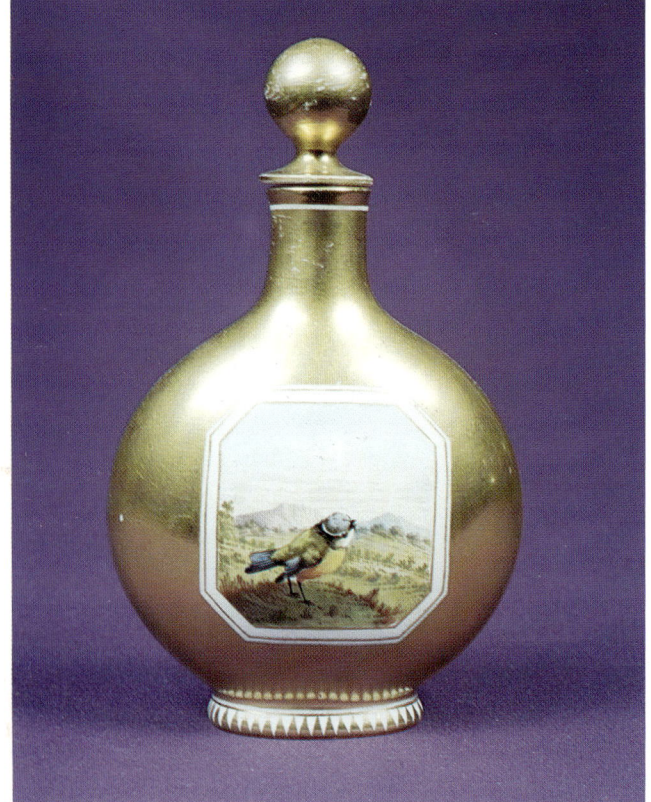 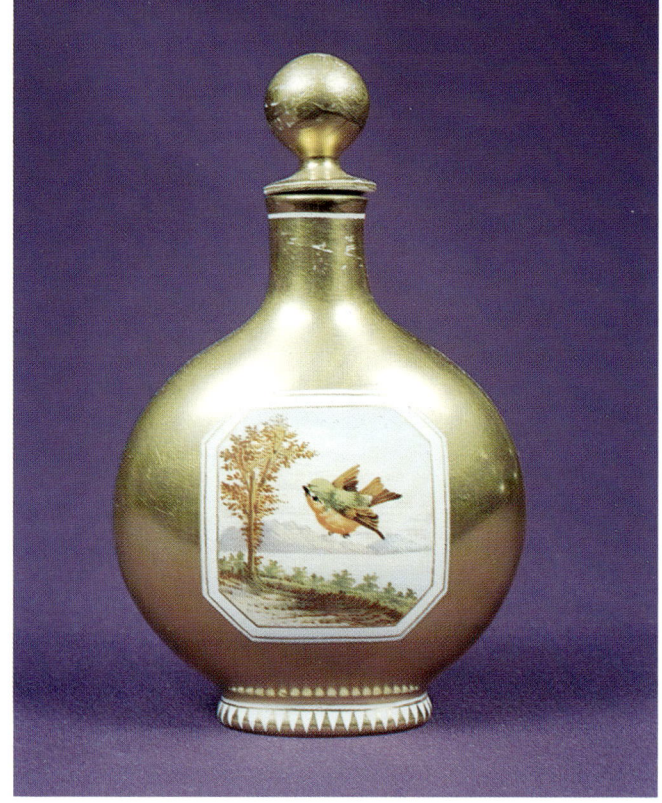

Lot #209. Coalport very fine bird portrait scent bottle and stopper, 5" [12.7 cm], a lovely oval shape made of hard paste porcelain, both the front and back handpainted with two different bird portraits in octagonal frames, the bottle entirely covered in gold enamel which is in superb condition, ball stopper with some re-gilding, bottom signed *Coalport* with crown emblem marked *AD 1780*, numbered *A5675*. These bird portraits are unusual stylistically in that the bird is depicted in much larger proportion than the surrounding landscape so that the beauty of each bird can be better seen and appreciated. Cf. Pavia [1995] for a similar example. [Both sides of this bottle are shown.] Est. $800.00-$1,200.00.

ART GLASS - BACCARAT - RICHARD - SABINO - STEUBEN

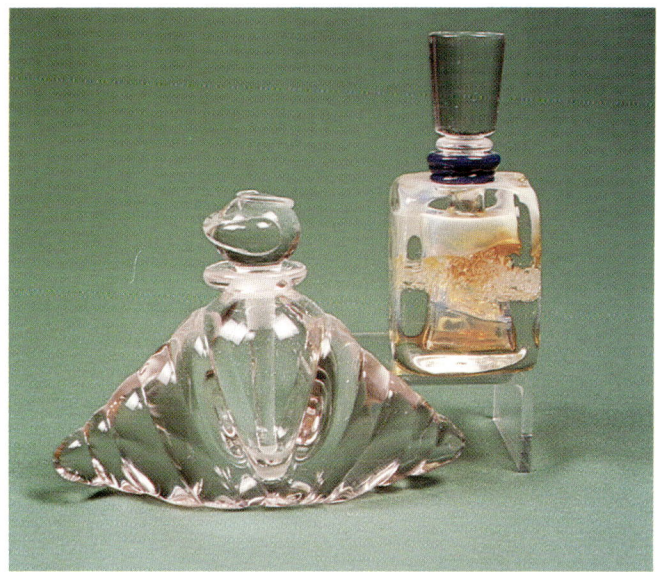

Lot #210. Pair of contemporary art glass perfume bottles: clear glass bottle and stopper with long dauber, 2.8" [7.1 cm], signed *Michael Small 1986;* clear glass bottle [with blue glass neck] and stopper, 3.2" [8.3 cm], internally decorated with amber and opalescent inclusions, stamped on the side with the initial *R*. Two bottles. Est. $100.00-$175.00.

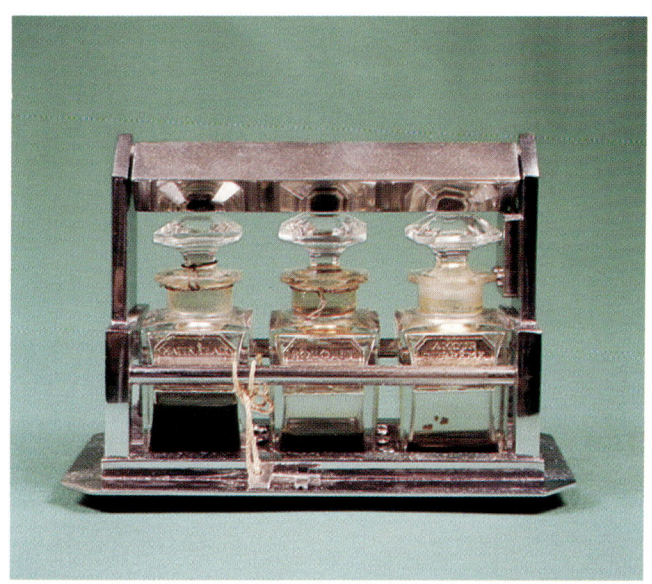

Lot #211. Brajan *Amour Suprême, Bouquet, Matin Clair* set of three clear crystal bottles/stoppers, each 3" [7.7 cm], some perfume, gold metallic labels, in an Art Deco chrome tantalus holder, with its key, each signed *Baccarat* with the acid-etched emblem. Bacc. #111 [1911 and later]. Est. $500.00-$600.00.

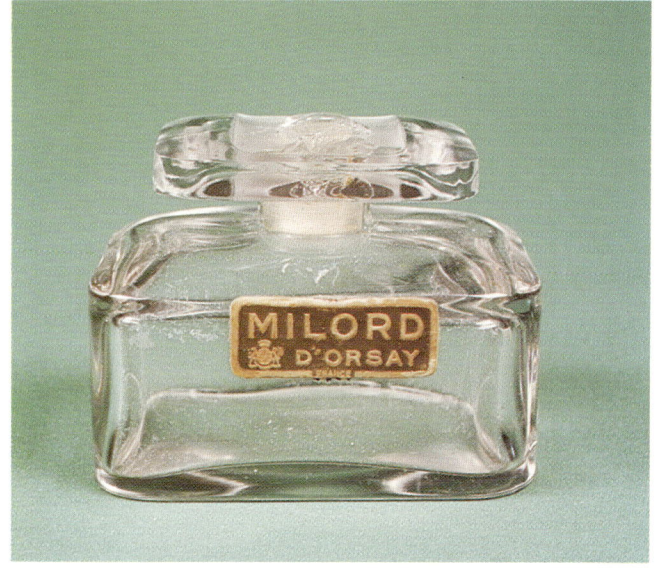

Lot #212. D'Orsay *Milord* clear crystal bottle and stopper, 2.2" [5.6 cm], of short rectangular form, the portrait of Le Conte d'Orsay in 19th century attire molded] into the stopper, empty, unsigned. Bacc. #793 [1944]. Est. $125.00-$175.00.

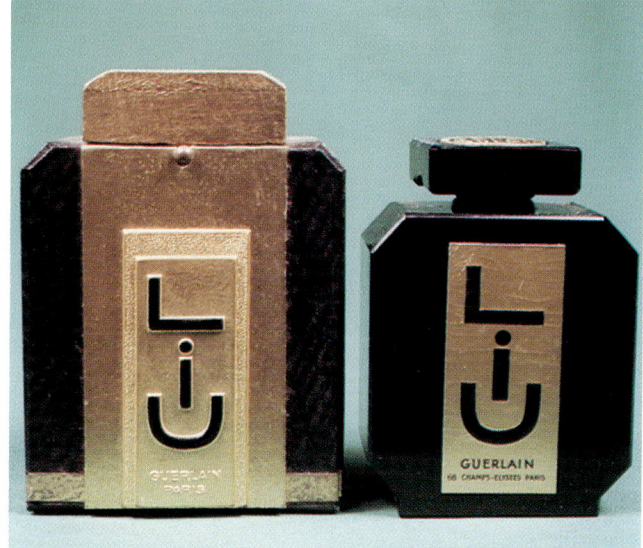

Lot #213. Guerlain *Liu* large size black crystal bottle and stopper of square shape, 3.5" [8.9 cm], gold and black labels in excellent condition on front of bottle and top of stopper, Guerlain labels on bottom, empty, in its elegant black and gold presentation case of similar shape, unsigned. Bacc. #679 [1929]. Est. $500.00-$650.00.

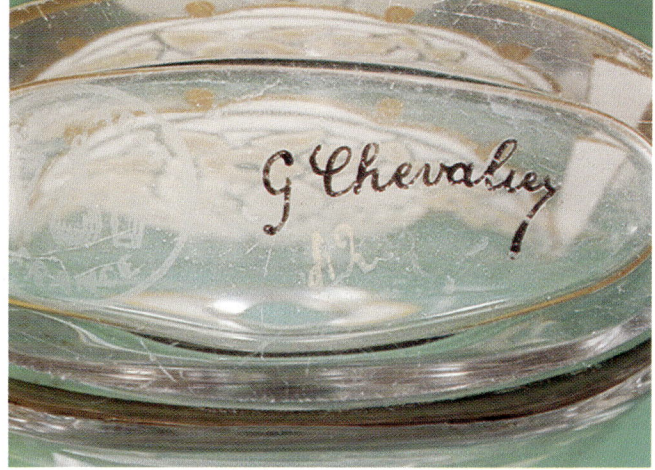

A closeup photograph of the bottom of the Baccarat bottle shown in the following Lot #214 on page 84. The acid-etched Baccarat emblem can be seen to the left, and the signature of *G. Chevalier* in black enamel to the right.

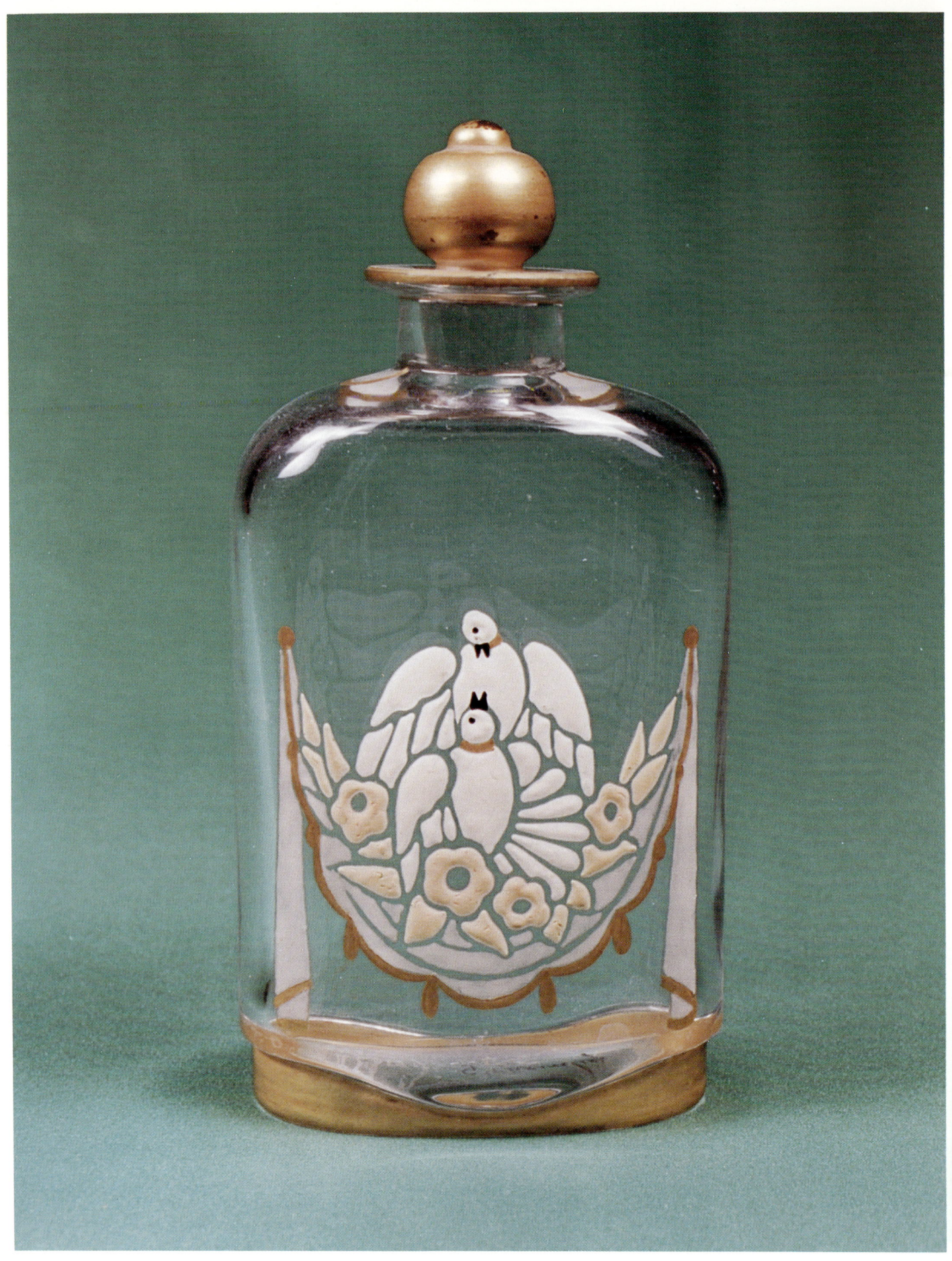

Lot #214. Extremely rare experimental clear crystal bottle and stopper, 5.4" [13.7 cm], of flask shape with rounded shoulders, beautifully decorated with doves in a nest of flowers surrounded by drapery in white and gold enamel by Georges Chevalier, empty, bottom signed with Baccarat emblem and *G. Chevalier* in gold. Chevalier was an important artist of the Art Deco era and worked for Baccarat beginning in the early 1920's. He was considered the greatest expert in the technique of enameling on glass. The bottle is shown here larger than actual size. This bottle is not catalogued in the existing literature. Est. $1,500.00-$2,000.00.

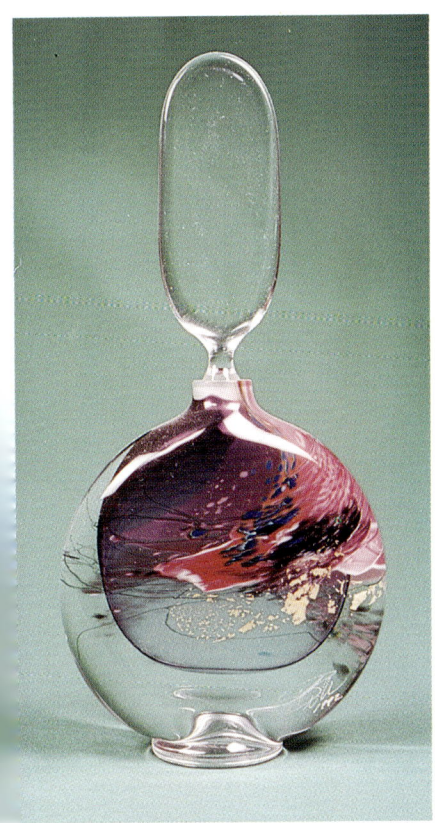

Lot #215. Very large contemporary art glass perfume bottle and stopper, 9.3" [23.6 cm], oval stopper, the flat bottle with mauve, pink, gold, and blue inclusions, signed on the side and dated 1992, the bottom engraved SFSV2060 - N. W. G. 1992. Est. $100.00-$175.00.

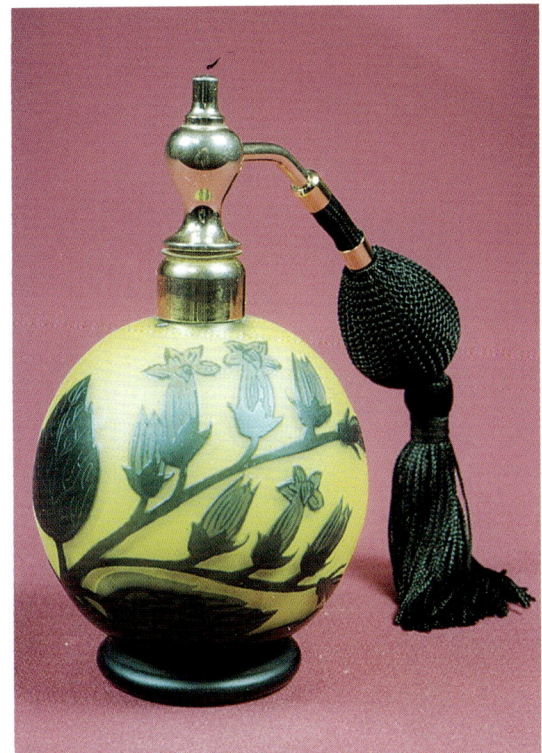

Lot #216. Richard cameo glass perfume bottle and metal atomizer attachment, 4.7" [11.9 cm], dark teal green over lemon yellow glass, with a design of flowers and leaves on one side and a moth on the other side, new atomizer ball, signed *Richard* in cameo, of Czechoslovakian manufacture. *Richard* was a name used by Loetz Witwe in the mid 1920's. Est. $500.00-$750.00.

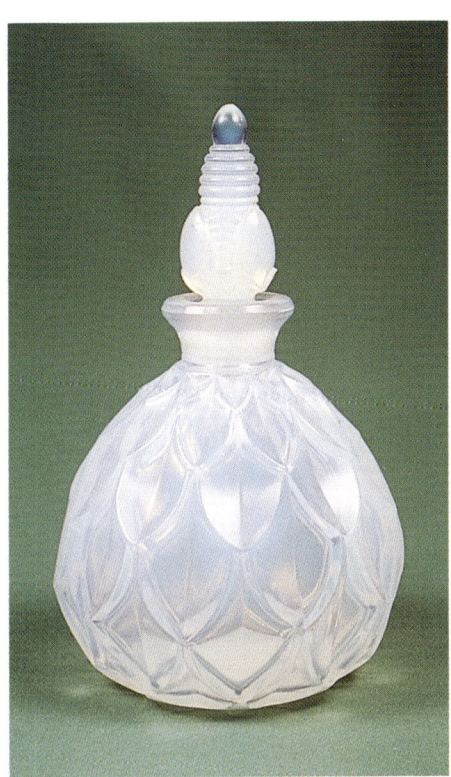

Lot #217. Sabino opalescent glass bottle and stopper, 5.3" [13.5 cm], the bottle molded entirely of rows of overlapping leaves, the stopper also designed with an abstract botanical motif, bottom signed *Sabino Paris*. Est. $200.00-$300.00.

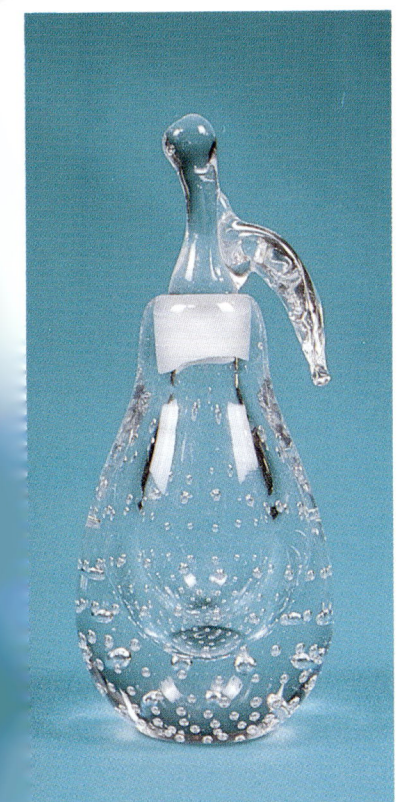

Lot #218. Pear shaped perfume bottle and stopper, 6" [15.2 cm], the heavy bottle decorated internally with controlled bubbles in a swirl, the stopper molded as a stem and a leaf, unsigned. Est. $100.00-$150.00.

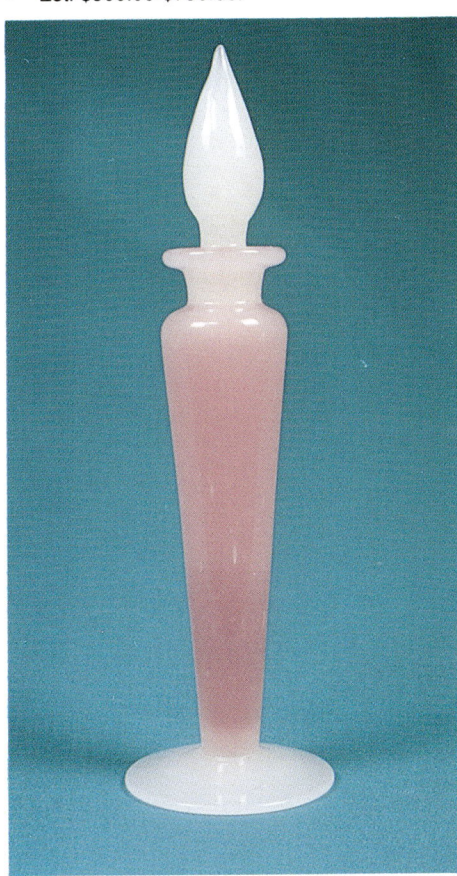

Lot #219. Steuben rosaline and alabaster white glass bottle and stopper, 7.8" [19.8 cm], the elegant long form on a round pedestal base, flame stopper [chip to tongue of stopper], polished pontil bottom, unsigned. Cf. Sloan, p. 54. Est. $400.00-$500.00.

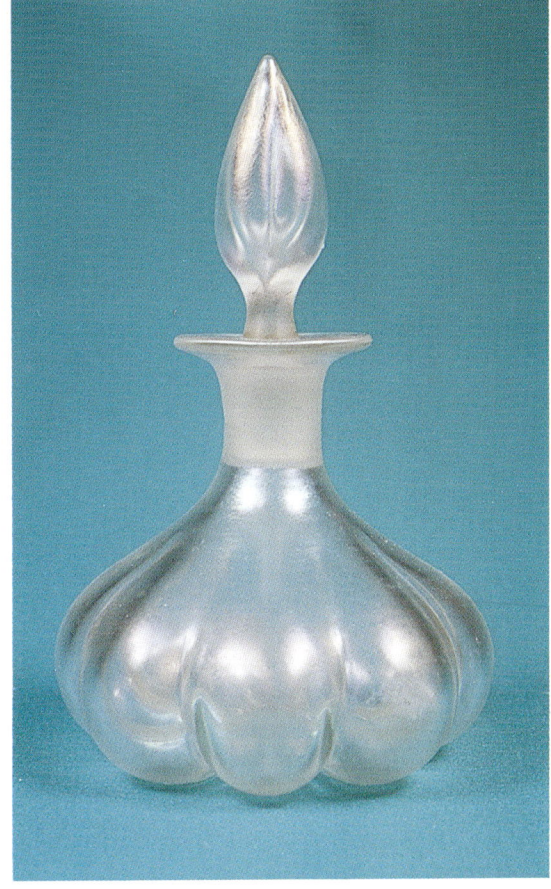

Lot #220. Steuben translucent and opalescent glass bottle and stopper, 4.6" [11.7 cm], of melon shape with 8 lobes and long neck, stopper with a similar design, unsigned. Est. $400.00-$500.00.

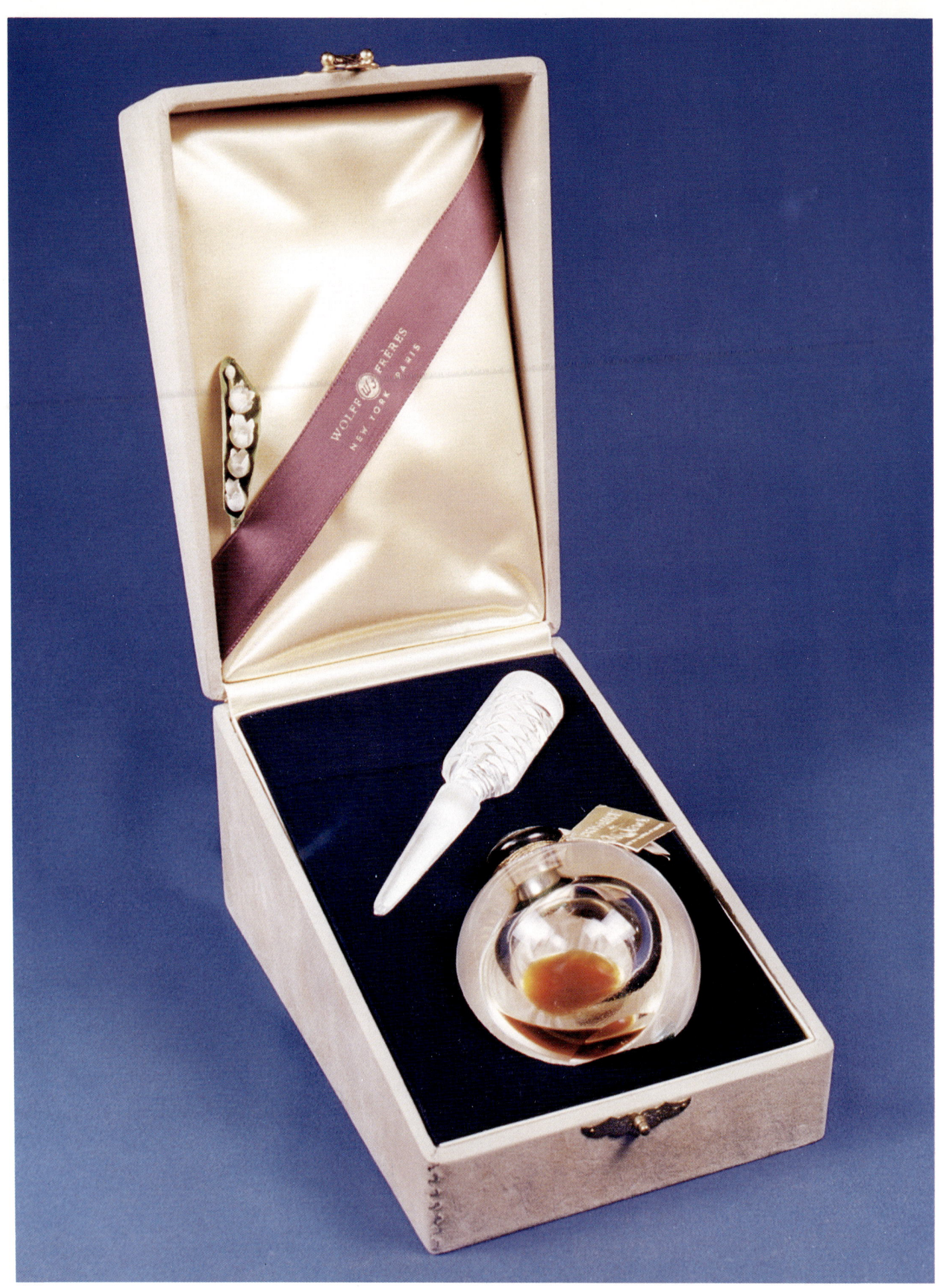

Lot #221. Wolff Frères *Crisance* very fine clear crystal bottle and stopper, 5" [12.7 cm], of ball shape with an elegant long dauber internally decorated with intertwined swirls, unopened condition [perfume evaporated], bottom signed *Steuben*, a tiny tag around the neck proclaims "Crisance, the rarest perfume in the world, in a pure crystal flacon by Steuben Glass"; in its elegant gray suede case lined with silk and blue velvet. Circa 1948. This American creation is in the finest tradition of luxury perfume. Est. $2500.00-$3500.00.

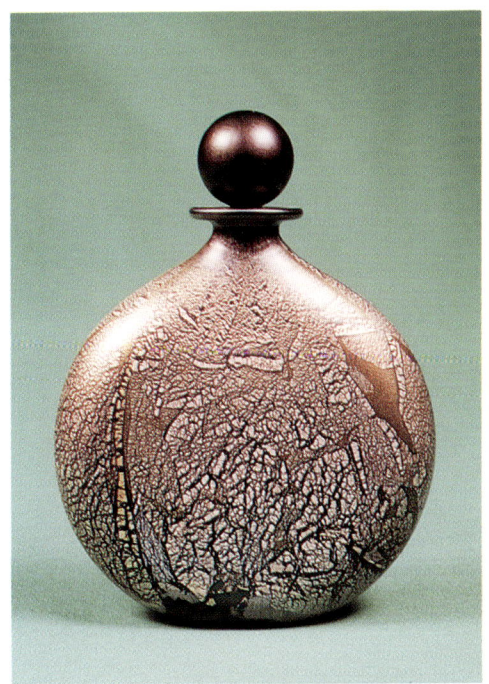
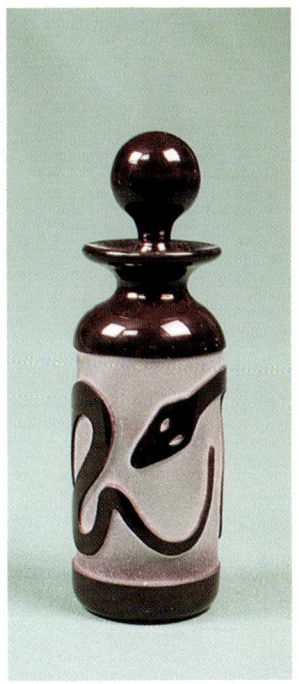
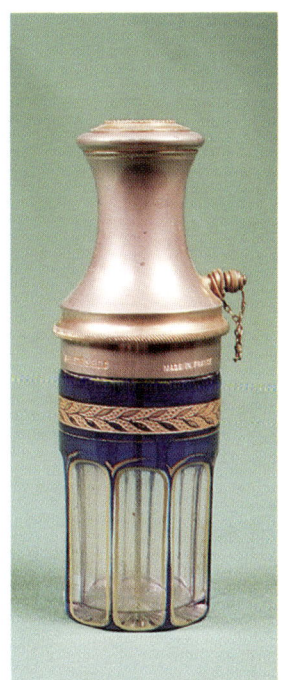
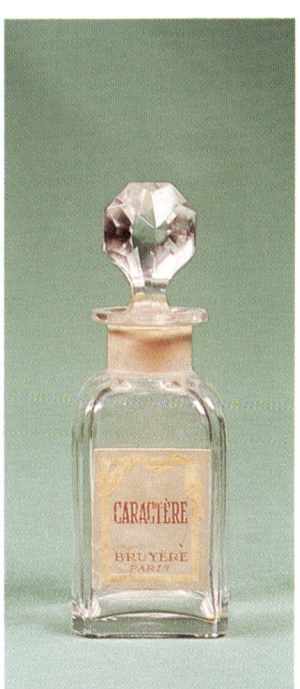

Lot #222. Isle of Wight glass bottle and ground stopper, 5.9" [14.9 cm], the blue glass bottle of flattened round shape and covered with a very pleasing textured gold irridescence, bottom signed with Isle of Wight label, of English manufacture. Est. $100.00-$200.00.

Lot #223. Modern artist scent bottle of black glass over clear, 4.9" [12.4 cm], of cylinder form with a ball stopper and long dauber, the bottle deeply acid etched with an undulating serpent in sharp relief, bottom signed B & B 1992. Est. $100.00-$200.00.

Lot #224. Perfume bottle of blue crystal over clear with metal atomizer pump, 5.2" [13.2 cm], eight rectangular windows and decorated with a band of gold leaves, signed *Le Parisienne, Made in France;* the atomizer functions and still has the tiny closure cap and chain. Est. $150.00-$250.00.

Lot #225. Bruyère *Charactère* clear crystal bottle and stopper, 4.5" [11.4 cm], a traditional decanter form with a faceted jewel-like stopper, empty, label on front, Baccarat emblem on bottom; this precise design is not referenced in the Baccarat book, but the bottle corresponds to #68 [1909] and the stopper to #51 [1909]. Est. $100.00-$200.00.

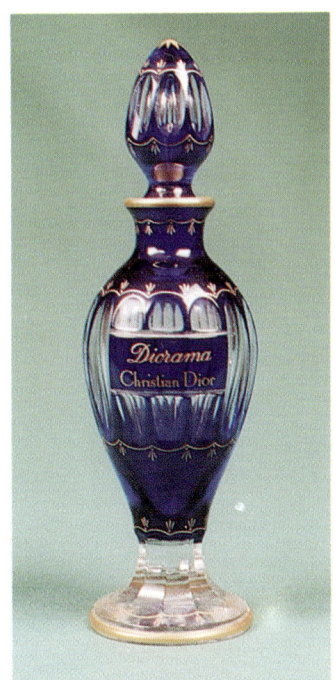
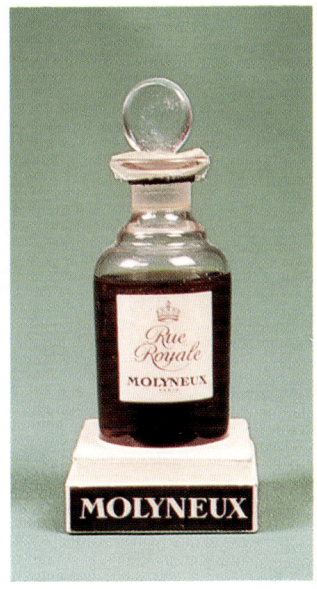
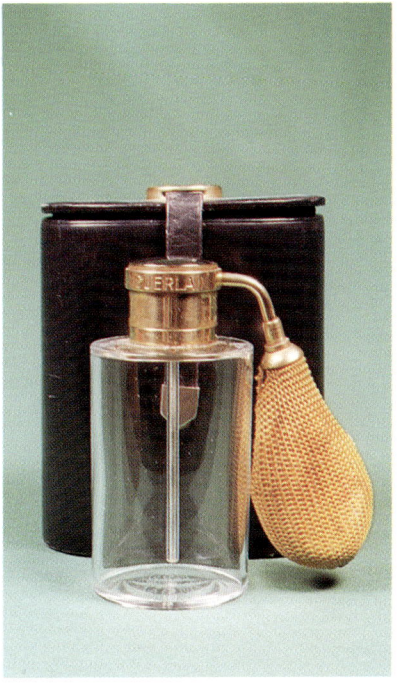
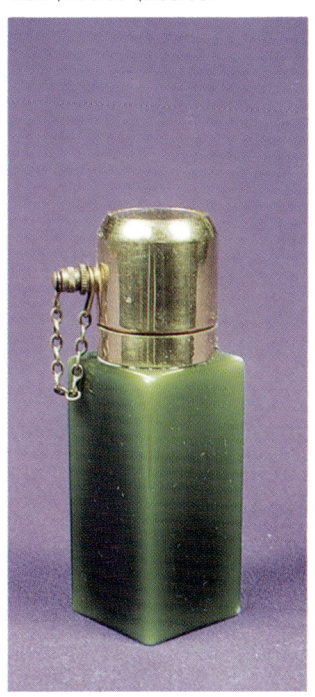

Lot #226. Christian Dior *Diorama* blue and clear crystal bottle and stopper of amphora shape, 7.1" [18 cm], empty, the blue glass cut with windows of clear crystal on both the bottle and stopper, names and decoration enameled in gold in superb condition, Baccarat emblem on bottom. Bacc. #814 [1949]. Est. $500.00-$650.00.

Lot #227. Molyneux *Rue Royale* clear crystal bottle and stopper in an apothecary shape, 3.5" [9 cm], square label, full and sealed, Baccarat emblem on base, probably made during World War II, since back label says: *Rapporter ce flacon vide à votre fournisseur est un devoir national et une nécessité vitale pour notre industrie* ['Returning this bottle when empty to the perfumer is a national duty and a vital necessity for our industry']. Bacc. #524 [1940]. Est. $100.00-$150.00.

Lot #228. Guerlain clear crystal bottle with a gold metal atomizer top, 3.9" [9.8 cm], of column shape, atomizer ball hardened with age, metal atomizer marked *Guerlain* around top, in its fitted black leather case the inside of which is also marked *Guerlain;* signed *Baccarat* in acid on bottom, circa 1930. Cf. Atlas & Monniot *Guerlain,* p. 297. Est. $75.00-$100.00.

Lot #229. Ybry *Femme de Paris* green over opaque white crystal bottle with metal atomizer top, 3.4" [8.5 cm], both the gold metal neck and the pump impressed *Made in France,* bottom signed in acid *Ybry Paris.* Est. $450.00-$600.00.

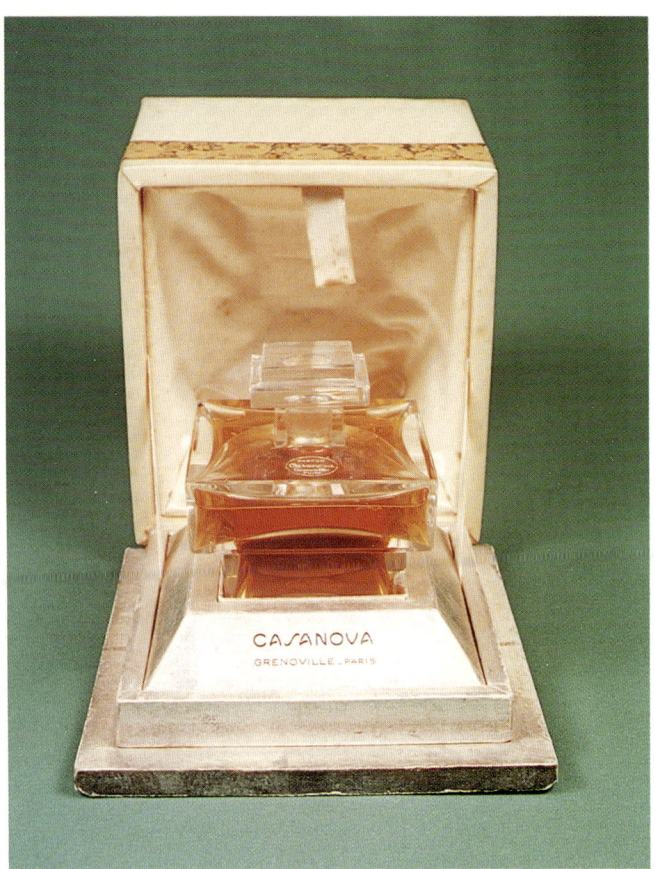

Lot #230. Grenoville *Casanova* clear crystal bottle and stopper, 2.6" [6.6 cm], an unusual Art Deco design made totally of rectangular and square facets, even the neck of the bottle is square, empty, decal label, [note multiple chips to the bottle], Baccarat emblem on bottom, in a beautiful presentation case decorated with flowers. This bottle is not catalogued in the Baccarat reference book. Est. $500.00-$600.00.

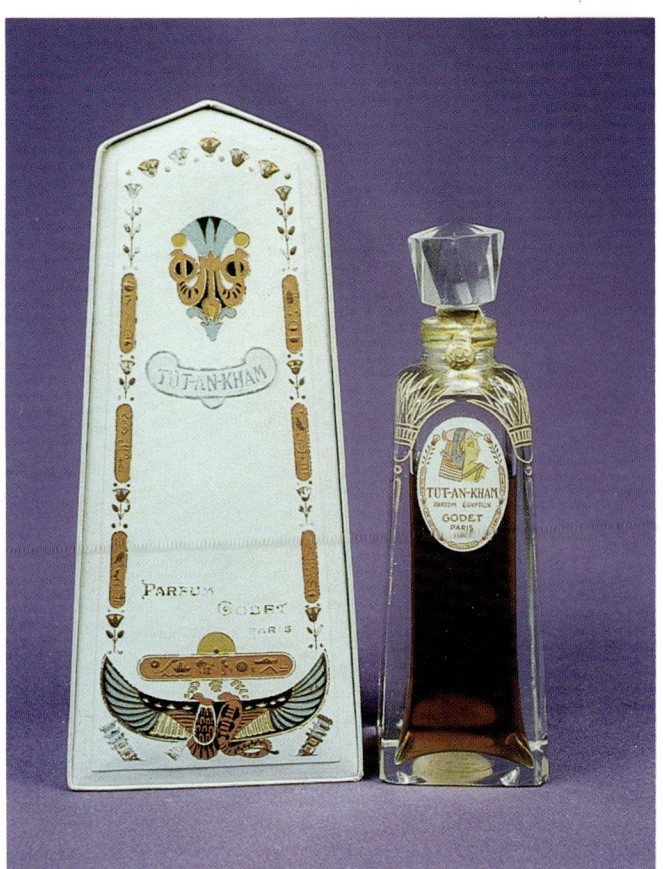

Lot #231. Godet *Tut-An-Kham* very rare clear crystal bottle and stopper, 4.6" [11.7 cm], of obelisk shape, the stopper with triangular facets, the shoulders of the bottle carved and gilded with stylized Egyptian lotus motifs, near full and with original seal bearing *Godet* tag, blue oval label, Baccarat emblem on bottom [miniscule flake to side, very small interior bruise on bottom], in its blue box lined with gold fabric and decorated with Egyptian motifs. Bacc #214 [1913]. Est. $800.00-$1,000.00.

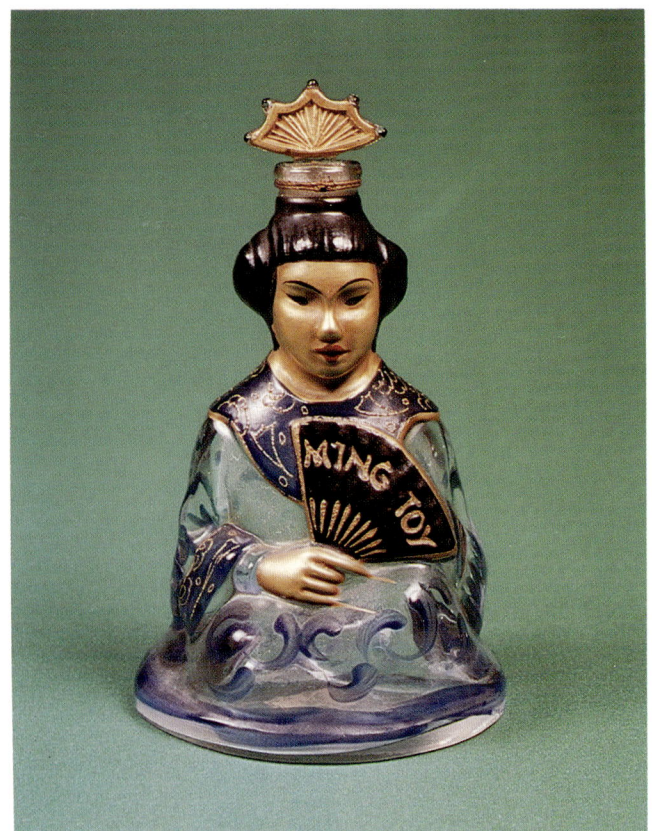

Lot #232. Forest *Ming Toy* very rare clear crystal bottle and stopper, 4.3" [11 cm], in the shape of an oriental lady seated and holding a fan with the words *Ming Toy*, beautifully enameled in blue, black, and gold, no wear to the enamel, empty, unsigned, bottom with small paper label *Made in France*. Bacc. #510 [1923]. Est. $3,000.00-$3,500.00.

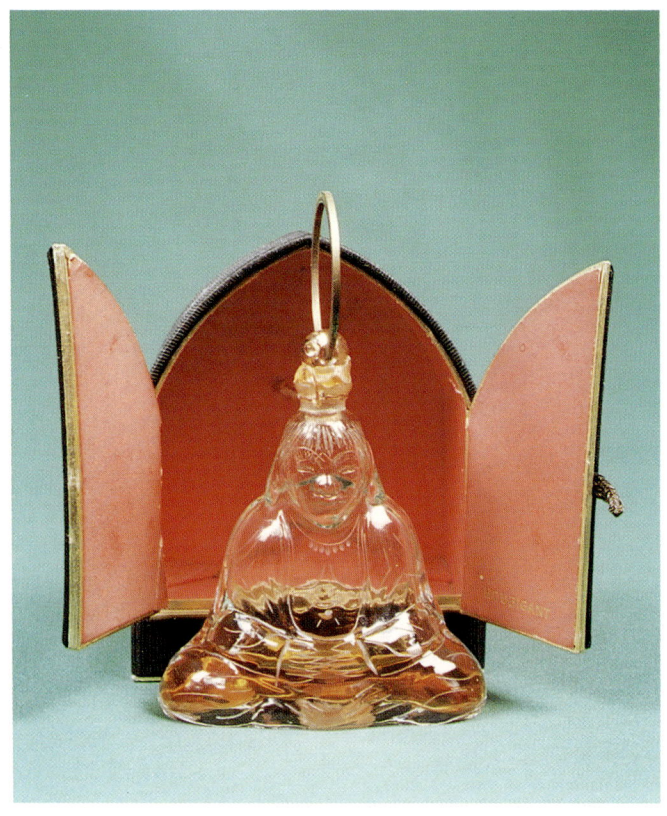

Lot #233. Houbigant *Subtilité* ['Subtlety'] clear crystal bottle and stopper molded entirely as a sitting Buddha, 3.3" [8.5 cm], gold label on back, some perfume, signed *Baccarat* in the circle emblem, in its altar-form box of black fabric with coral interior. Bacc #417 [1919]. Est. $500.00-$750.00.

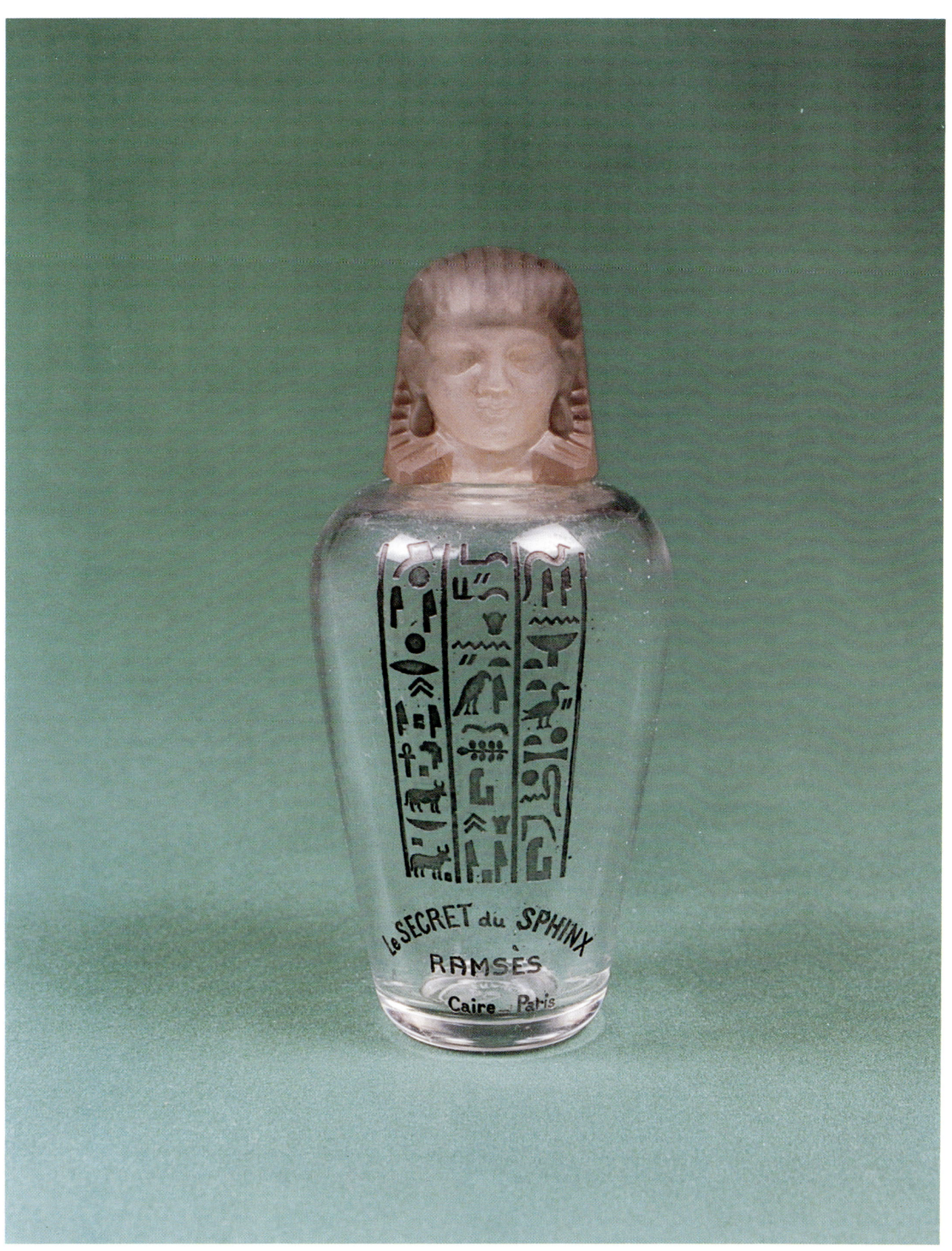

Lot #234. Ramsès *Le Secret du Sphinx* ['The Secret of the Sphynx'], extremely rare clear crystal bottle, inner stopper, and frosted overcap, 4" [10.2 cm], in the shape of an Egyptian canopic jar, the overcap molded as the head of the Pharoah, the body of the bottle etched with hieroglyphics below which are found the names of the perfume and the company, gray patina, bottom signed *Baccarat* in emblem. Bacc. #323 [1917]. This is possibly the rarest and most desirable of all the Egyptian motif bottles produced by Baccarat. Canopic jars, quite large and made of alabaster, were used in ancient Egypt to hold the internal organs of the deceased, for example, the heart. The bottle is shown here larger than actual size. Est. $8,000.00-$10,000.00.

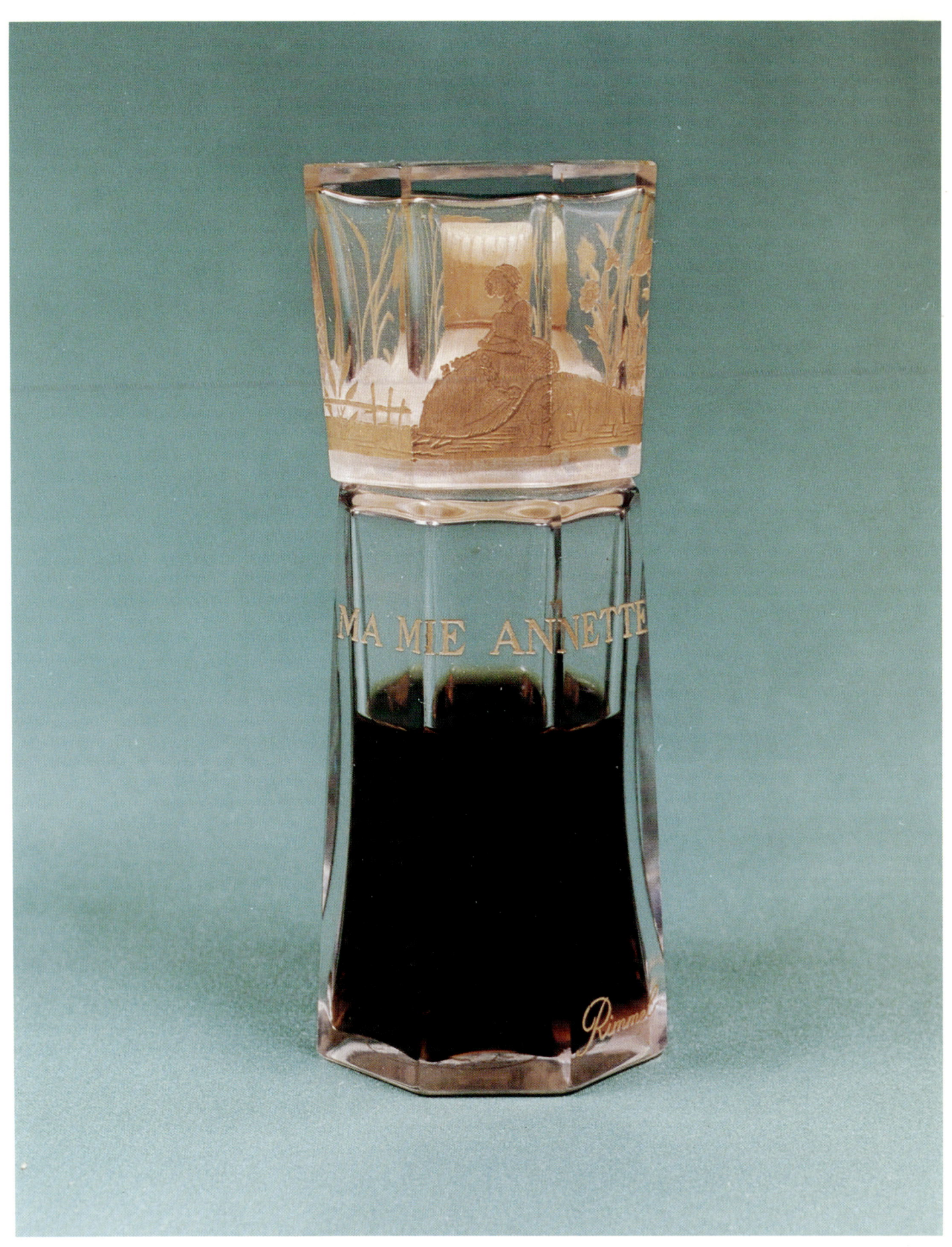

Lot #235. Rimmel *Ma Mie Annette* ['My Sweetheart Annette'] extremely rare and unusual perfume bottle, inner stopper and overcap, 4.3" [10.8 cm], designed as an octagonal tower, the translucent crystal overcap enameled in gold with a scene of a woman seated near a pond with flowers, the name enameled on the front of the bottle and signed *Rimmel* in gold near the base, unopened with most perfume, bottom with *E. Rimmel* paper label and signed *Baccarat* in circle emblem. Bacc #519 [1923]. This bottle has not been pictured in published sources; it is shown here larger than actual size. Est. $4,500.00-$5,500.00.

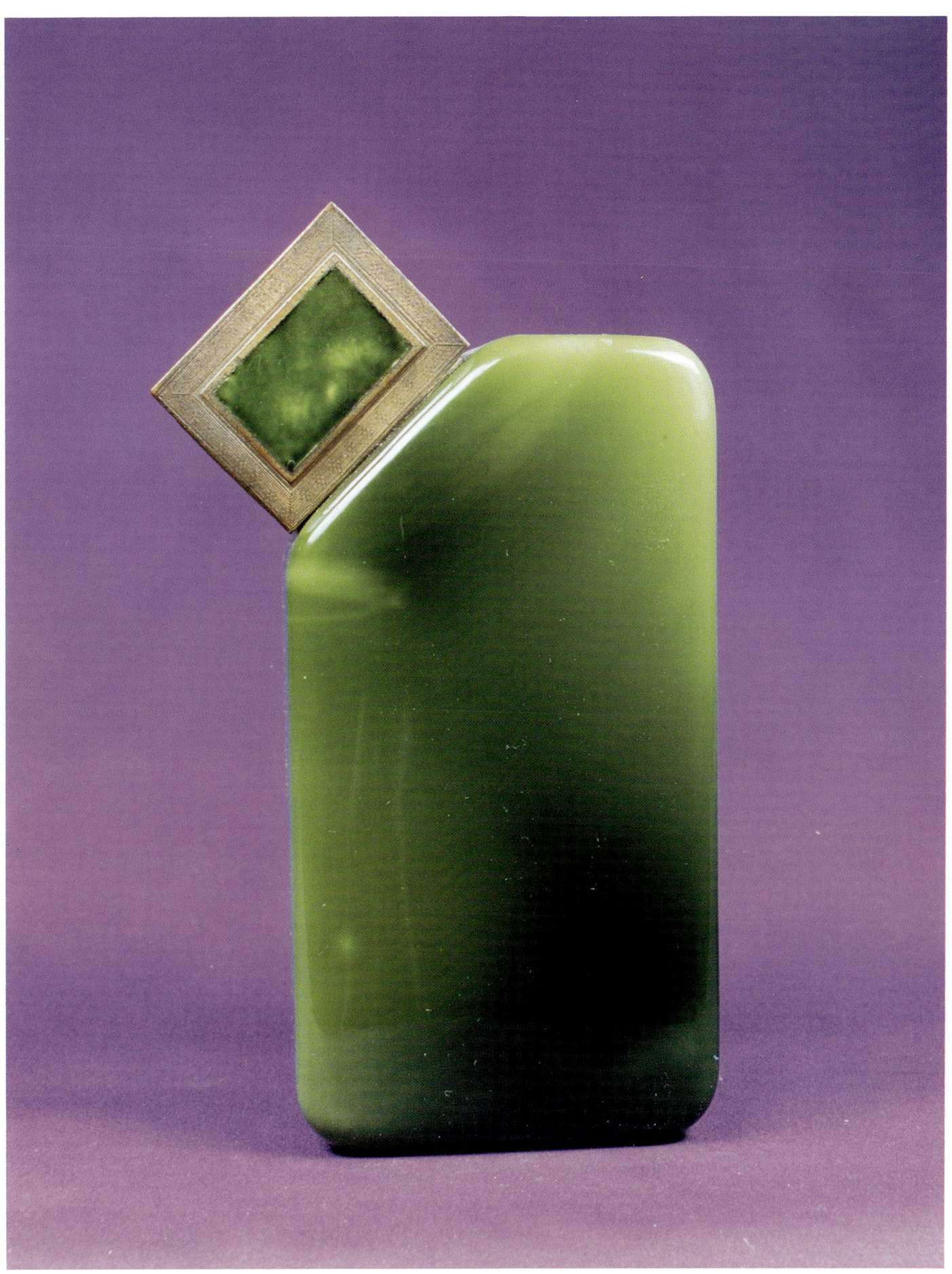

Lot #236. Ybry *Femme de Paris* green over white crystal bottle with clear glass inner stopper and metal overcap, 7.5" [19 cm] to top of overcap, no label, inner glass stopper with some chips, bottom signed *Ybry Paris* in a rectangle; the metal overcap is covered in green over white enamel and is in superb condition. This large size, possibly for bath salts or merely for display, is quite rare. Est. $1,000.00-$1,200.00.

COMMERCIAL PERFUME BOTTLES

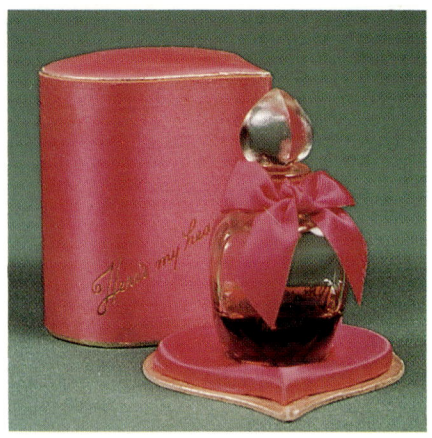

Lot #237. Avon *Here's My Heart* clear glass bottle and stopper, 2.5" [6.4 cm], the bottle molded with hearts on four sides, the name in gold enamel on front, in its pink heart-shaped box lined with gold foil. A truly adorable perfume presentation. Est. $175.00-$250.00.

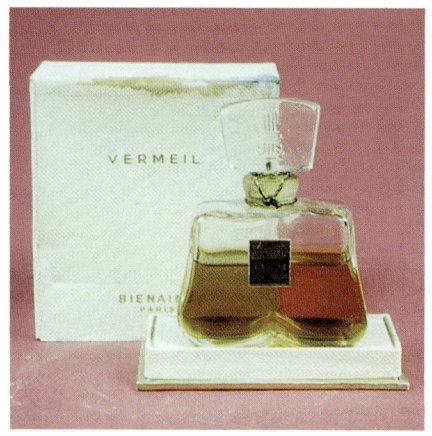

Lot #238. Bienaimé *Vermeil* ['Vermillion'] clear glass bottle and stopper, 3" [7.8 cm], the bottle almost a butterfly shape, the stopper molded with lines, near full and unopened, gold metallic label, in its cream box [some stains], circa 1936. Est. $100.00-$150.00.

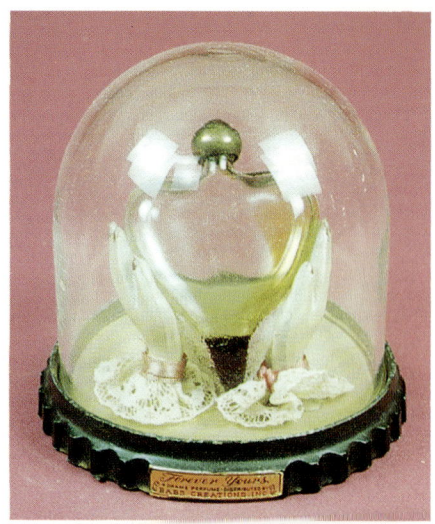

Lot #239. Babs Creations *Forever Yours* clear glass bottle and brass ball cap, 3" [7.6 cm], shaped as a heart, some perfume, held by two metal hands under a glass bell, gold label at bottom of metal holder. Est. $150.00-$250.00.

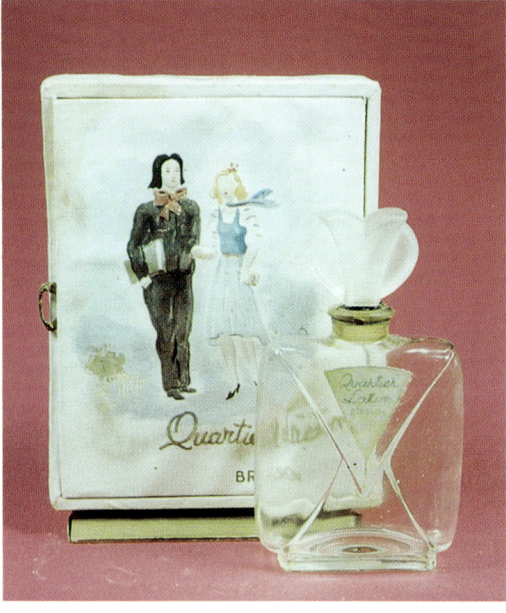

Lot #240. Brisson *Quartier Latin* ['Latin Quarter'] clear glass bottle and frosted glass stopper, 4.3" [10.9 cm] the bottle shaped like an envelope, the stopper of heart form, empty, label [faded] on front, in an adorable box [some stains] decorated with university motifs with two students on front and the masks of comedy and tragedy on top of the box, circa late 1940's. Est. $200.00-$250.00.

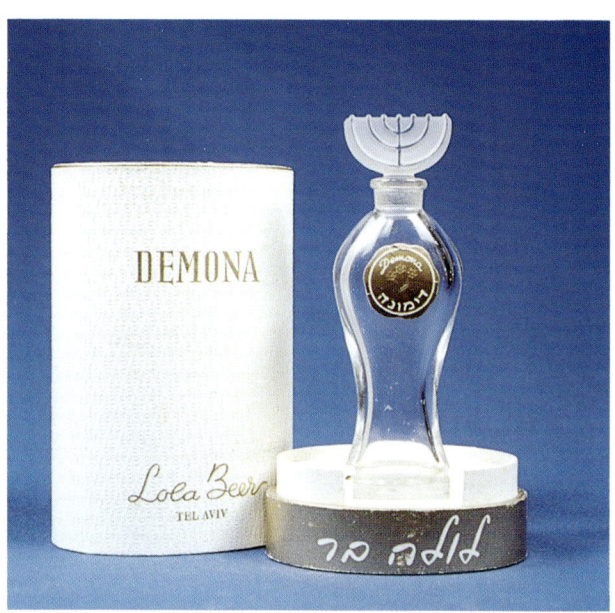

Lot #241. Lola Beer *Demona* [a city in the Negev in Israel] clear glass bottle and frosted glass stopper, 4.4" [11.2 cm], the bottle of inverted baluster form, the stopper shaped as a Menorah, empty, gold label on front, in its oval box, names also in Hebrew on the label and on the box, marked *Made in Israel*. Not pictured or referenced in existing publications. Est. $150.00-$250.00.

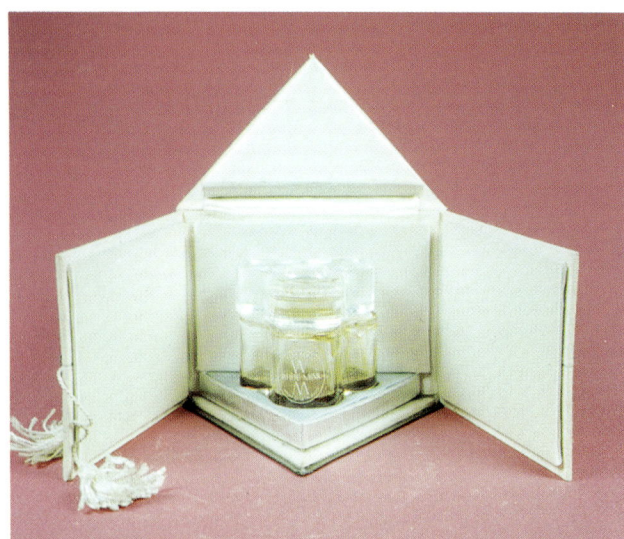

Lot #242. Cara Nome *White Mink* clear glass bottle, inner glass stopper, and heavy glass overcap, 1.9" [4.8 cm], the bottle a very unusual triangular form with broadly rounded indented sides, some perfume, label on bottle, in its very unusual box of white satin which opens from the front. Not pictured or referenced in existing publications. Est. $350.00-$450.00.

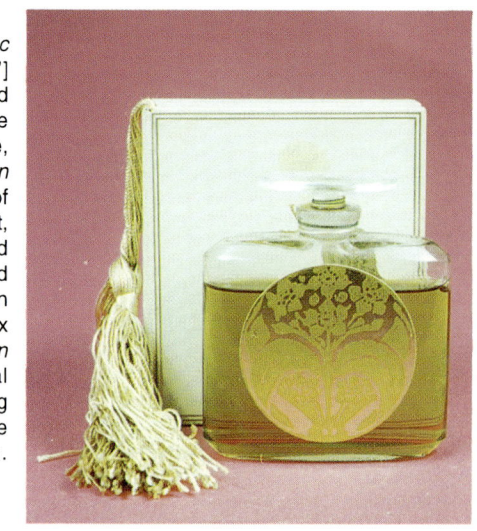

Lot #243. Caron *Le Tabac Blond* ['Blond Tobacco'] clear glass bottle and stopper, 3.3" [8.5 cm], the bottle of flat oval shape, stopper molded *Caron* and frosted, gold label of a tobacco flower on front, label also on base, full and sealed, in its tasseled book-form box [small stain on outside], inside of box marked *Présentation Provisoire* ['Provisional Presentation'] indicating that this was among the earliest examples. Est. $175.00-$250.00.

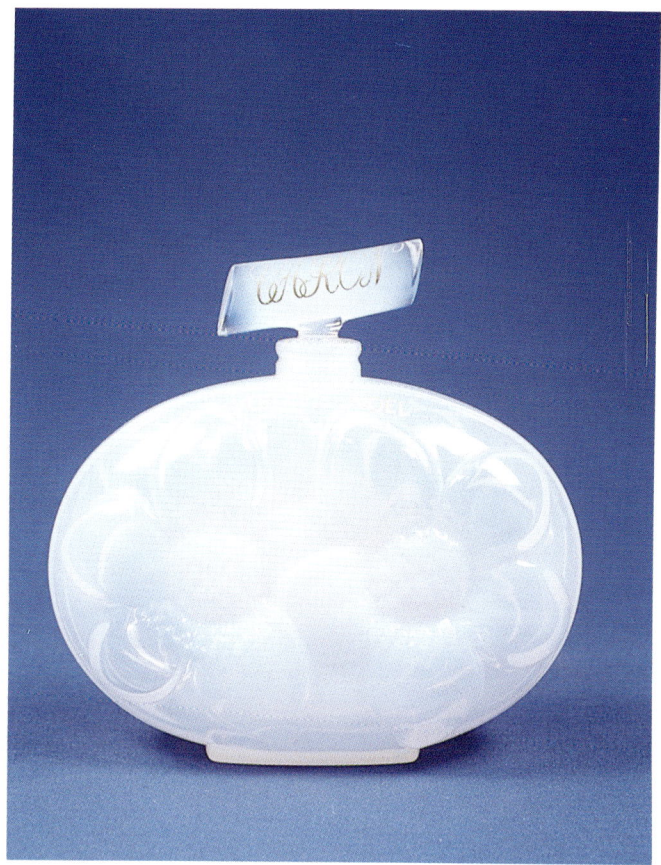

Lot #244. Caron *Voeu de Noel* ['Christmas Wish'] opalescent white glass bottle and stopper, 3.6" [9.1 cm], empty, the front molded with a pair of open flowers, the stopper as a small bar, name and company enameled in gold on front; circa late 1940's. Est. $600.00-$750.00.

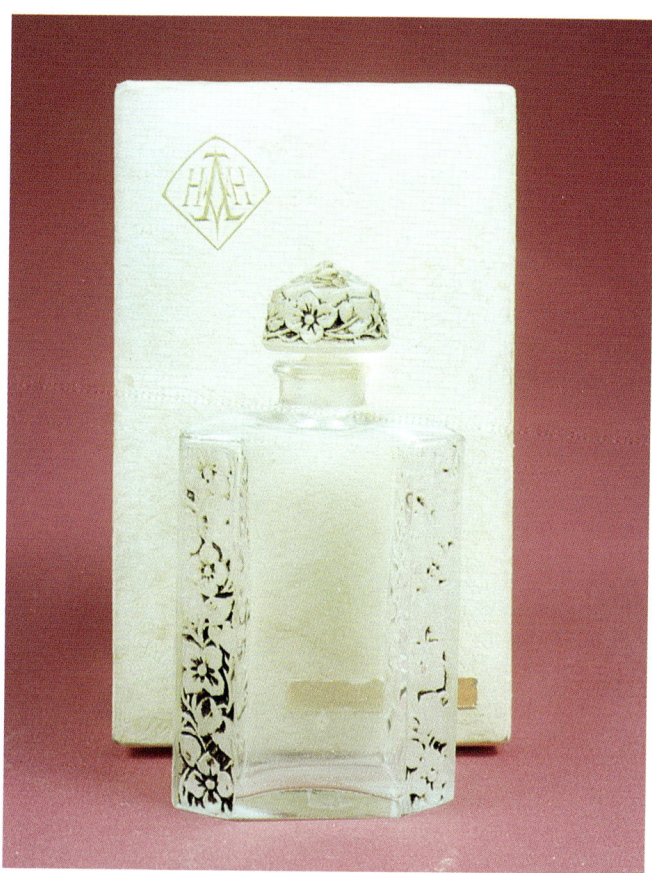

Lot #245. Harriet Hubbard Ayer *Lilas* fine quality clear glass bottle and stopper, 4.2" [10.7 cm], of rectangular form with panels of flowers molded and frosted on the sides and in a border on the stopper, the flowers heightened with brown patina, empty, bottom acid-etched *Made in France* in circle, in its cream-colored satin-lined box; circa 1934. Est. $600.00-$750.00.

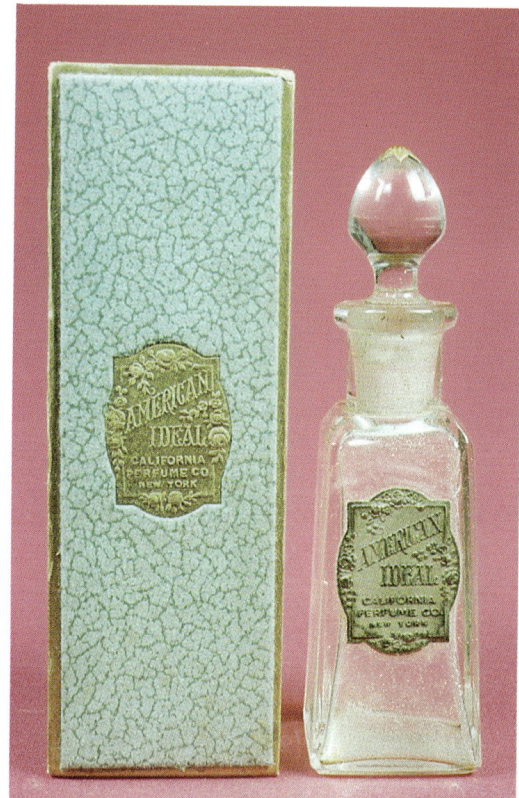

Lot #246. California Perfume Company *American Ideal* clear glass bottle and stopper, 4.5" [11.4 cm], the bottle with gently sloping sides, stopper with a gold enameled flower, empty, metallic label, in its green box also with a gold label; circa 1918. Est. $150.00-$250.00.

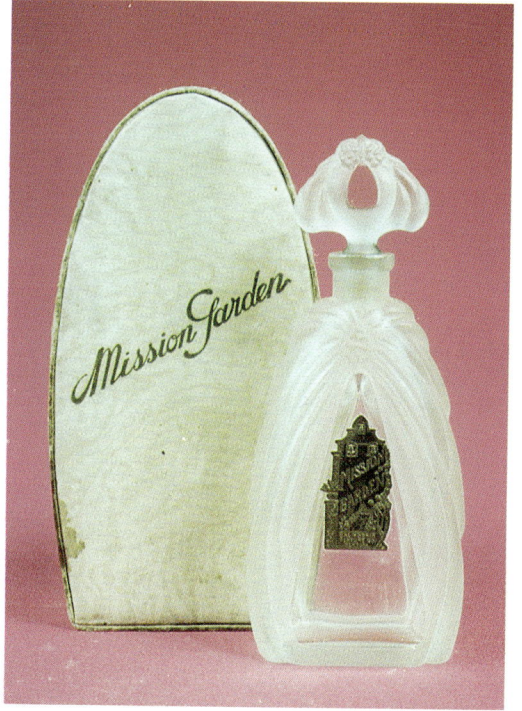

Lot #247. California Perfume Company *Mission Garden* clear and frosted glass bottle and stopper, 4.9" [12.4 cm], the bottle designed with a clear triangular window in the center surounded by berries and leaves in frosted glass, stopper of conforming design, empty, pretty gold label shaped as a California Mission, in its satin lined box, the glass probably of Bohemian manufacture; circa 1916. Est. $350.00-$450.00.

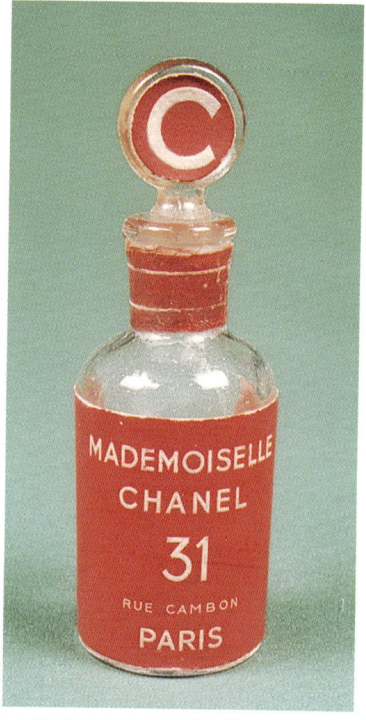

Lot #248. Mademoiselle Chanel *31* rare and important clear glass bottle and stopper of apothecary shape, 4" [10.2 cm], red and white label around most of bottle and neck, label states: *Mademoiselle Chanel, 31, rue Cambon*, label with *C* also on stopper, bottom molded with a star. Est. $400.00-$500.00.

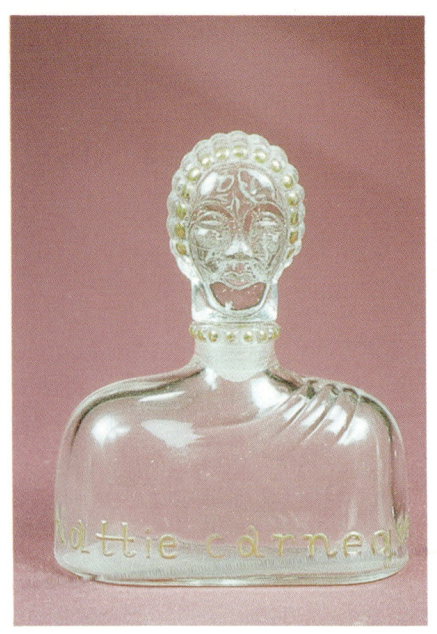

Lot #249. Hattie Carnegie large size clear glass bottle and stopper, 4.2" [10.7 cm], in the shape of a woman's head and shoulders in Art Deco style, name spelled out in raised letters at bottom, label lacking, empty. Est. $300.00-$450.00.

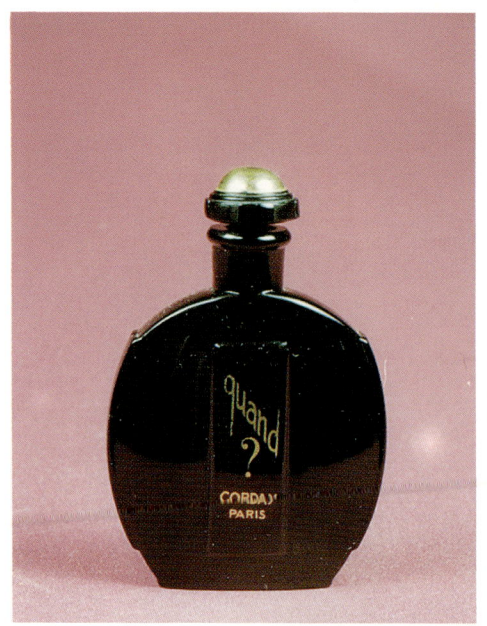

Lot #250. Corday *Quand?* ['When?'] black glass bottle and stopper, 3.4" [8.6 cm], of round form with a rectangular panel molded on the front, stopper enameled in gold, names also in gold on front, empty, bottom signed in acid *Made in France;* circa 1935. Est. $400.00-$500.00.

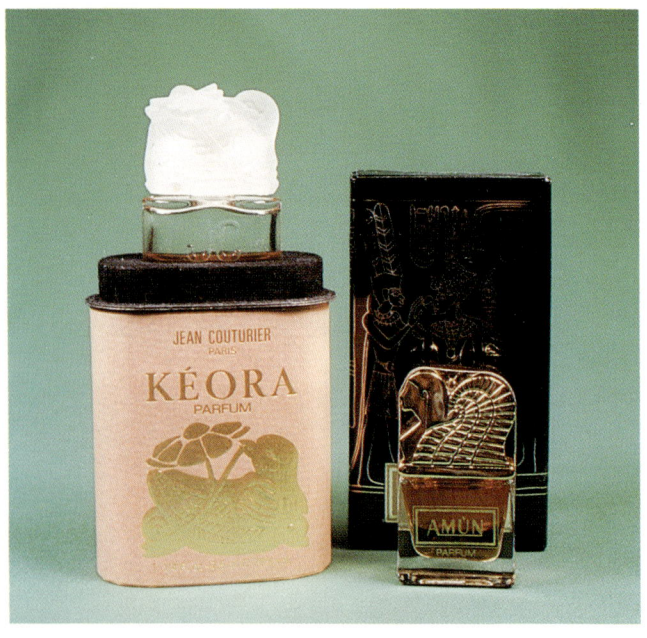

Lot #251. Jean Couturier *Kéora* clear glass bottle and frosted glass stopper, 2.2" [5.7 cm] the stopper with a bird and the Indian flower Kéora, some perfume, in its peach and gold box; Cantilène/Payot *Amün* clear glass bottle and gold metal overcap, 2.5" [6.4 cm], the stopper molded in the form of a Sphynx, full and sealed, in its black box with a picture taken from a trumpet found in Tutankhamen's tomb. Two items. Est. $100.00-$150.00.

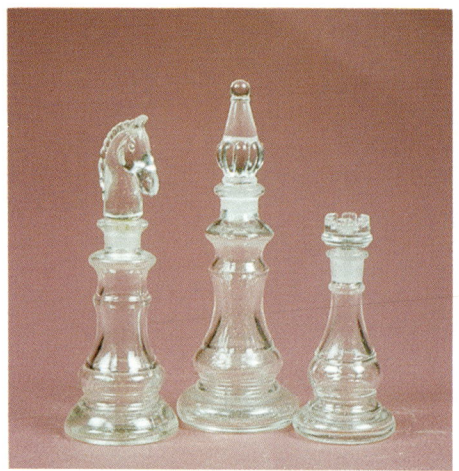

Lot #252. Mary Chess group of three clear glass figural bottles used for various scents, all empty and without decal labels: Knight 4.2" [10.7 cm]; King 4.6" [11.7 cm]; Rook 3" [7.6 cm]. Three bottles. Est. $75.00-$125.00.

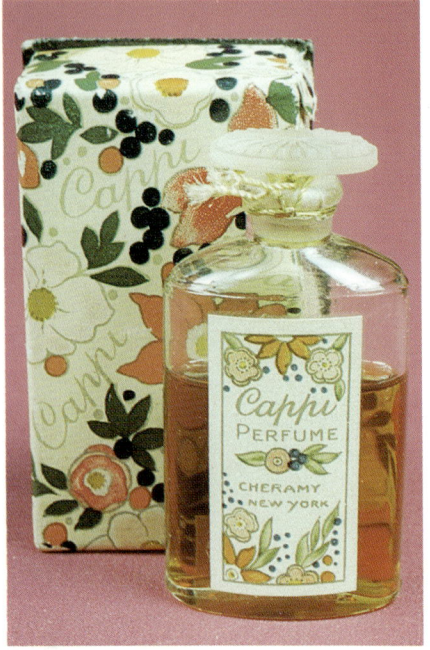

Lot #253. Cheramy *Cappi* clear glass bottle and frosted glass stopper, 2.6" [6.6 cm], of flask shape, the stopper molded as a flower, with perfume and sealed, pretty label on front, bottom molded *Cheramy,* in its colorful floral box. Est. $75.00-$125.00.

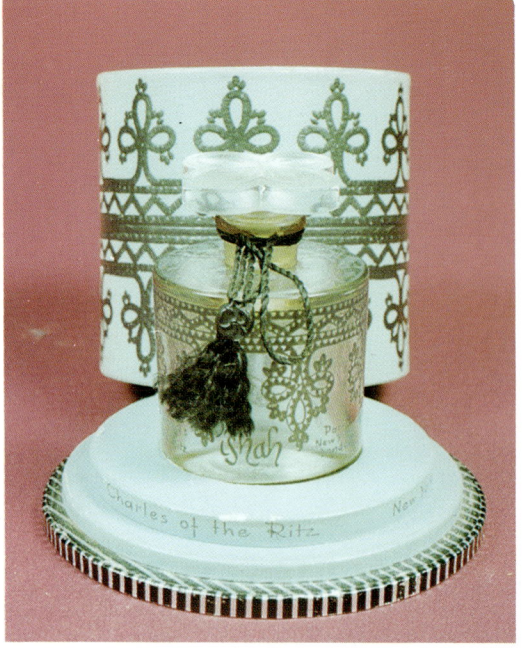

Lot #254. Charles of the Ritz *Ishah* clear glass bottle and frosted glass stopper, 2.2" [5.6 cm], the bottle of cylinder form and decorated with a lace design in black enamel, the stopper shaped as a stylized blossom, empty, in its aqua box also decorated with black lace, bottle signed *Made in France;* circa 1954. Est. $175.00-$250.00.

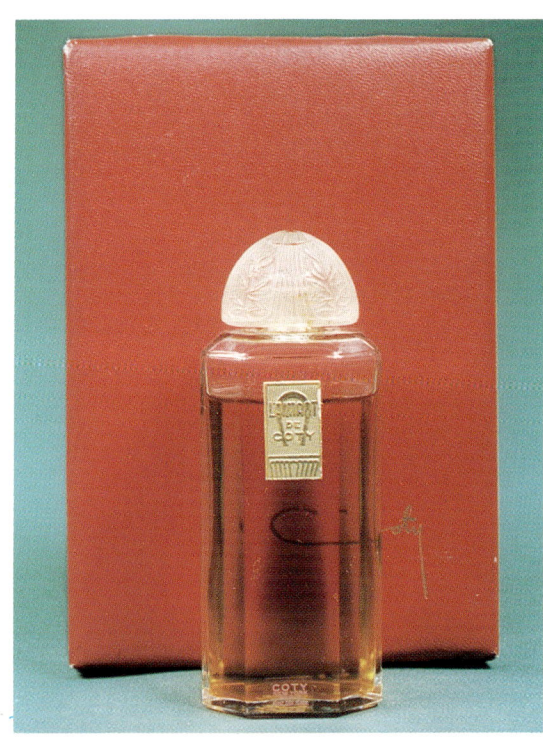

Lot #255. Coty *L'Aimant* ['The Magnet'] clear glass bottle and frosted glass stopper, the bottle in the shape of an elongated octagonal column, the stopper molded with leaves, near full, gold label, bottom signed *Coty*, in its satin lined red leatherette box. Est. $250.00-$300.00.

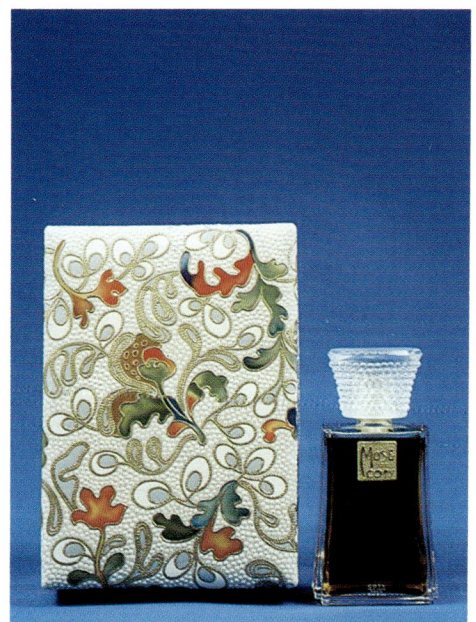

Lot #256. Coty *Muse* large size [2 oz.] clear glass bottle and inner stopper with frosted glass overcap, 4.1" [10.4 cm], full and sealed, gold label on front, in its satin lined box with a beautiful embossed gold Florentine exterior. Est. $200.00-$300.00.

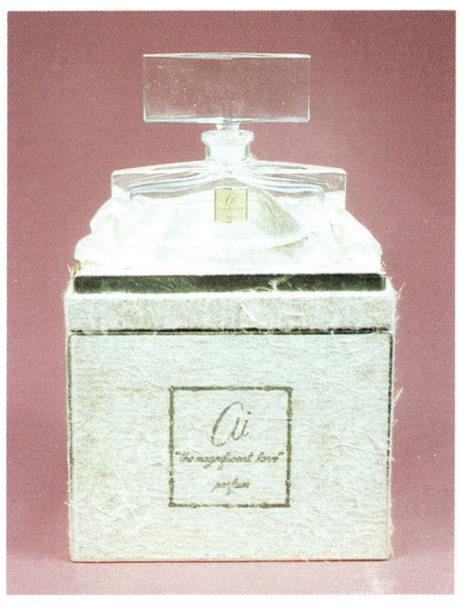

Lot #257. Cosmetic Chemicals Co. *Ai* [Hawaiian for "the magnificent love"] fine quality hand-cut clear crystal bottle and stopper, both of diamond shape, 4" [10.2 cm], empty, gold label on front, in its satin-lined box [with separate compartments for both bottle and stopper] covered with Hawaiian tapa paper; not pictured or referenced in existing publications. Est. $200.00-$300.00.

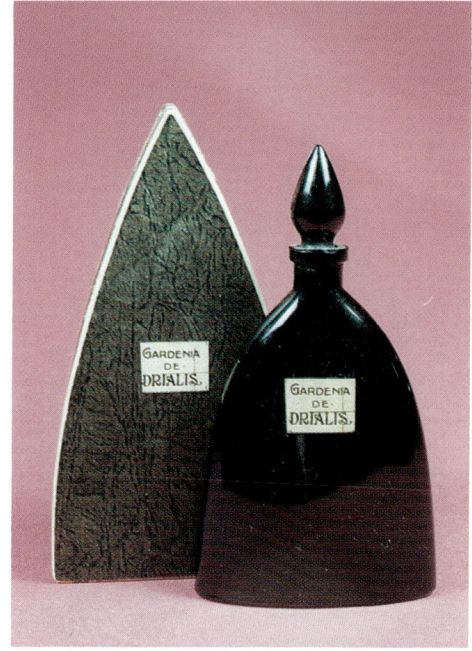

Lot #258. Drialis *Gardenia* black glass bottle and stopper, 4.8" [12.2 cm], the stopper of teardrop form, the bottle of similar shape but flat, empty, label on front, in its brown box also with a label on front. Est. $200.00-$300.00.

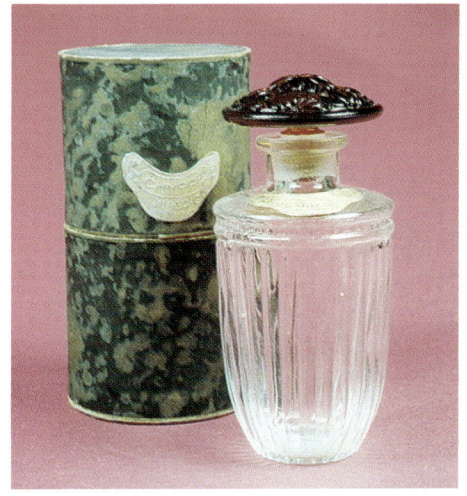

Lot #259. De Valois *Chypre* clear glass bottle and amber glass stopper, 4" [10.2 cm], the bottle molded all around with vertical ribs, the stopper molded with flowers in relief, empty, in its black and gold box. Est. $100.00-$150.00.

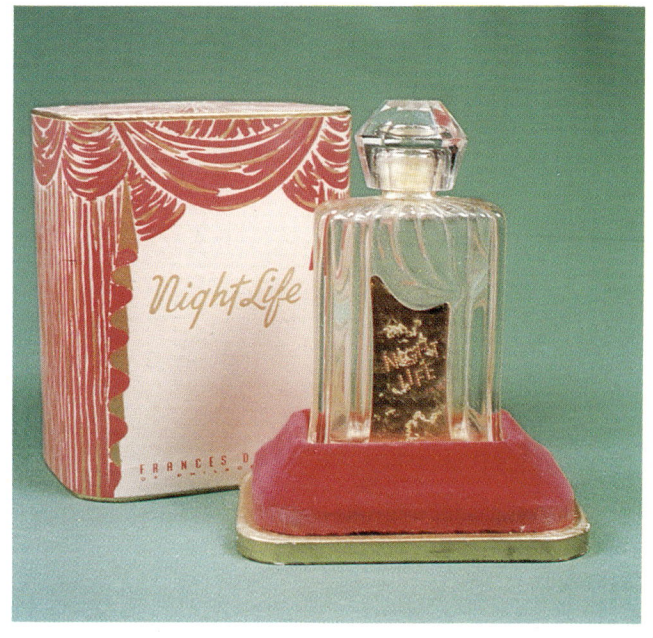

Lot #260. Frances Denney *Night Life* clear glass figural bottle and stopper, 3.5" [8.9 cm], the bottle shaped as a stage on which the curtain is rising, faceted stopper, empty, gold label which fits into the open part of the stage, in its beautiful pink and gold box also decorated as an open stage; circa 1940's. Est. $400.00-$500.00.

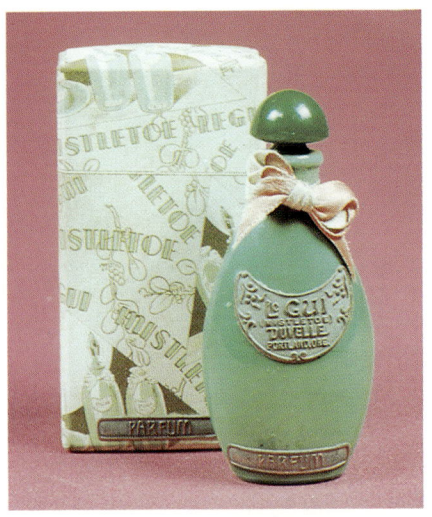

Lot #261. Duvelle *Le Gui* ['Mistletoe'] green glass bottle and stopper, 3.2" [8.1 cm], of teardrop shape with a button stopper, empty, pretty metallic labels on front of bottle which is also decorated with pink bows, in its box covered with a graphic of Duvelle perfumes. Est. $250.00-$300.00.

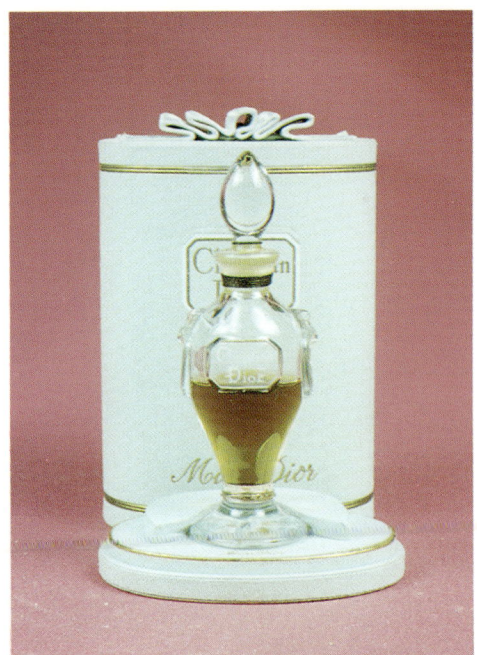

Lot #262. Christian Dior *Miss Dior* clear glass bottle and stopper, 3.7" [9.4 cm], the bottle shaped as an urn with two molded rings on either side, with some perfume and sealed, name in white enamel on front, in its gray box decorated with ribbon. This is the 1/4 oz. size. Est. $150.00-$250.00.

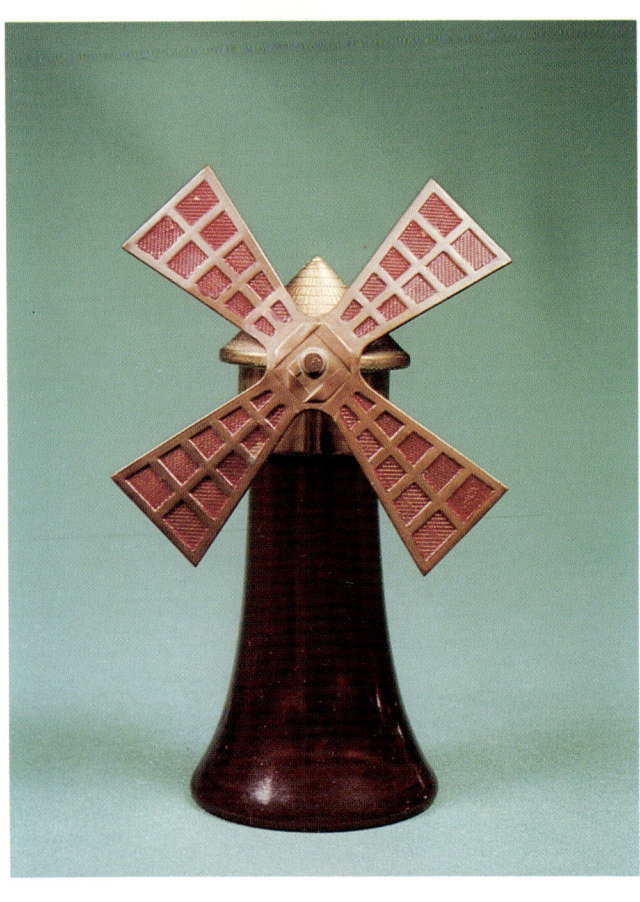

Lot #263. Deroc *Gai Monmartre* red glass bottle and clear glass inner stopper with a brass metal overcap in the shape of the Moulin Rouge ['Red Mill'], 5.5" [14 cm], the metal blades of the windmill decorated with red enamel and fully capable of turning; this bottle is circa 1925 and is very rare. Est. $800.00-$1,200.00.

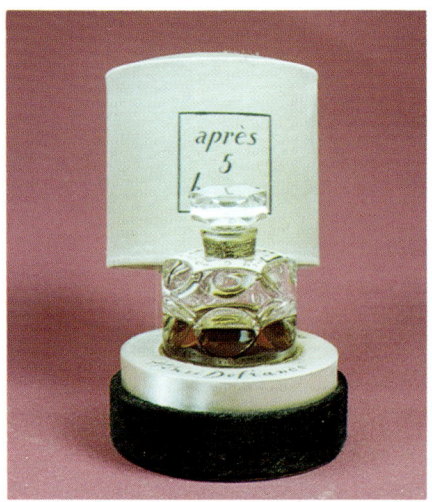

Lot #264. Henri Defrance *Après 5 Heures* ['After 5 O'Clock'] clear glass bottle and stopper, 2" [5.1 cm], the bottle designed with indented oval facets, with perfume, star-shaped label around shoulders of the bottle, in its cream satin and black velvet box. Est. $150.00-$200.00.

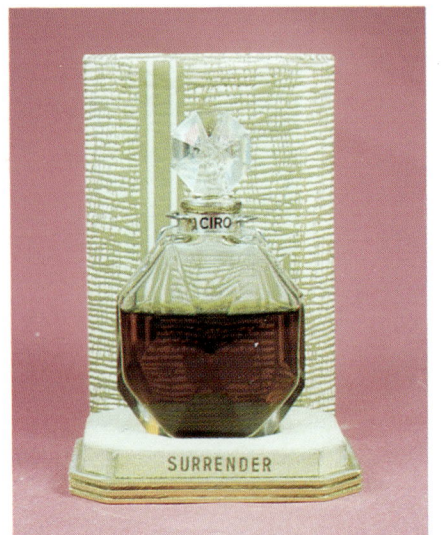

Lot #265. Ciro *Surrender* clear glass bottle and stopper, 4.1" [10.5 cm], designed to resemble a faceted gemstone, labels on the shoulders of the bottle, sealed, in its original beige and gold box. Est. $200.00-$275.00.

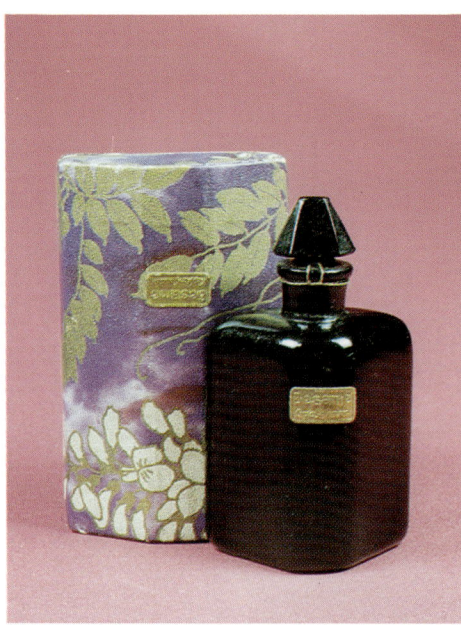

Lot #266. Crusellas *Besame* ['Kiss Me'] black glass bottle and stopper, 3.4" [8.6 cm], of unusual rounded triangular shape, sealed, gold label on front, in its beautiful purple box decorated with wisteria in gold, also with a gold label; uncatalogued in existing reference works. Est. $250.00-$300.00.

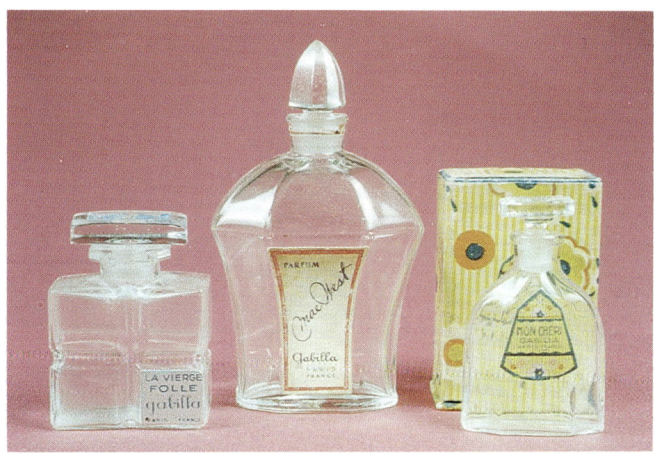

Lot #267. Gabilla *Mae West* rare clear glass bottle and stopper, 3.9" [9.9 cm], of basket shape, empty, with label; *La Vierge Folle* clear glass bottle and stopper, 2.1" [5.3 cm], silver label, empty, signed *Gabilla*; *Mon Chéri* clear glass bottle and stopper, 2.4" [6.1 cm], stopper molded *Gabilla*, empty, with label, in its colorful box. Three items. Est. $200.00-$300.00.

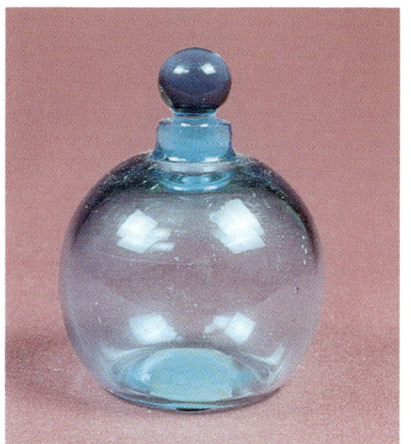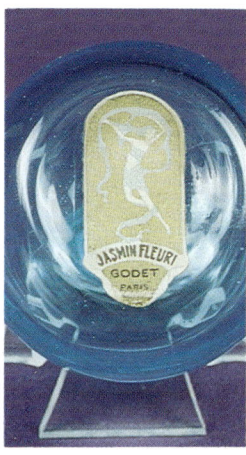

Lot #268 Godet *Jasmin Fleuri* ['Flowering Jasmin'] turquoise glass bottle and stopper of ball shape, 2.7" [6.9 cm], empty, beautiful turquoise and gold label on bottom; the lovely turquoise color of this bottle renders its simple shape a thing of beauty. Est. $100.00-$150.00.

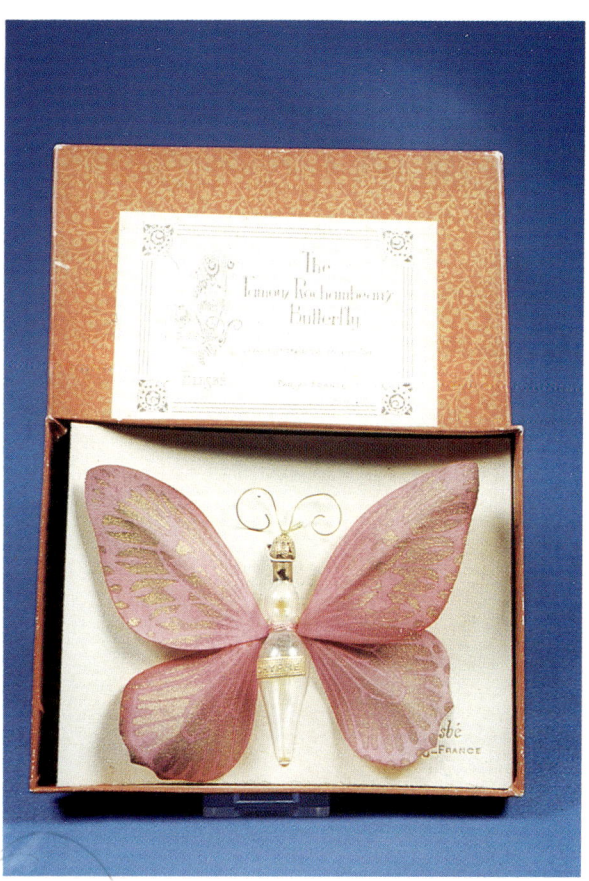

Lot #269. Elesbé - Rochambeau *Chypre* clear glass perfume vial with metal filagree cap in the shape of a butterfly's body, approximately 2.7" [6.8 cm], with crimson and gold fabric butterfly wings attached to the bottle, gold label, unused but evaporated, mounted on a card signed *Elesbé Paris*, in its red box marked *The Famous Rochambeau Butterfly*. Because of their fragility, the marvelous perfume presentations of Rochambeau are rarely seen today in excellent condition such as this. Est. $400.00-$600.00.

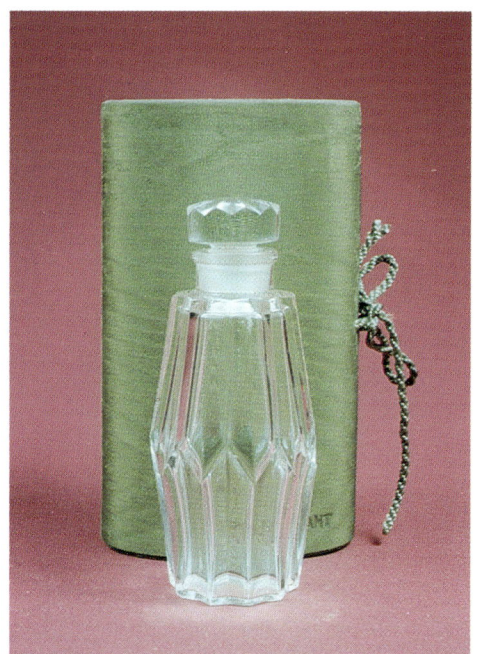 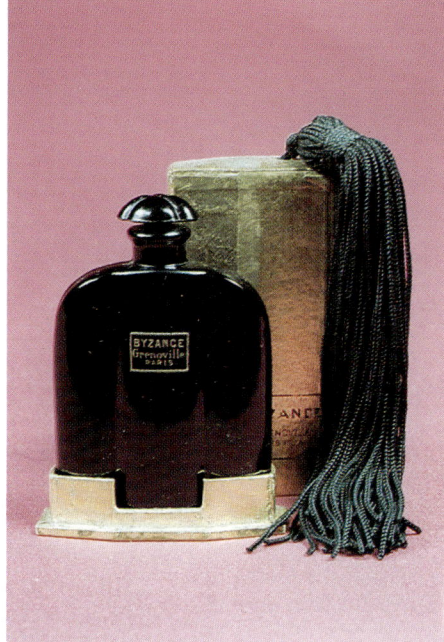 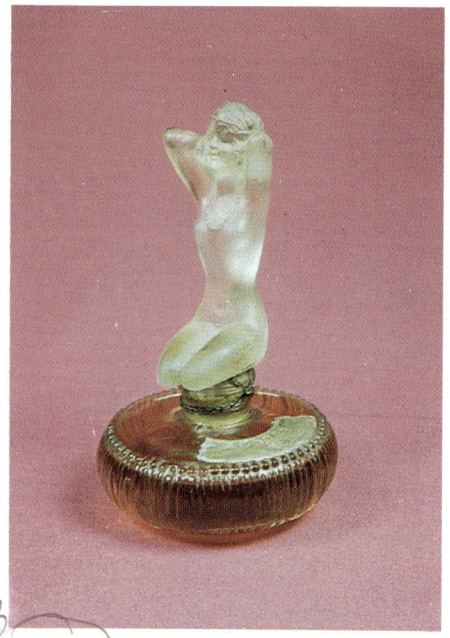

Lot #270. Houbigant *Présence* clear glass bottle and stopper, 4.1" [10.4 cm], the bottle designed with indented vertical pleats which intersect at the middle and create a zig-zag design, stopper with a conforming design, empty, in its green moiré box with rope ties, circa 1930's. Est. $250.00-$350.00.

Lot #271. Grenoville *Byzance* ['Byzantium'] black glass bottle and stopper, 2.4" [6.1 cm], of flask shape, empty, label on front, in a beautiful gold foil box with a black tassel, circa 1930's. Est. $200.00-$300.00.

Lot #272. Eroy *Adorée* clear glass bottle and frosted glass stopper, 4.2" [10.7 cm], the bottle shaped as a cushion, the stopper as a kneeling nude woman, with perfume and sealed, gold label; this figure is often thought of as Isadora Duncan. Est. $200.00-$250.00.

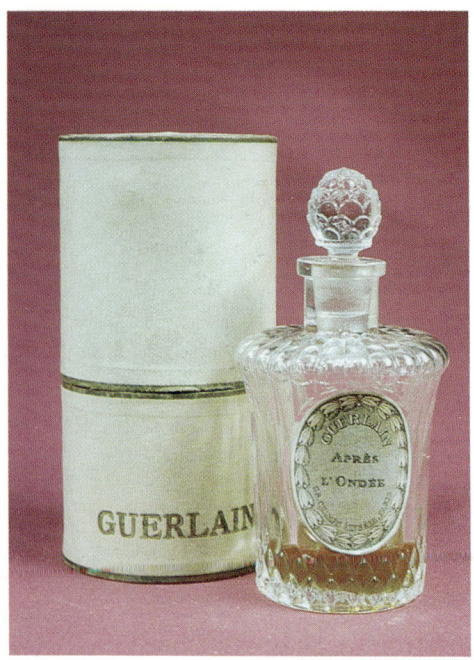
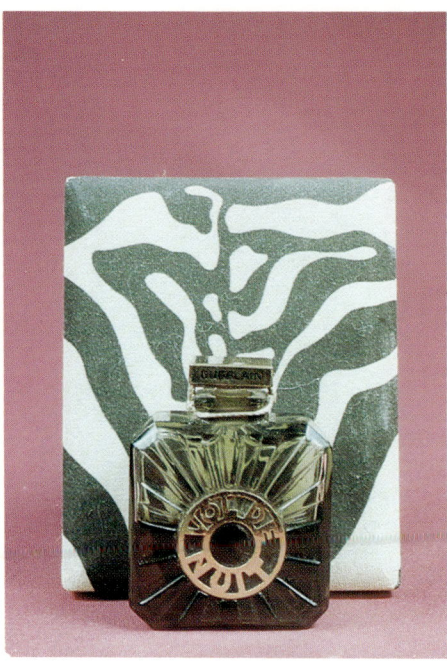
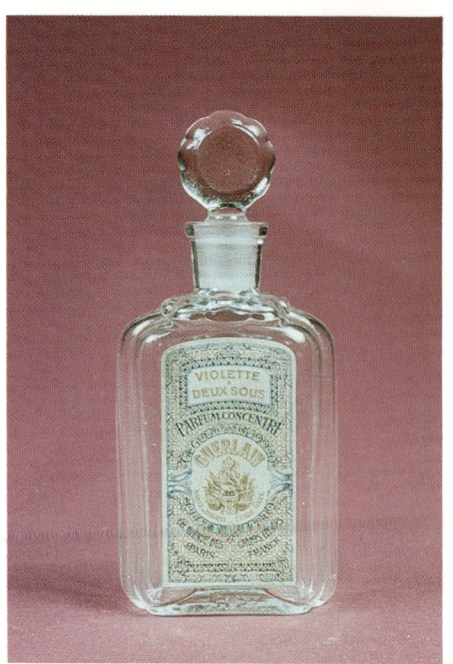

Lot #273. Guerlain *Après L'Ondée* ['After the Rain'] clear glass bottle and stopper, 4.5" [11.4 cm], the sides and shoulders of the bottle designed with rounded ribs, the stopper shaped as a pinecone, some perfume, oval label on front, in its original box. Est. $100.00-$150.00.

Lot #274. Guerlain *Vol de Nuit* ['Night Flight'] dark olive green glass bottle and stopper, 2.7" [6.8 cm], the brass-covered cap impressed *Guerlain,* the bottle molded with rays emanating from the central brass medallion, unopened with some perfume, in its zebra-motif box. Est. $200.00-$300.00.

Lot #275. Guerlain *Violette à Deux Sous* ['Violets for Tuppence'] rare clear glass bottle and stopper, 5.3" [13.5 cm], an early flask shape with rounded corners, beautiful old label on the front, molded *Guerlain Paris* on back with unusual flag display, bottom also signed *Guerlain Paris* in the mold, empty; circa 1910. Cf. *Guerlain*, p. 180. Est. $250.00-$400.00.

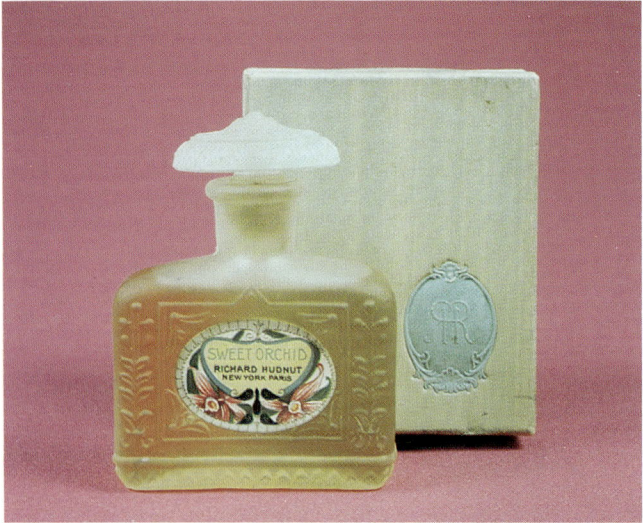

Lot #276. Richard Hudnut *Sweet Orchid* frosted glass bottle and stopper, 3" [7.8 cm], of rectangular form molded with leaves and an oval indentation at center, unused, colorful label, in its box with a blue medallion with the *RH* logo. Est. $100.00-$150.00.

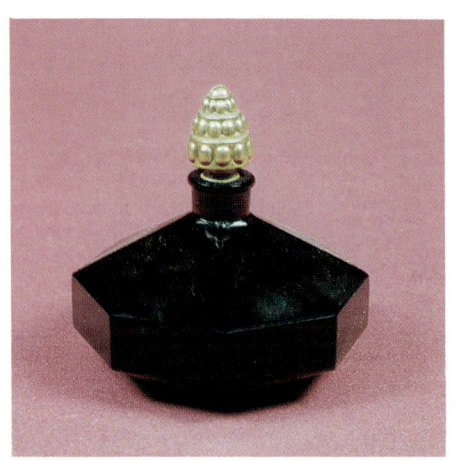

Lot #277. Richard Hudnut *Le Début Noir* black glass bottle and stopper, 2.5" [6.4 cm], a rather large size for this fragrance, of flat octagonal shape, the stopper molded with tiers of tiny cabochons and brilliantly gilded, empty, label lacking. Est. $400.00-$500.00.

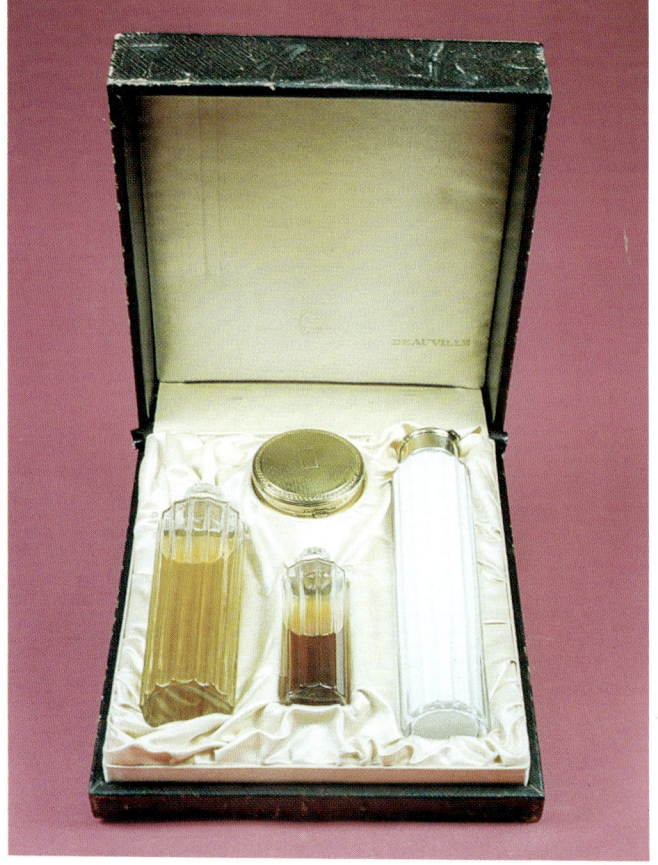

Lot #278. Richard Hudnut *Deauville* set of four items: clear glass bottle and stopper with scalloped sides for perfume, 3.3" [8.4 cm]; similar clear glass bottle for eau de toilette, 4.8" [12.2 cm]; similar clear glass bottle with brass cap for dusting powder, 6.4" [16.3 cm]; brass compact marked *Doublette;* the glass bottles acid-stamped with the *Hudnut* logo on the bottom and the names in gold enamel on top; all items in unused condition, in their black leather box with a *D* logo in gold. Est. $200.00-$300.00.

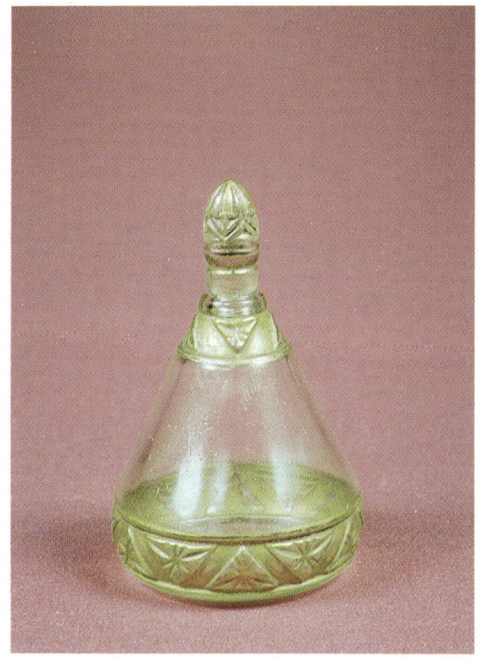

Lot #279. Richard Hudnut *La Rêverie* ['Daydream'] clear glass bottle and stopper, 2.7" [6.9 cm], of inverted cone shape, molded with a band of triangular motifs around the base and top of the bottle and enameled in gold, stopper of conforming design, empty, no label. Est. $250.00-$350.00.

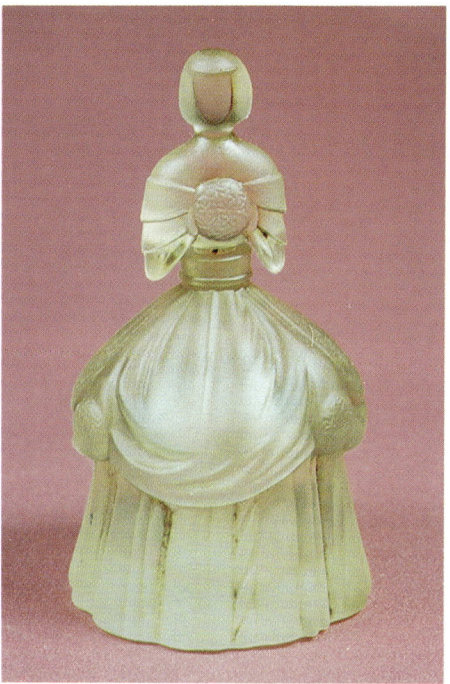

Lot #280. Eisenberg *847-A* frosted glass bottle and stopper, 3.5" [8.9 cm], in the shape of a lady in formal gown holding a bouquet of flowers at her bosom, empty, traces of brown patina, label on bottom; circa 1938. Est. $700.00-$850.00.

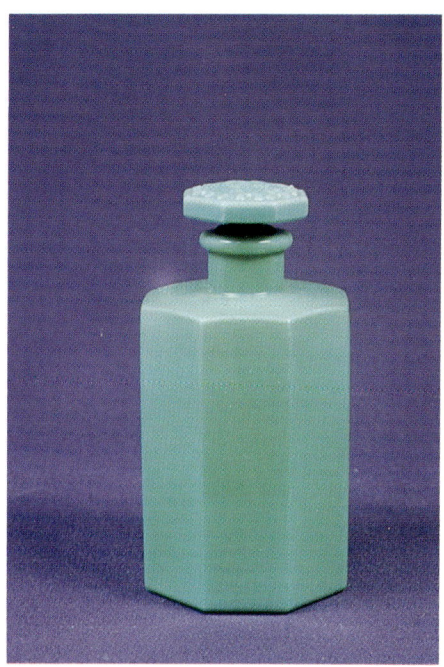

Lot #281. Langlois unidentified fragrance opaque green glass bottle and stopper, 3.1" [8 cm], in the shape of an octagonal column, stopper also octagonal and molded with mistletoe, empty, bottom signed *Langlois Made in France* in enamel. Est. $200.00-$275.00.

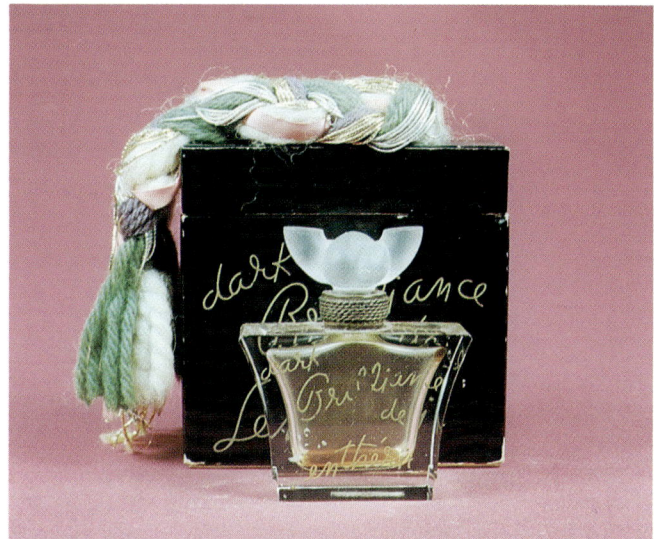

Lot #282. Lenthéric *Dark Brilliance*, clear glass bottle and frosted glass stopper, 3.1" [7.8 cm], base of heavy glass, names in gold enamel [some letters worn], stopper in the form of a knot of yarn, in its drop-front black box with a braid of multicolor yarn, empty. Est. $150.00-$225.00.

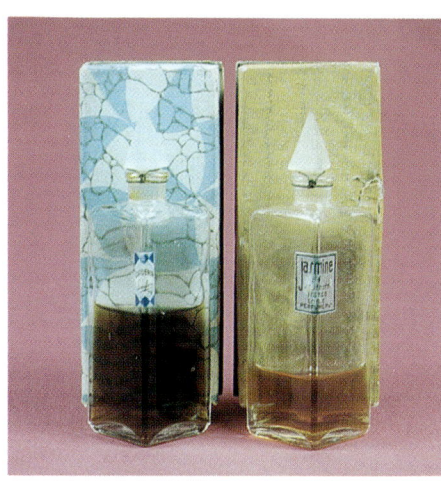

Lot #283. Langlois *Gardenia* clear glass bottle and frosted glass stopper, 4.6" [11.7 cm], of unusual triangular form, near full and sealed, blue label, in its blue box; Lorie Perfumers *Jasmine of Southern France*, identical bottle, silver label, sealed with some perfume, orange box [tear to box cover]. Two items. Est. $150.00-$225.00.

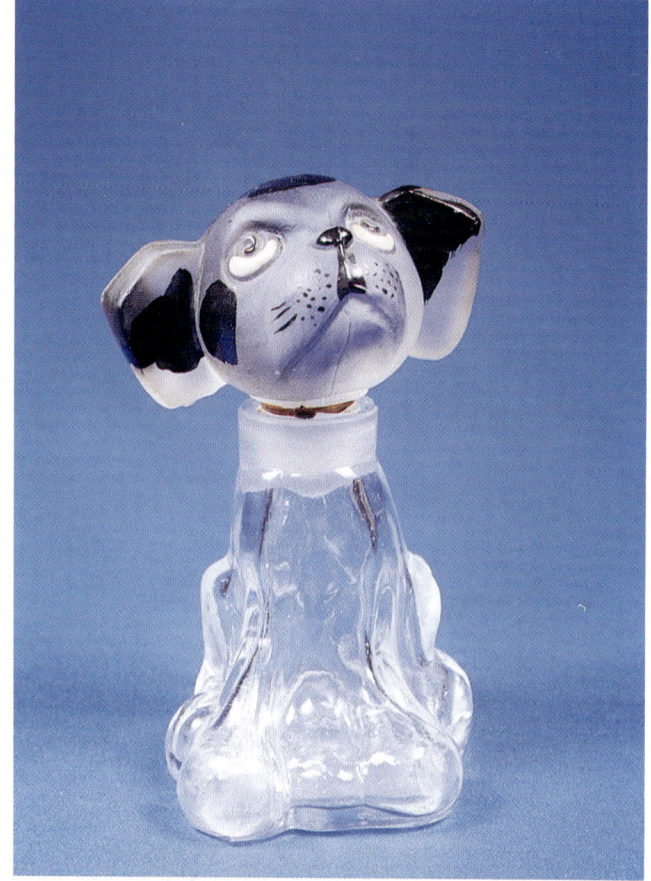

Lot #284. Jovoy *Allez...Hop!* ['Up We Go!'] clear glass perfume bottle and frosted glass stopper, 4.2" [10.7 cm], molded as a big puppy with very large paws, the stopper forming the puppy's head, enameled in black and white, small chip on the neck and on tongue of stopper, bottom signed *Jovoy Paris,* circa 1924. Jovoy later became Corday. Est. $600.00-$750.00.

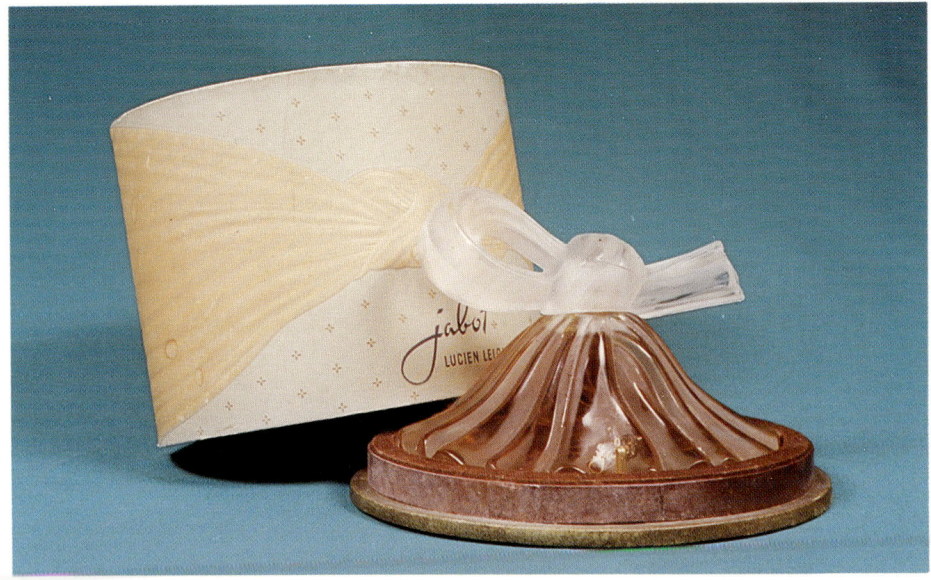

Lot #285. Lucien Lelong *Jabot* frosted glass bottle and stopper with overcap, 2.3" [5.8 cm], the entire bottle in the shape of an elaborate bow, inner stopper, decal label on front and on bottom, empty, in its seldom seen elegant hatbox. Est. $1,000.00-$1,250.00.

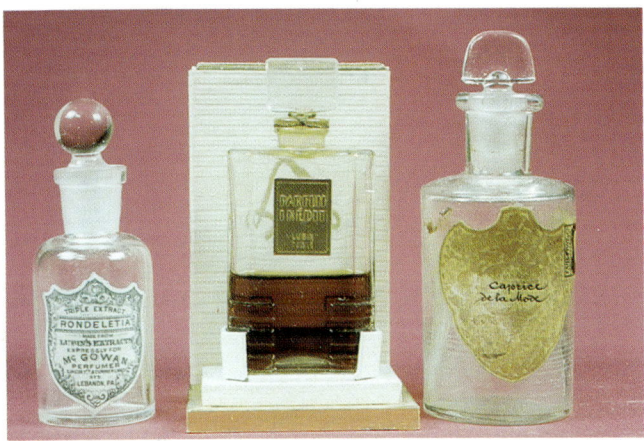

Lot #286. Lubin *Parfum Inédit* ['Unpublished Perfume'] clear glass bottle and stopper, 3.5" [8.9 cm], of rectangular form with molded geometric motifs, gold label in its white and gold box and outer box; *Caprice de la Mode* ['Fashion's Whim'] very old clear glass bottle and stopper, 4.5" [11.4 cm], of apothecary form, empty, label on front [stained] with additional label marked *Paul Prot Successeurs*, back of bottle molded *Lubin Parfumeur;* McGowan *Rondeletia* [made from Lubin's extracts], clear glass bottle and stopper, 3.6" [9.1 cm], shield label, empty. Three items. Est. $150.00-$250.00.

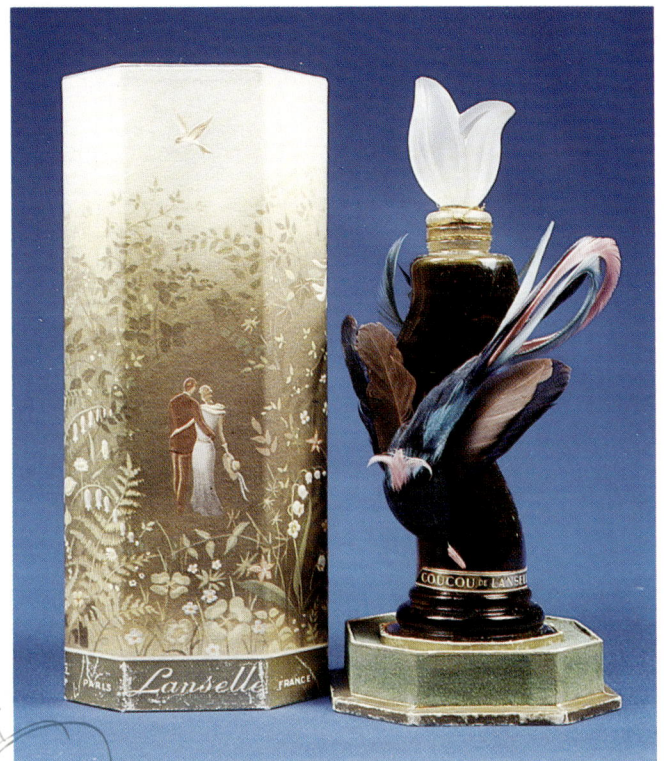

Lot #287. Lanselle *Coucou* clear glass bottle with frosted glass stopper, 7" [17.8 cm], the bottle shaped as an undulating column on an octagonal base, the stopper shaped as two leaves, full and sealed, gold label near base and decorated with a blue and pink cuckoo made of feathers, molded *Lanselle* on bottom, in a beautiful multicolored box signed F. Guerycolas which depicts two lovers walking deep into a lush garden. A rare and superb perfume presentation, circa 1940's. Est. $1,200.00-$1,500.00.

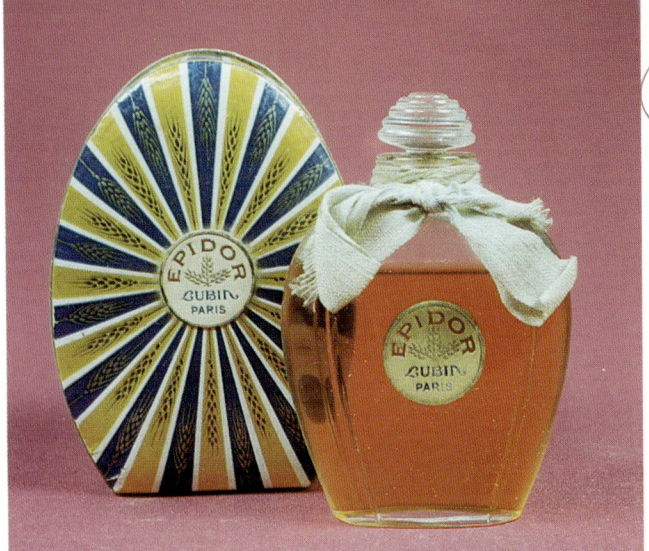

Lot #288. Lubin *Epidor* rare clear glass bottle and stopper, 3.2" [8.1 cm], the bottle of horseshoe shape with a button stopper, label on front, in its beautiful box of blue and yellow decorated with blades of wheat, empty, bottom signed in acid *Lubin Paris*. During the French Revolution, the months of the year were renamed; *Epidor*, based on *épi* ['blade of wheat'] was the new, revolutionary name for August. Est. $700.00-$850.00.

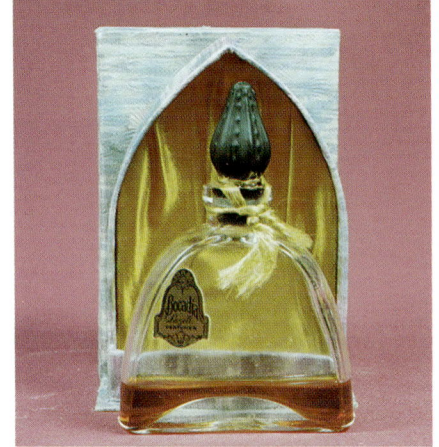

Lot #289. Lazell *Bocadia* clear glass bottle and stopper with black enamel, 3.9" [9.9 cm], unopened but with little perfume, gold label on front, in its colorful silk-lined box; circa 1920's. Est. $100.00-$150.00.

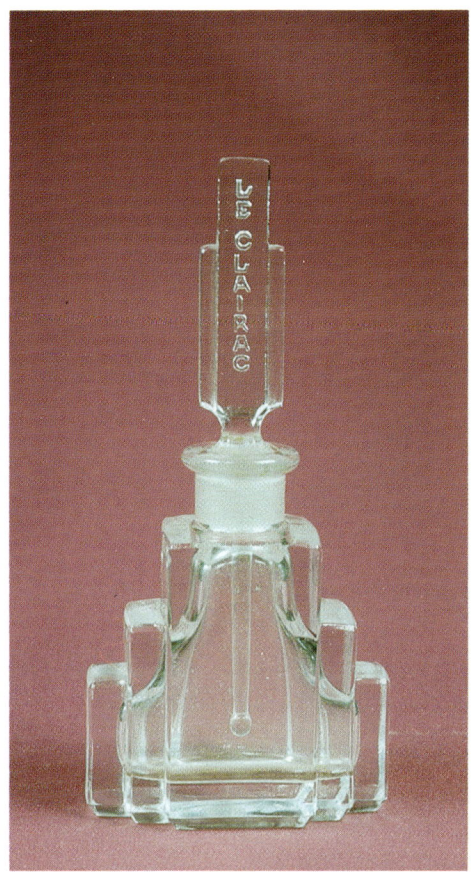

Lot #290. Le Clairac clear glass bottle and stopper, 5" [12.7 cm], in an Art Deco architectural design, name molded into the stopper, long dauber, empty. Est. $75.00-$100.00.

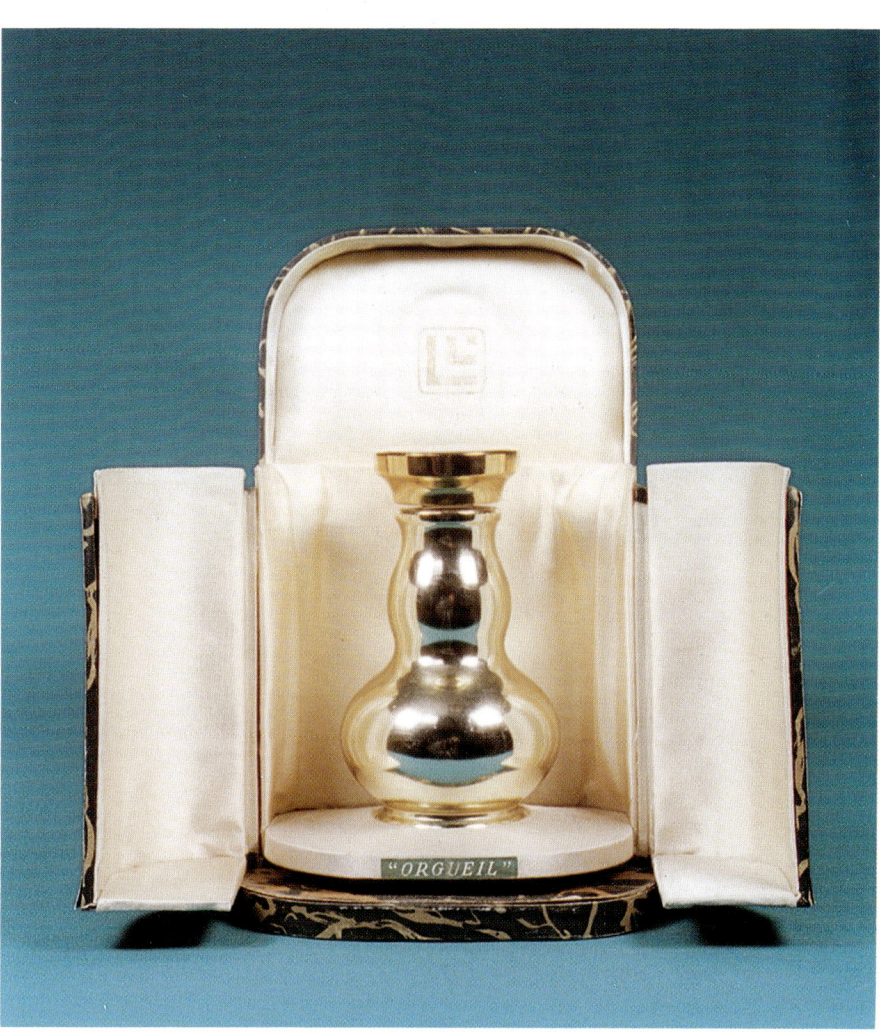

Lot #291. Lucien Lelong *Orgueil* ['Pride'] glass bottle and gold cap, 4.7" [11.9 cm], an interesting curvaceous shape somewhat resembling a chess piece, the entire bottle encased in gold [internal bruise to the glass invisible from the outside], empty, gold label on bottom, probably the largest size made for this bottle [label states 4 fl oz.], bottom marked *dummy*, in its box lined in white satin and covered with paper in *faux marbre*. Est. $500.00-$600.00.

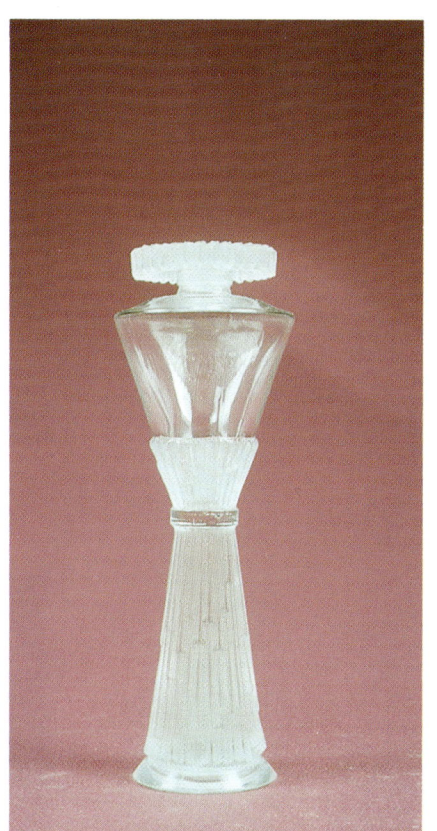

Lot #292. Lucien Lelong *Impromptu* large clear and frosted glass bottle in the shape of a futuristic tower, 6.5" [16.5 cm], no label, empty. Est. $200.00-$300.00.

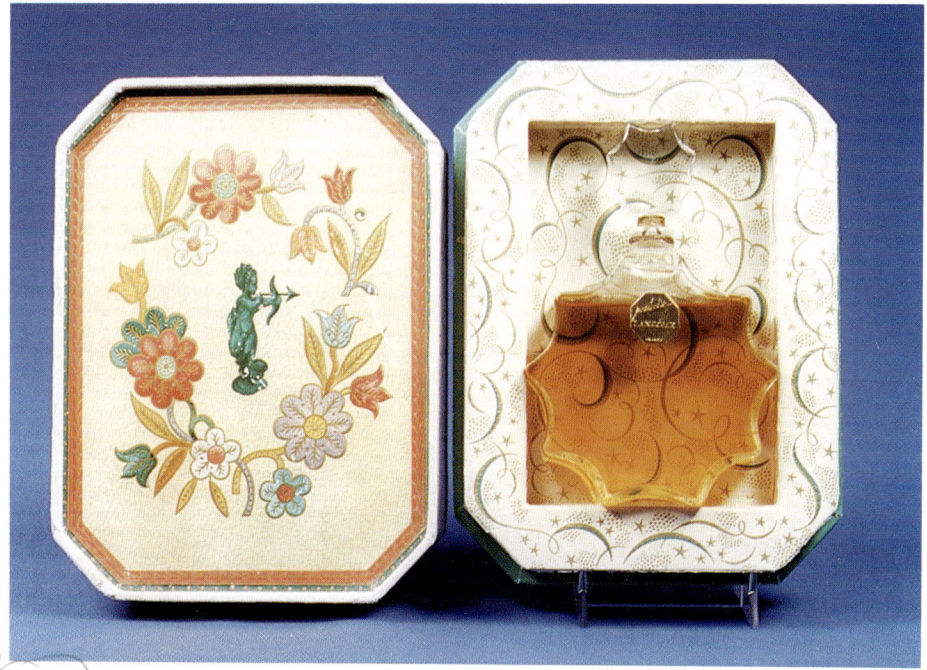

Lot #293. Lancôme *Peut-Etre* ['Perhaps' but translated in Lancôme publicity as 'Who Knows...'] clear glass bottle and stopper, 1.9" [4.8 cm], both bottle and stopper in a star shape with eight points, full and sealed, gold metallic label at center, in a beautiful box decorated with a 17th century Florentine motif and a cupid and printed by Draeger; this was designed by Jean Sala and produced as a limited edition in 1943, the very darkest year of World War II. Est. $1,200.00-$1,500.00.

Lot #294. Jeanne Lanvin large size black glass bottle and stopper, 4.3" [11.4 cm], ribbed stopper with gold enamel, the famous logo of the designer and her daughter on the front in gold enamel, signed *Jeanne Lanvin* in gold enamel below the logo, empty. Est. $250.00-$350.00.

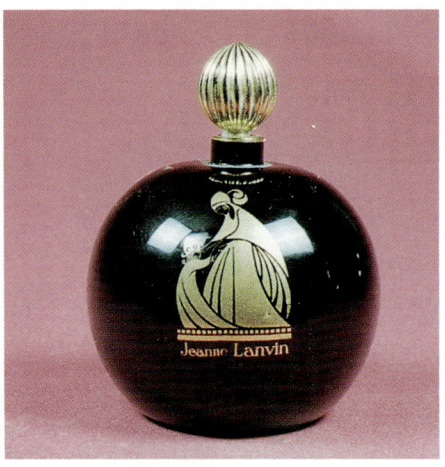

Lot #295. Mury *Caresse d'Amour* ['Love's Caress'] clear glass bottle and frosted glass stopper, 3.5" [8.9 cm], stopper molded with tiny flowers and with green patina, some perfume, gold label on center front, in its dark red box, circa 1917. Est. $300.00-$400.00.

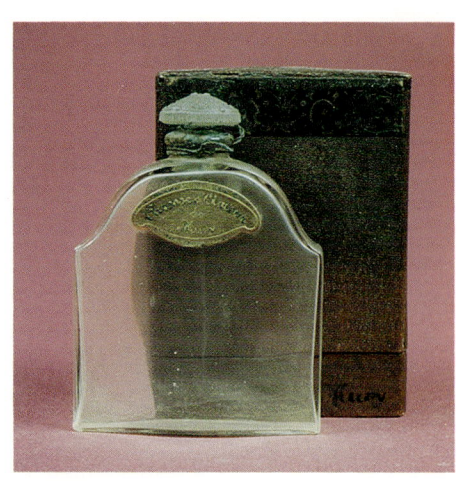

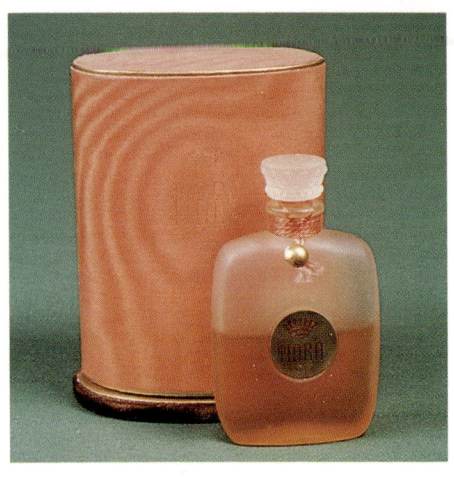

Lot #296. Alexandra de Markoff *Tiara* frosted glass bottle and stopper, 2.7" [6.9 cm], of flask shape with a circular indentation on both sides for the label, stopper shaped as a crown, full and sealed, gold labels front and back, in its coral moiré box signed on the front *Alexandra de Markoff*. Est. $150.00-$225.00.

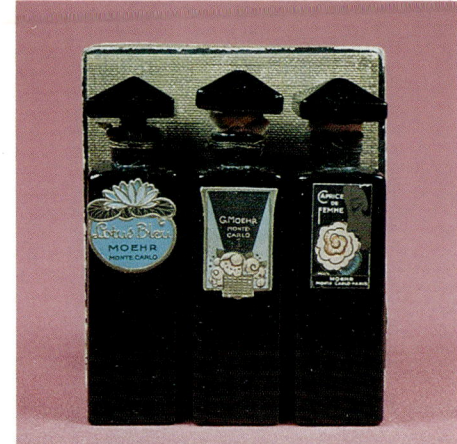

Lot #297. Moehr *L'Aimée* ['Beloved'], *Lotus Bleu*, *Caprice de Femme* set of three black glass bottles and stoppers, each 3.1" [7.9 cm], two opened and empty, one sealed, each with a beautiful graphic label, in their gold box [worn]. Est. $200.00-$275.00.

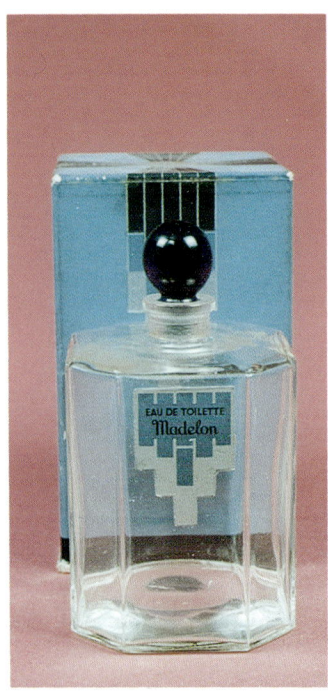
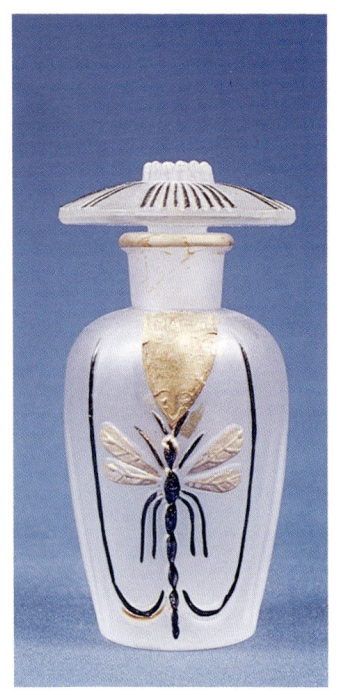
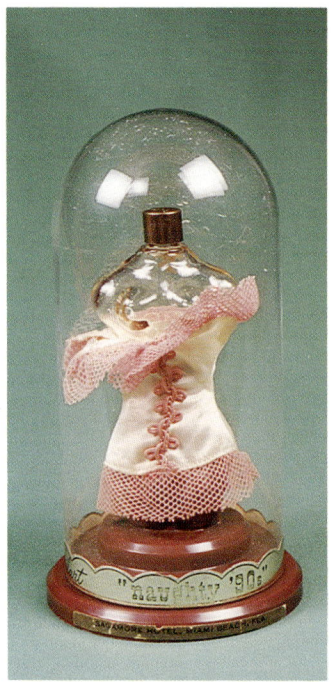
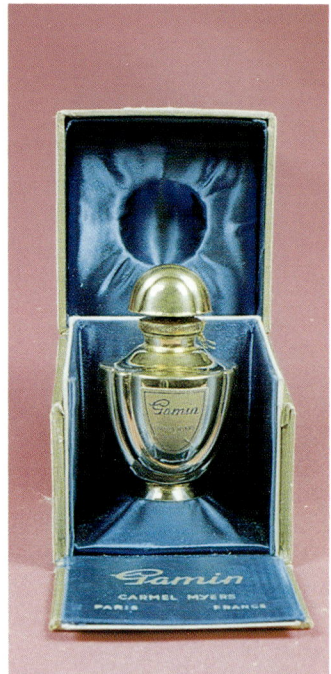

Lot #298. Madelon *Eau de Cologne* clear glass bottle and blue glass ball stopper, 4" [10.2 cm], the bottle of octagonal form, empty, interesting label in blue and silver with geometric motifs, in its box of conforming design [stain to box];not pictured or referenced in existing publications.. Est. $125.00-$200.00.

Lot #299. Marvo Beauty Laboratories [New York] unidentified fragrance, frosted glass bottle and stopper, 3.5" [8.9 cm], the bottle molded with a flying insect in relief on two sides, the stopper molded abstractly as a flower, the design highlighted with gold and black enamel, gold label on front, empty, maker of bottle unidentified. Est. $400.00-$500.00.

Lot #300. Milart *Naughty Nineties Perfume Fantasy* clear glass perfume bottle in the shape of a woman's figure with gold cap on a black plastic stand with glass dome, 5.5" [14 cm] with stand, dressed in a pink bustier, some perfume, decal label on bottle, gold label under plinth, around bottom marked *Sagamore Hotel, Miami Beach Florida*. Est. $125.00-$175.00.

Lot #301. Myers Carmel Myers *Gamin* ['Mischievous'] glass bottle and stopper encased in gold, 3" [7.8 cm], of urn shape decorated with a drapery motif, empty, gold label on front, in its drop-front box lined in blue satin whose exterior is also decorated with drapery motifs in gold. Est. $300.00-$400.00.

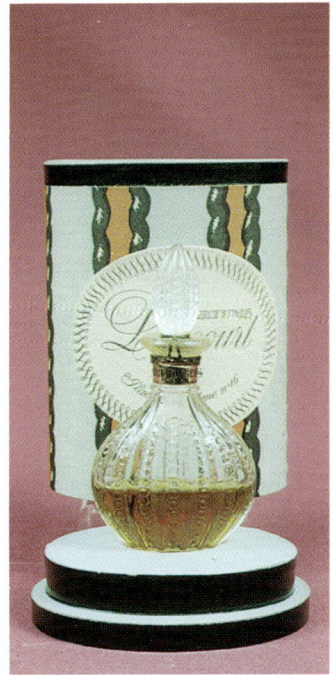
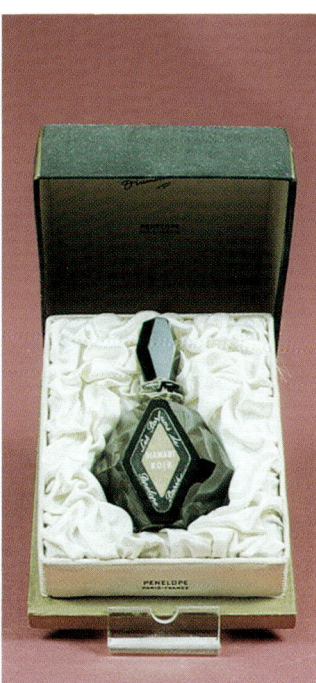
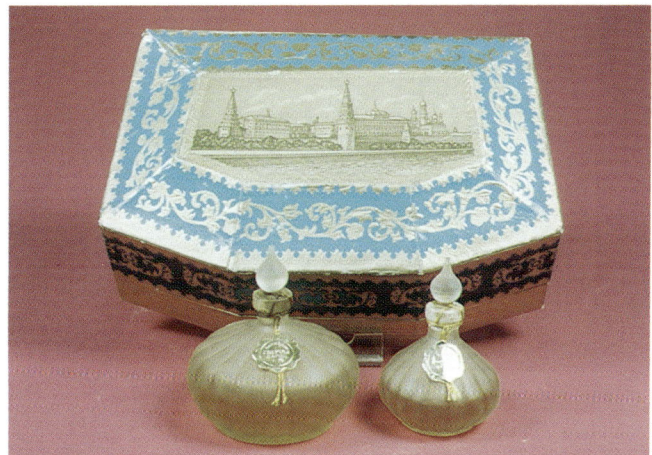

Lot #304. Nóvaya Zaryá ['New Dawn'] *Golubói Laryétz* ['Blue Treasure Chest'] pair of frosted glass bottles and stoppers, 3.3" and 3.1" [8.5 and 8 cm], in the shape of an onion dome seen in Kremlin architecture, both full and sealed, gold labels, in their blue and gold box decorated with a panoramic scene of the Moscow Kremlin; of Russian manufacture during the Soviet era. Est. $350.00-$450.00.

Lot #302. Lincourt [Place Vendôme #16] *Pour Toi Seul* ['For Thee Alone'] clear glass bottle and stopper, 3.4" [8.6 cm], the oval bottle molded with vertical strands of beads, half-full and sealed, gold label around neck, in its pretty oval boxl circa 1945. Est. $150.00-$250.00.

Lot #303. Penelope *Diamant Noir* ['Black Diamond'] black glass bottle and stopper, 3.2" [8.1 cm], both bottle and stopper designed with diamond-shaped facets, full and sealed, in its satin-lined black case; unreferenced in existing literature. Est. $200.00-$300.00.

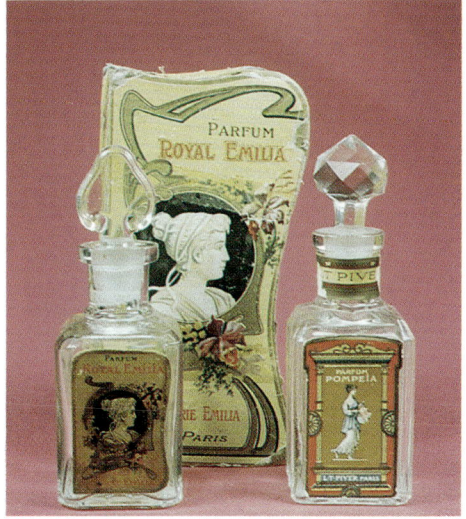

Lot #305. Parfumerie Emelia *Parfum Emelia* clear glass bottle and stopper, 4.5" [11.4 cm], decanter form, empty, label on front, in its colorful but very worn and fragile box in the Art Nouveau style; L. T. Piver *Pompeia* clear glass bottle and stopper, 4.6" [11.7 cm], empty, label with a classical maiden holding flowers. Two items. Est. $150.00-$250.00.

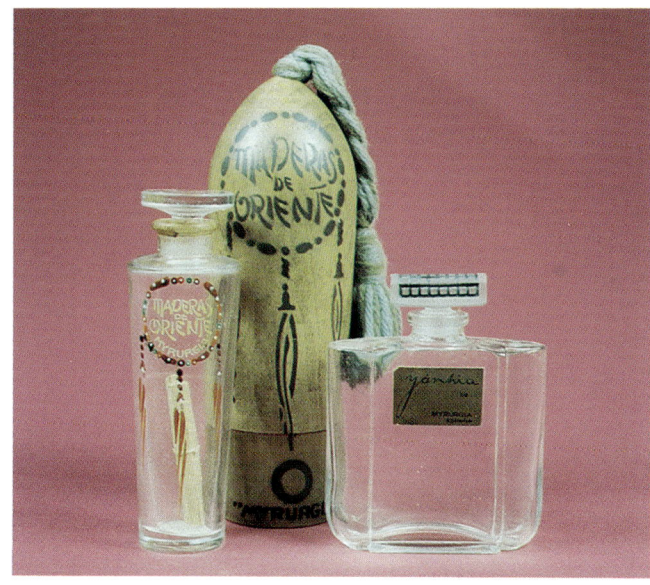

Lot #306. Myrurgia *Maderas de Oriente* ['Oriental Wood'] clear glass bottle and stopper, 4.4" [11.2 cm], of cylinder shape, names and decoration in red and green enamel, empty but with a tiny bundle of scented wood inside the bottle, in its wooden box marked with the names burned into the wood and decorated with a green wool braid; *Yánhia* rare clear glass bottle with frosted stopper, 3.4" [8.6 cm], the stopper molded with squares and the recesses enameled in black, empty, gold label, bottom signed *Myrurgia*. Two items. Est. $250.00-$350.00.

Lot #307. Princess Pat Ltd. *Princess Pat* black glass bottle and button stopper, 3.4" [8.6 cm], rectangular shape, stopper molded with tiny flowers, empty, pretty label on front, in its very lovely green and red box lined with red and yellow silk. Est. $300.00-$375.00.

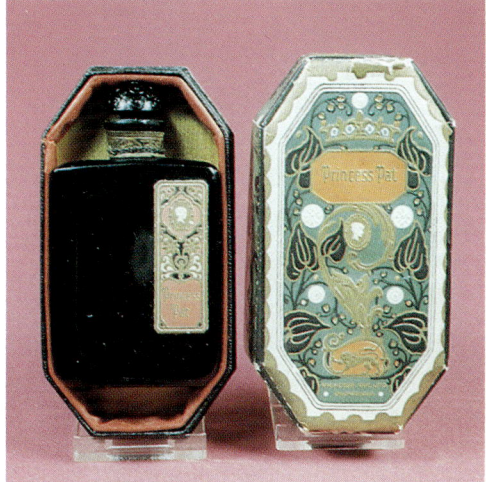
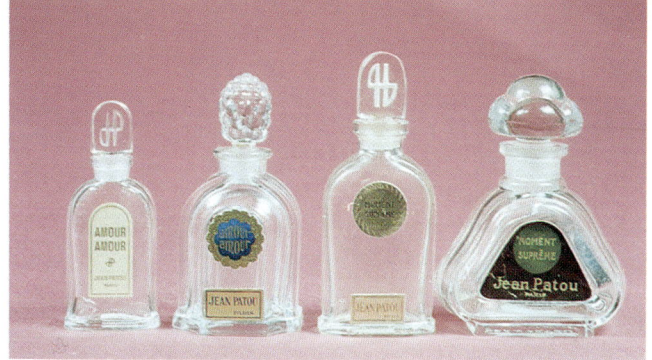

Lot #308. Jean Patou *Amour Amour* clear glass bottle and 'berry' stopper, 3.5" [8.9 cm], empty, gold labels on front; *Amour Amour* clear glass bottle and stopper, 3.1" [7.9 cm], empty, gold label, *JP* logo on stopper; *Moment Suprême* clear glass bottle and stopper, 3.9" [9.9 cm], empty, gold label, *JP* logo on stopper; *Moment Suprême* clear glass bottle and stopper, 3.5" [8.9 cm], empty, brown label, bottom signed *Jean Patou*. Four items. Est. $150.00-$250.00.

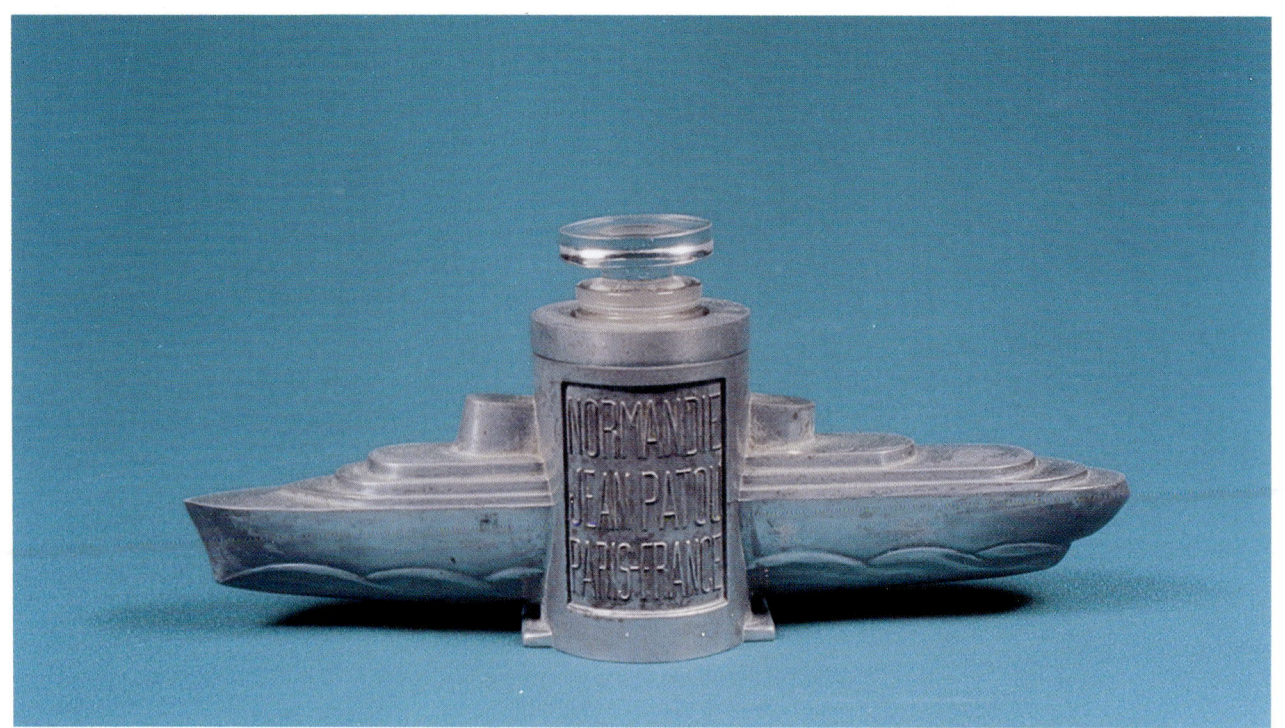

Lot #309. Jean Patou *Normandie* unusual and rare clear glass bottle and stopper with long dauber, set into a metal base [whose cap can be unscrewed] in the form of the liner Normandie, total height 3" [7.6 cm], empty, *Normandie Jean Patou Paris France* molded on front of ship, the bottle itself signed *Jean Patou*; circa 1935. Est. $1,750.00-$2,250.00.

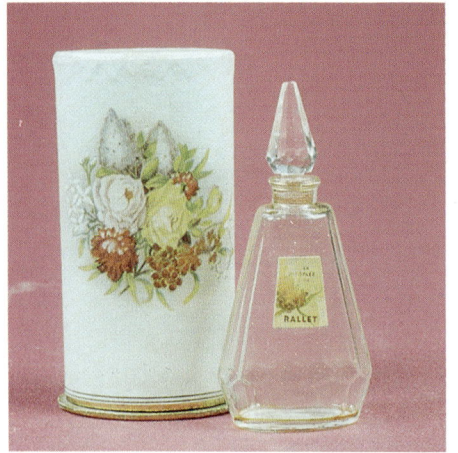

Lot #310. Rallet *La Giroflée de Rallet* ['The Wallflower of Rallet'] clear glass bottle and stopper, 3" [7.6 cm], both bottle and stopper molded with vertical facets, empty, pretty label on front and in its box decorated with roses and lilacs. Est. $100.00-$150.00.

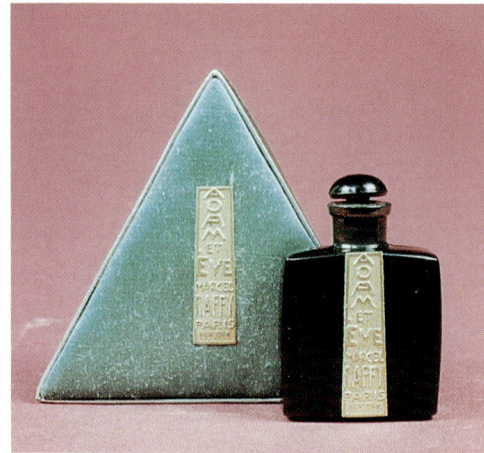

Lot #311. Raffy *Adam et Ève* black glass bottle and stopper, 2.5" [6.4 cm], of rectangular shape with a long label shaped as an Egyptian cartouche, in its triangular box covered in turquoise silk with an identical gold label; circa 1925. Est. $500.00-$600.00.

Lot #312. Pinaud *Scarlett* clear glass bottle with white cap and gold plastic overcap, 7" [17.8 cm], the bottle molded as the pleats of the woman's skirt, the overcap as her upper body, empty, bottom signed *Pinaud* in the mold; this is circa 1937, and refers to Scarlett O'Hara in *Gone with the Wind;* circa 1938. Est. $75.00-$125.00.

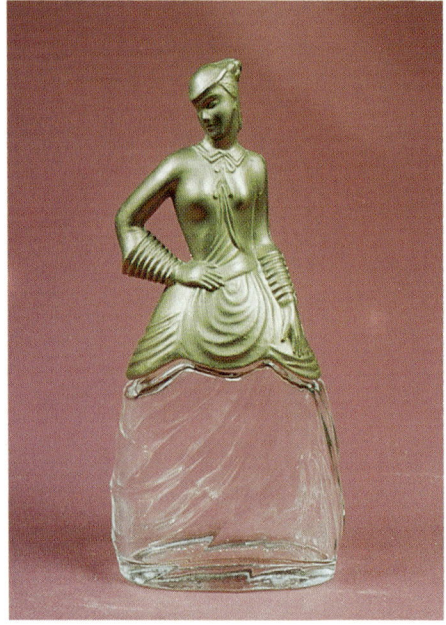

Lot #313. Raffy *Parfum Riche* frosted glass bottle and stopper, 3" [7.6 cm], the bottle of unusual shape with three sides resembling butterfly wings, the stopper molded with the words *Petals of Brittany*, in its triagular box [exterior stain] with silver label; not referenced in existing literature. Est. $450.00-$600.00.

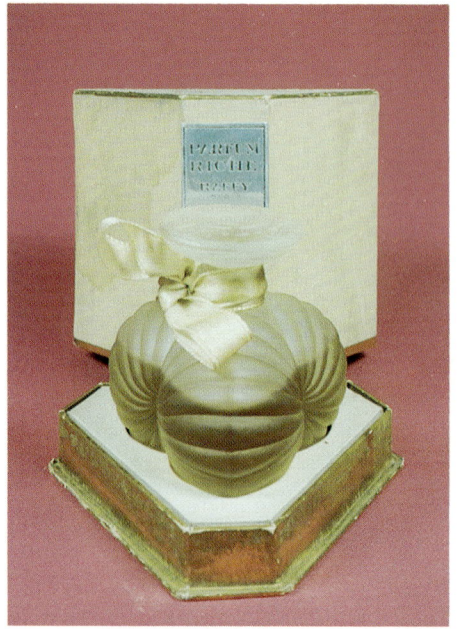

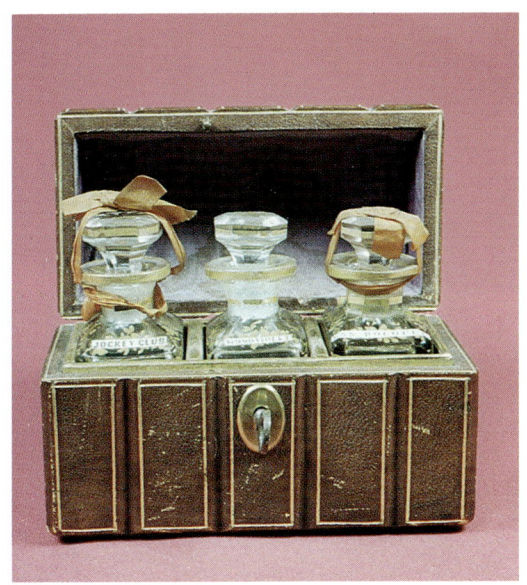
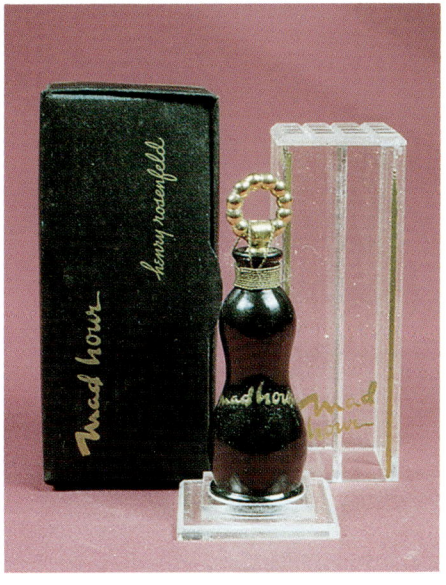
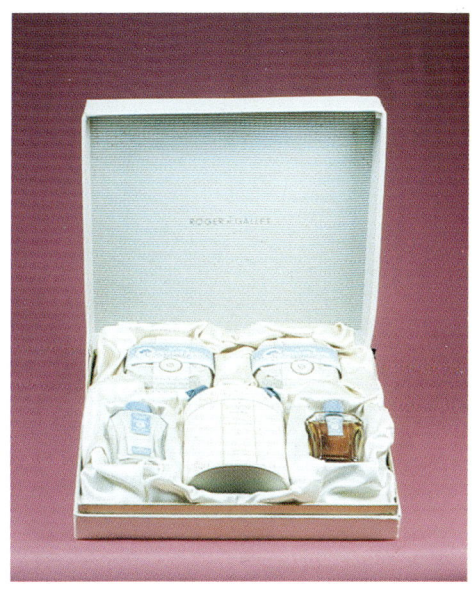

Lot #314. Rimmel *Essence Bouquet, Jockey Club, Wood Violet*, clear glass bottles and stoppers of rectangular form, each 3" [7.6 cm], the shoulders and stoppers of each bottle decorated with floral motifs in gold, labels on side, two empty, one unopened, in their red leather humpback trunk tooled in gold. Est. $250.00-$350.00.

Lot #315. Henry Rosenfeld *Mad Hour* black enameled glass bottle and gold enameled stopper, 3.5" [9 cm], the bottle shaped like an hourglass, the stopper as a loop of rope, full and sealed, name in gold enamel on front, gold label on bottom, mounted on a plinth in a lucite box, in its black box; circa 1950. Est. $100.00-$175.00.

Lot #316. Roger & Gallet *Oeillet Bleu* ['Blue Carnation'] set of two round soaps, *Aftabath Powder, Dry Perfume* and *Eau de Cologne* in clear glass bottles with blue caps, all in superb, unused condition, in a cream colored box lined with satin. Est. $100.00-$125.00.

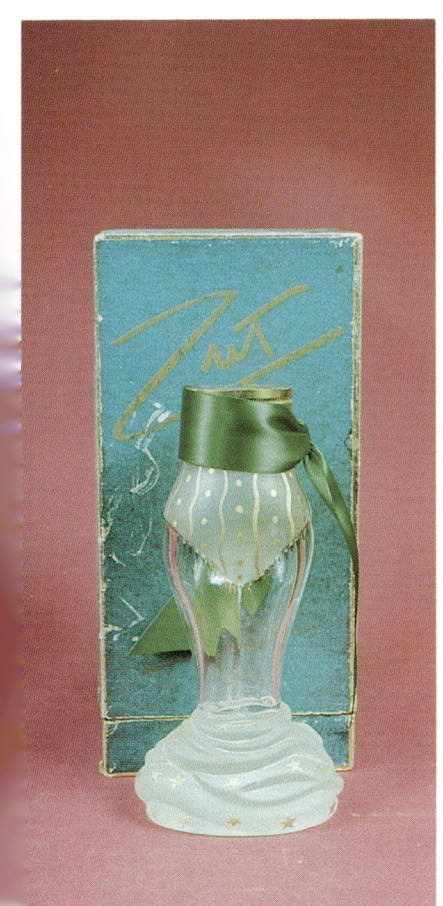
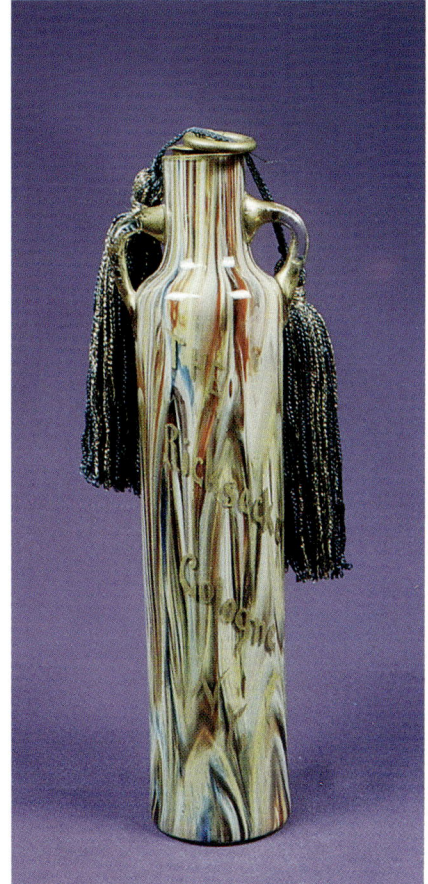
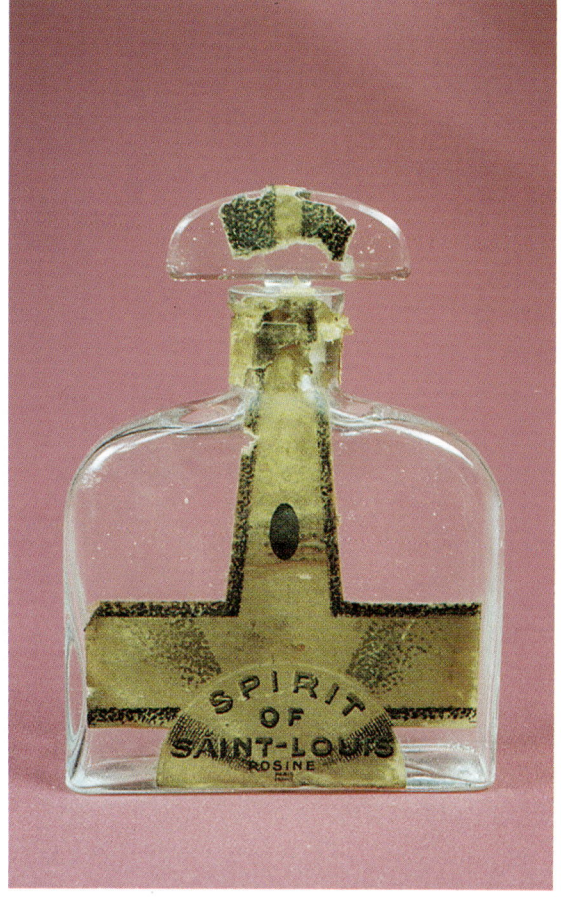

Lot #317. Schiaparelli *Zut* ['Damn!!'] large size glass bottle and stopper in the shape of a woman's torso from the waist downward 5.6" [14.2 cm], panties and base frosted, detail enameled in gold, gold enameled stopper, waist tied with green ribbon, empty, in its seldom seen green box lined with violet silk [material faded, box with some scratches], bottom signed *Schiaparelli Paris*. Est. $800.00-$950.00.

Lot #318. Ricksecker *The Ricksecker Cologne* rare and unusual cased glass bottle, 8.5" [21.6 cm], the inner layer of glass marbelized with green, red, blue, and white, two applied glass handles at the top and partially gilded, name in gold enamel on front, with a metal and cork cap [with tassels] signed *Ricksecker Perfumer New York*. The glass is of American manufacture, circa late 1800's. Est. $250.00-$400.00.

Lot #319. Rosine *The Spirit of Saint Louis* extremely rare clear glass bottle and stopper, 4.6" [11.7 cm], covered with a label depicting Lindberg's airplane *The Spirit of St. Louis,* with the red and white stripes of the American flag wrapped around the neck of the bottle, empty, parts of the label frayed, circa 1928, bottom with fragment of red paper label signed *Paul Poiret*. This was a limited edition [of very small quantity] produced soon after Lindberg's arrival in Paris in 1927, and very few examples of it are known to have survived. Est. $1,000.00-$1,200.00.

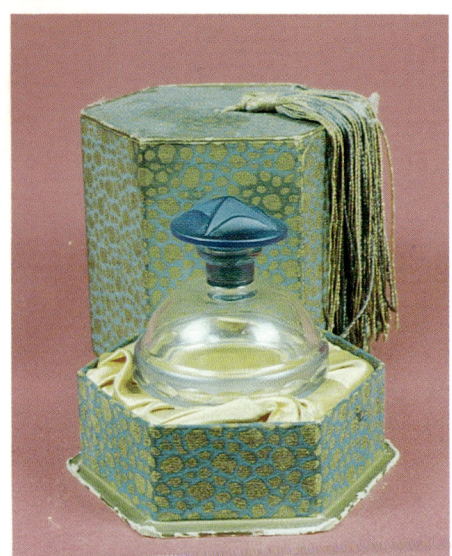

Lot #320. Unidentified perfumer *Narcisse* clear crystal bottle with bright blue glass stopper, 3.4" [8.6 cm], the bottle of ball shape with a decorative band around the center enameled in blue, empty, in its tasseled silk-lined box, circa 1920's; bottom signed *Czechoslovakia* in a line. Est. $300.00-$400.00.

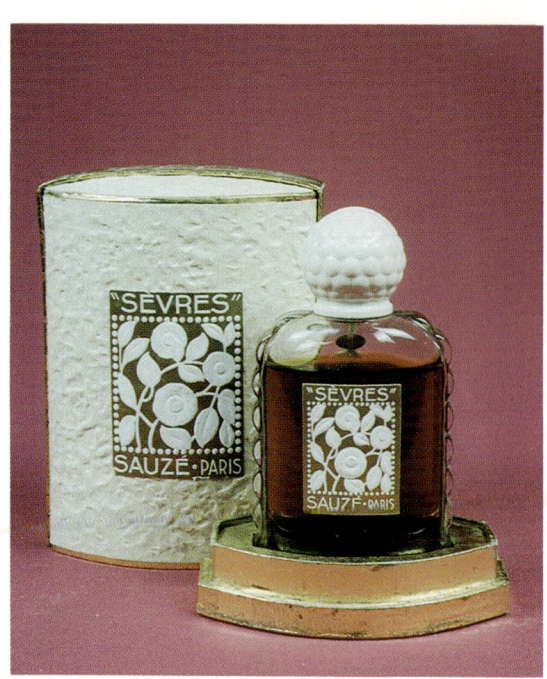

Lot #321. Sauzé *Sèvres* clear glass bottle, inner stopper, and ivory plastic overcap, 3.2" [8.1 cm], the sides of the bottle molded with scallops, near full and sealed, beautiful gold and ivory label on front, in its cream and gold box; circa late 1930's. Est. $150.00-$250.00.

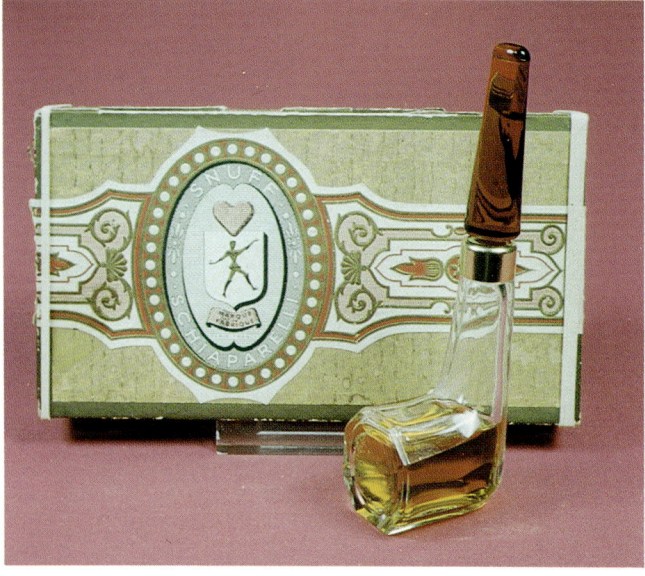

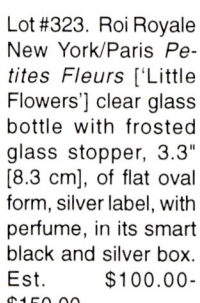

Lot #323. Roi Royale New York/Paris *Petites Fleurs* ['Little Flowers'] clear glass bottle with frosted glass stopper, 3.3" [8.3 cm], of flat oval form, silver label, with perfume, in its smart black and silver box. Est. $100.00-$150.00.

Lot #322. Schiaparelli *Snuff* clear glass bottle and amber glass stopper in the form of a pipe, 5.4" long [13.7 cm], near full of perfume, in its original box designed as if for cigars, with the Schiaparelli label made in the form of a cigar band. Est. $275.00-$375.00.

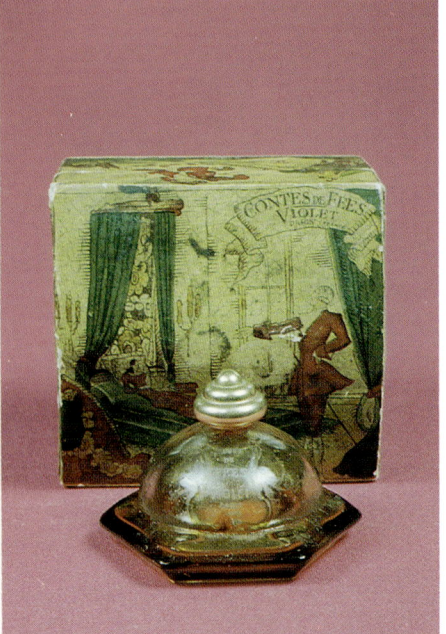

Lot #324. Violet *Contes de Fées* ['Fairy Tales'] clear glass bottle with gold cap, 1.7" [4.3 cm], the bottle of flat bell-shape with a hexagonal base, some perfume, decal label, in an adorable box shaped as a toy chest, with illustrations of famous tales: *La Belle au Bois Dormant* ['Sleeping Beauty'], *Le Petit Chaperon Rouge* ['Little Red Riding Hood'], *Barbe Bleue* ['Bluebeard'], *Le Petit Poucet* ['Jack in the Beanstalk'], *Le Chat Botté* ['Puss in Boots']. Circa 1939. Est. $400.00-$500.00.

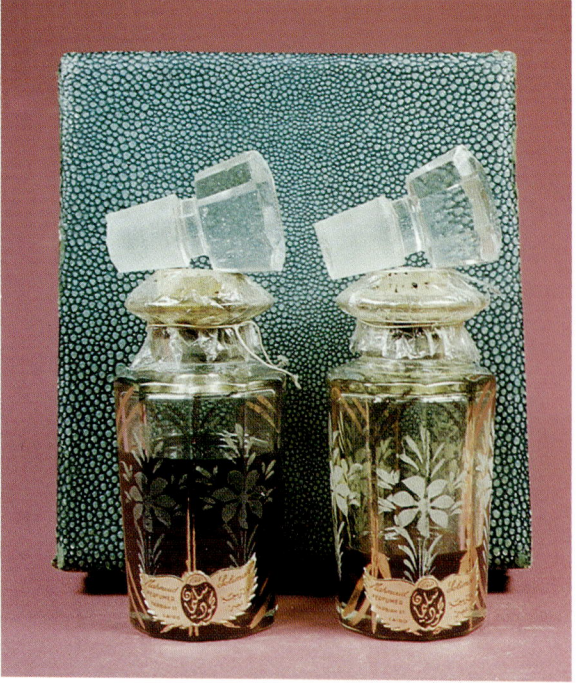

Lot #325. Mahmoud Soliman *Arabian Night* and *Queen of Egypt* clear glass bottles of decanter shape, cork-sealed, and with separate stoppers, height with stoppers 5.2" [13.2 cm], decorated with gold enamel, both with Soliman labels on the front and fragrance labels on the reverse, small chips on the stoppers, in their fabric-lined faux shagreen box with brass clasp. Est. $250.00-$350.00.

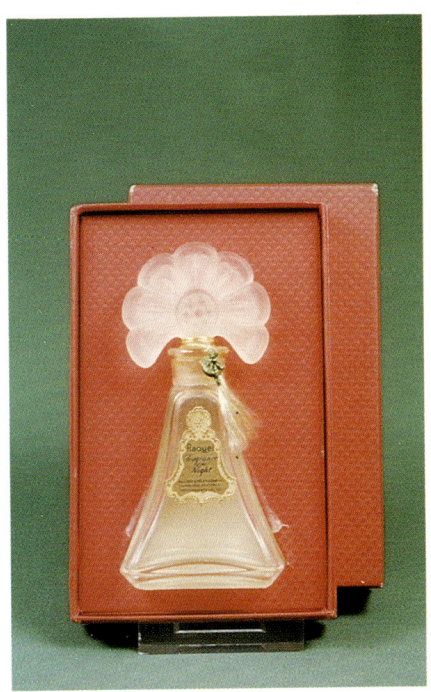

Lot #326. Raquel *Fragrance of the Night* clear glass bottle with frosted glass stopper, 4.5" [11.4 cm], the bottle of triangular shape, the stopper a tiara-form resembling a flower, empty, gold label, in its red box; circa 1930. Est. $275.00-$375.00.

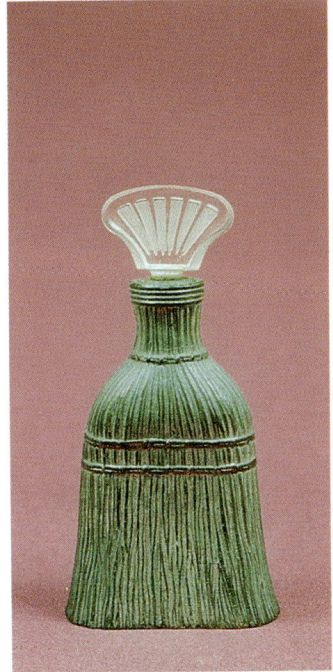

Lot #327. Tappan's *Clean Sweep* very early metal bottle with clear and frosted glass stopper, 3.3" [8.4 cm], designed as a whisk broom, with the metal intricately molded to show the broom's fibers, empty, label on bottom, circa 1890's. This is a wonderful American perfume presentation with a charming sense of humor that is undiminished by the passage of time. Est. $250.00-$350.00.

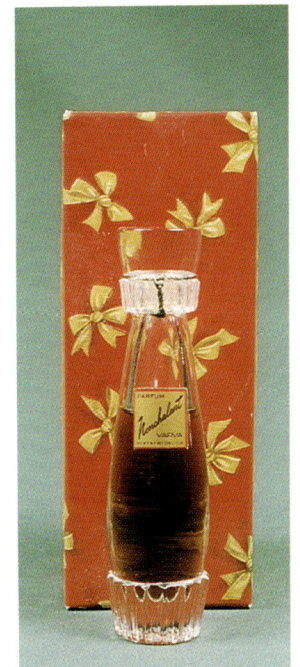

Lot #328. Varva *Nonchalant* clear glass bottle and stopper, 4.6" [11.7 cm], the bottle tall and columnar but with a molded scalloped border around the base of the bottle and the stopper, full and sealed, gold label on front, in its pretty red box decorated with yellow bows; not pictured in existing literature. Est. $150.00-$250.00.

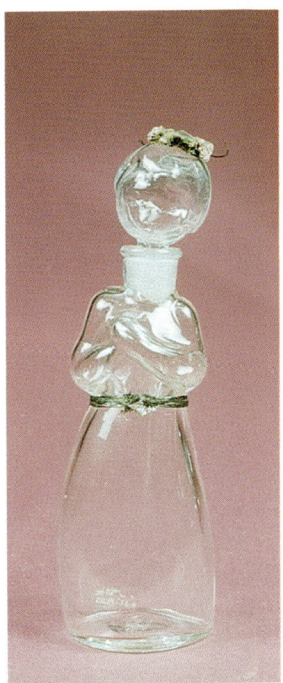

Lot #329. Helena Rubenstein *Slumber Song* clear glass bottle and stopper, 6.4" [16.2 cm], in the shape of an angel with her hands clasped at her breast and with a halo of flowers, empty; this was also called *Night Perfume*. Est. $300.00-$400.00.

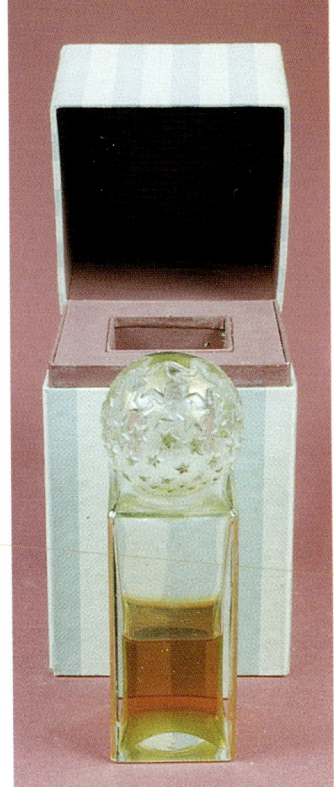

Lot #330. Saint Cyr *Flêches d'Amour* ['Love Arrows'] clear glass bottle, inner stopper, and heavy glass overcap, 4" [10.2 cm], the bottle of rectangular shape with gold enamel on its edges, the stopper molded with stars of differing size and enameled in gold, in its box which totally conceals the bottle and allows only the overcap to be displayed. Est. $350.00-$450.00.

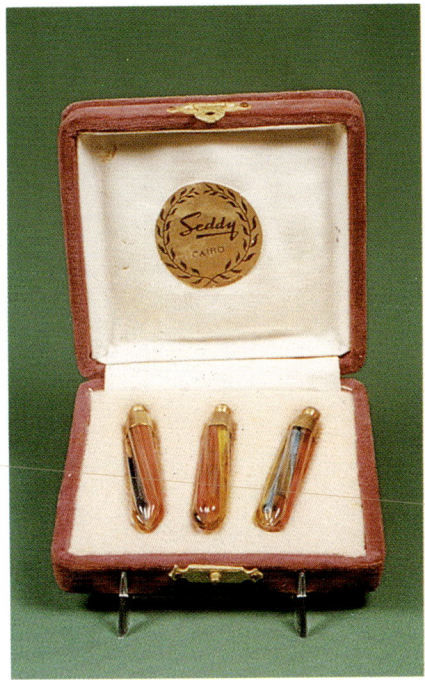

Lot #331. Seddy [Cairo] set of three Czechoslovakian glass perfume bottles with metal mounted applicators, each 2.7" [6.9 cm], the bottles molded with a swirled design and internally decorated with pink, yellow, and blue which create a rainbow effect when turned, metal mounts signed *Czechoslovakia*, gold label inside their case of purple velvet. Est. $500.00-$600.00.

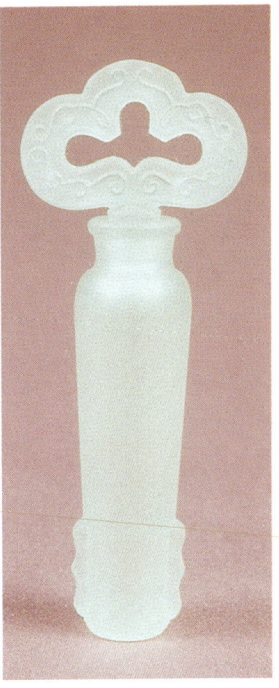

Lot #332. Unidentified perfumer unusual frosted glass perfume bottle and stopper in the shape of a large key, 4" [10.2 cm], stopper molded with a scroll design and with a long glass dauber; cf. North p. 13 #6. Est. $200.00-$250.00.

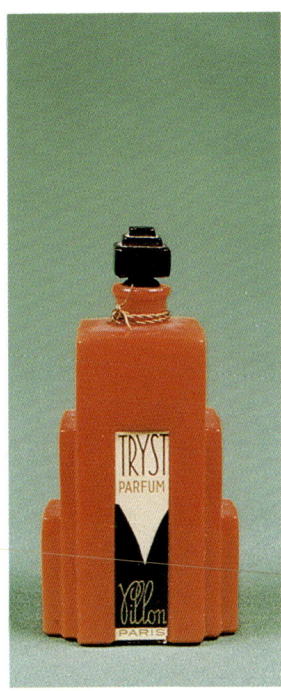

Lot #333. Villon *Tryst* red glass bottle and black stopper, 3.3" [8.3 cm], the entire design resembling that of a modern skyscraper, empty, original label on front; circa 1940's. Est. $250.00-$350.00.

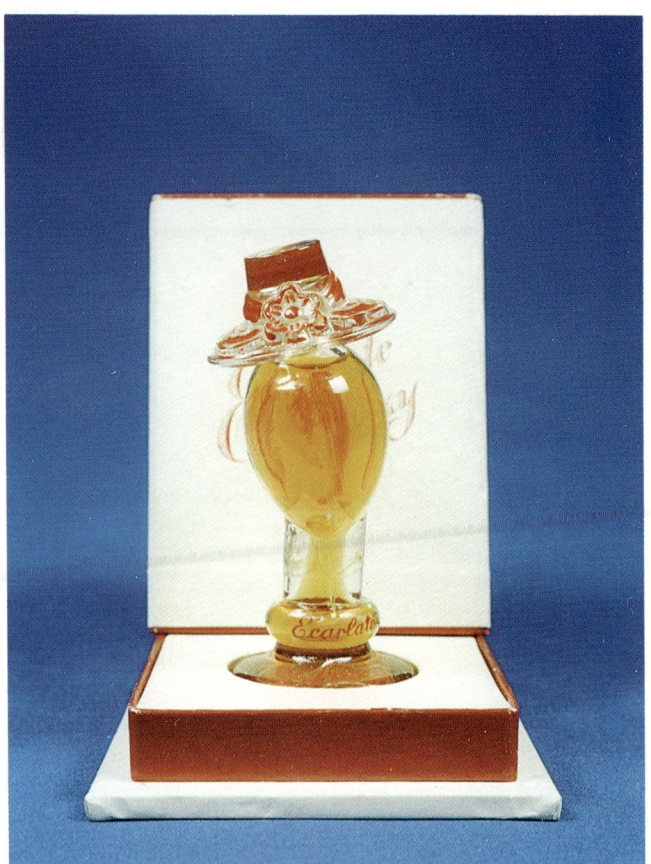

Lot #334. Suzy *Ecarlate de Suzy* ['Scarlet...'] very small size clear glass bottle and stopper in the form of a lady's head with a chapeau, 3" [7.6 cm], with perfume, names and decoration in red enamel, gold label on bottom [marked 1/4 oz.] in its red and cream box. Est. $450.00-$550.00.

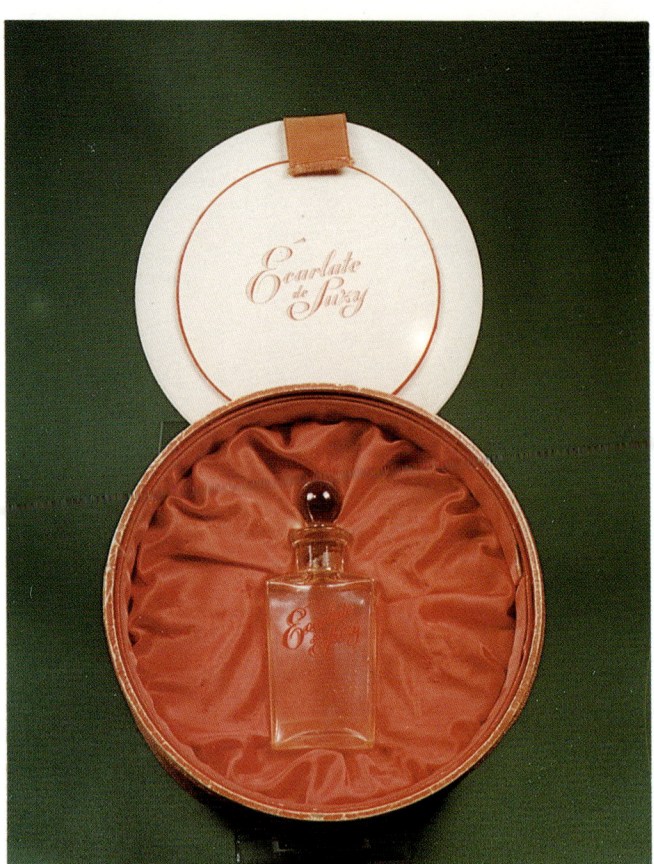

Lot #335. Suzy *Écarlate* ['Scarlet'] *de Suzy* clear glass rectangular bottle and ball-shaped stopper, 3.4" [8.6 cm], empty, names in enamel on front, in a round 'hatbox' presentation lined with red satin. Est. $125.00-$175.00.

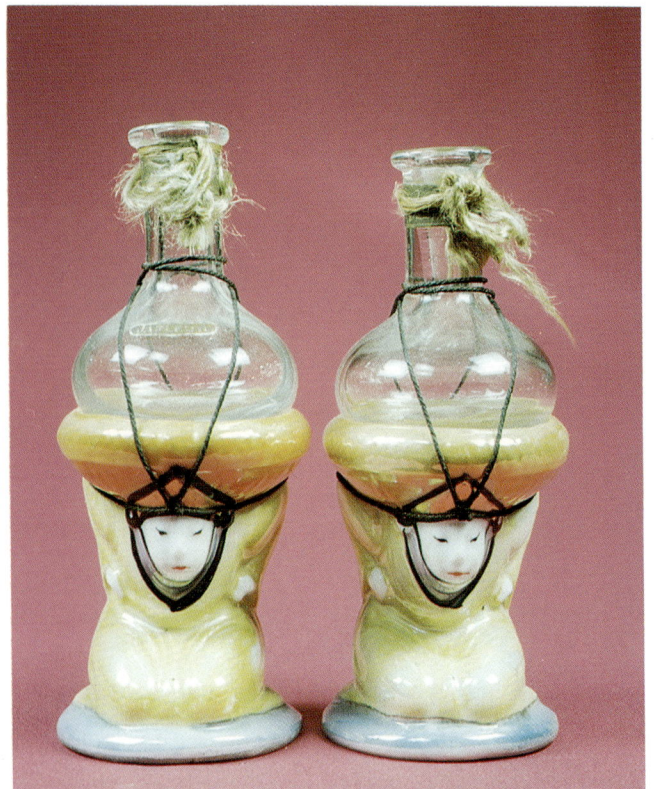

Lot #336. Vantine's *La Fleur* ['The Flower'] an adorable pair of clear glass bottles [which would have originally have had cork stoppers] attached by cord to two porcelain holders, total height 5.6" [14.2 cm], one with perfume label, both empty and with Vantine's label around neck; the porcelain holders designed as oriental women supporting the bottles on their heads and shoulders, painted in orange, yellow, and blue luster, signed *Vantine's 665 Made in Japan*. Two items. Est. $350.00-$450.00.

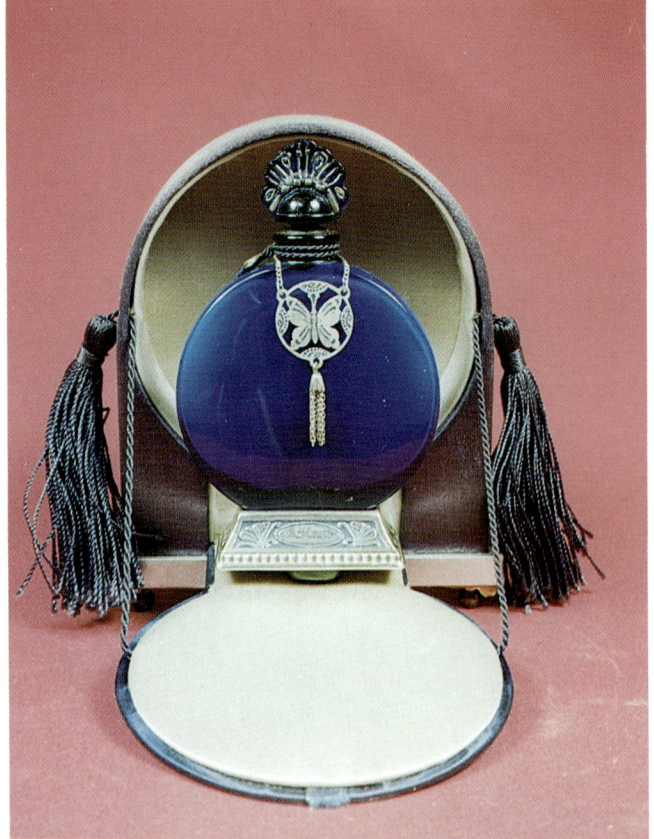

Lot #337. Lucretia Vanderbilt cased blue-over-white glass bottle and blue glass stopper, 4" [10.2 cm], the bottle mounted on a silver metal base, sealed, butterfly medallion around the neck, in its beautiful drop-front box of blue and cream satin on four metal feet; the box is in very well-preserved condition. Est. $1,200.00-$1,500.00.

THE FRENCH MASTERS OF PERFUME BOTTLE DESIGN:
DAILLET - DEPINOIX - GAILLARD - JOLLIVET - LALIQUE - VIARD

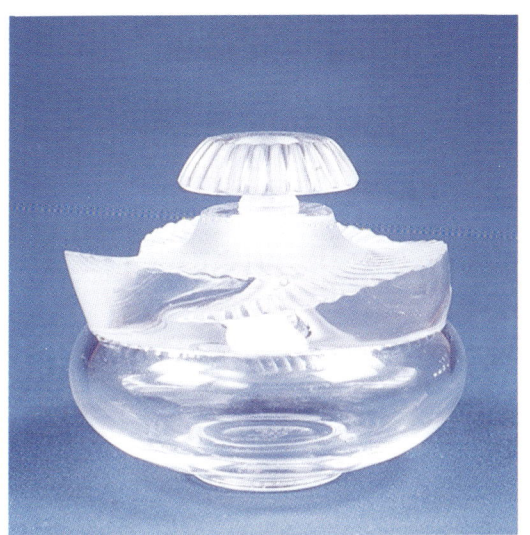

Lot #338. Cristal Lalique *Baptiste* clear crystal bottle and stopper, 2.5" [6.4 cm], an unusual form designed with a clear perfume well and three waves of spirals above and on the stopper, bottom signed *Lalique* in script. Utt #CL-199. Est. $200.00-$300.00.

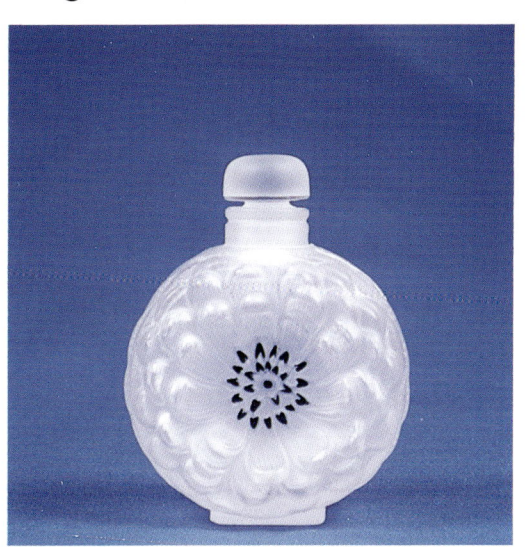

Lot #339. Cristal Lalique *Dahlia* very petite size frosted glass bottle, 3.4" [8.6 cm], designed with a large open flower on both sides of the bottle, button stopper, centers of the flower enameled in black, paper label on side of bottle, bottom signed *Lalique France* in script. Utt #ML-617/CL-105. Est. $150.00-$250.00.

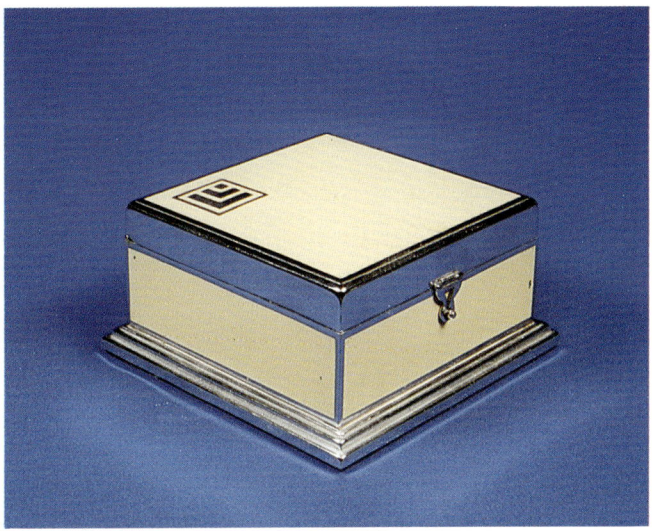

Lot #340. Lucien Lelong [for various fragrances such as *Parfum N, Parfum L*, etc.] rare chrome powder box enameled in cream color, the base 3.7" square [9.4 cm], 1.8" tall [4.5 cm], empty, mirror inside, the Lelong logo on the upper left corner; this powder box matched the perfume bottle and chrome case designed by René Lalique for Lucien Lelong. Est. $200.00-$300.00.

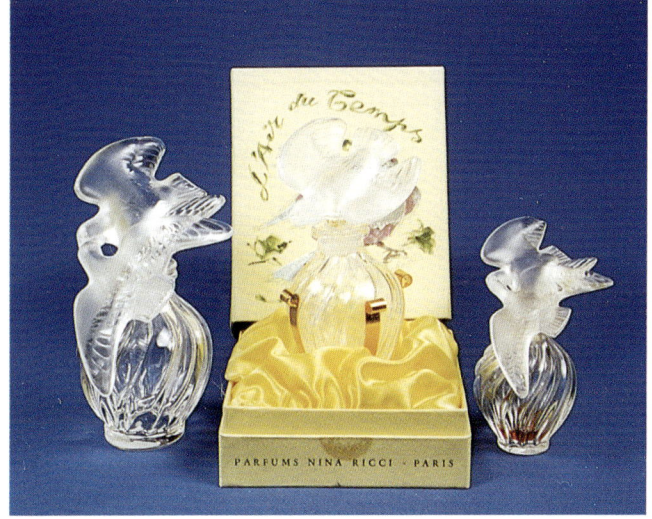

Lot #341. Nina Ricci *L'Air du Temps* clear and frosted crystal bottle, 3.6" [9.1 cm], the bottle with a swirled design, the all-glass stopper molded in the shape of a single dove, empty, unsigned, in its yellow box; bottle and stopper with double doves, 3.2" [8.1 cm], empty; identical larger size bottle with double dove stopper, 4.3" [10.9 cm], empty, bottom signed *Lalique*. Three items. Est. $125.00-$200.00.

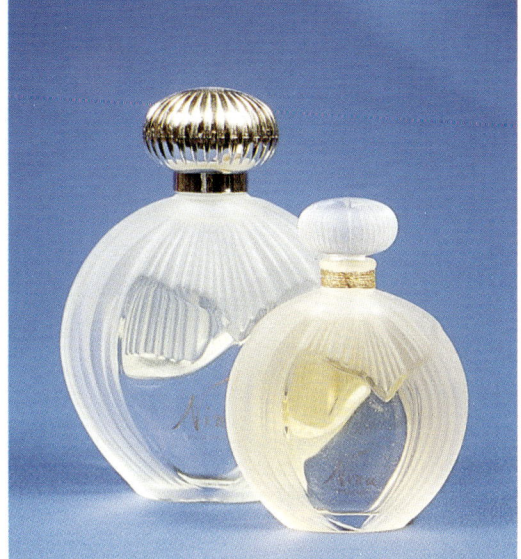

Lot #342. Nina Ricci *Nina* clear and frosted glass bottle and stopper, 3.4" [8.6 cm], the bottle designed with folds of material in frosted glass on the sides and a clear heart-shaped window in front and back, with perfume, name in gold enamel, unsigned; eau de toilette bottle with a gold cap, 4.4" [11.2 cm], full, name in gold enamel, bottom molded *Lalique*. Utt #NR-116. Two items. Est. $100.00-$150.00.

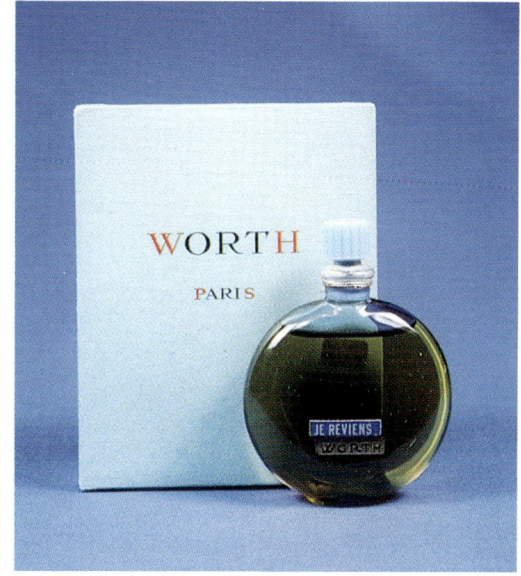

Lot #343. Worth *Je Reviens* ['I Will Return'] smoky blue glass bottle and opaque turquoise stopper, 3.7" [9.4 cm], this flat round form synonymous with Worth perfumes, *Worth* in molded block letters on front, full and sealed, bottom molded *R. Lalique*, in its turquoise box lined with white satin. Utt #W-2. Est. $250.00-$350.00.

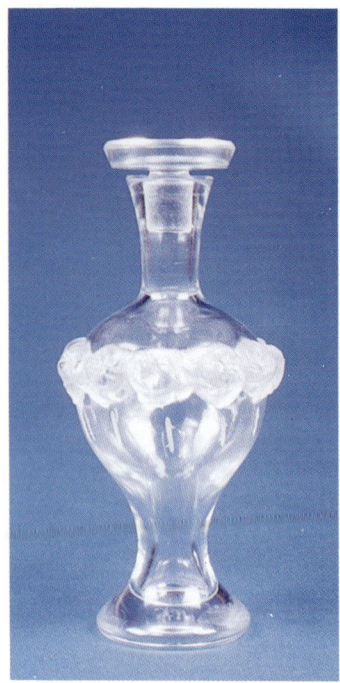 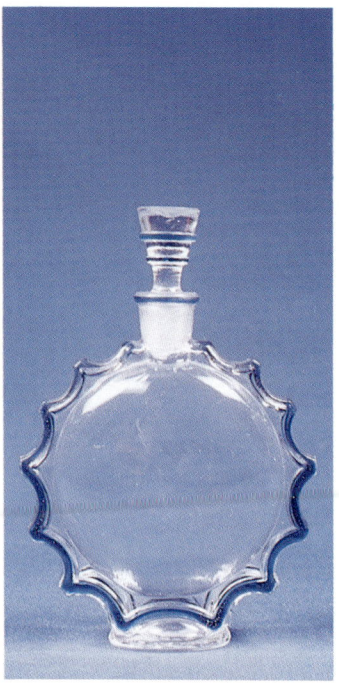 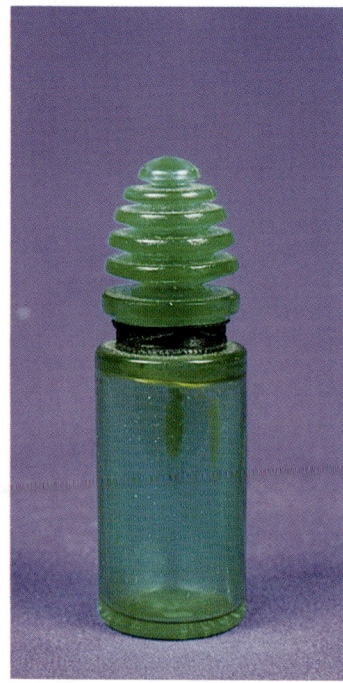 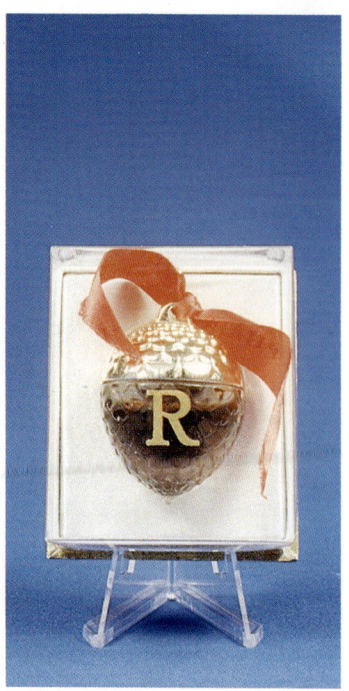

Lot #344. Cristal Lalique *Martine* clear and frosted glass bottle and stopper, 5.7" [14.5 cm], bottle of urn shape with a band of frosted roses and their etched stems, designed by Marc Lalique, bottom inscribed *Lalique France*. Utt #CL-114. Est. $200.00-$300.00.

Lot #345. Worth *Requête* ['Request'] clear glass bottle and stopper, 3.6" [9.1 cm], of flat round shape with a scallop motif enameled in blue, empty, initial *W* impressed in stopper, molded *Lalique*. Utt #W-105. Est. $350.00-$450.00.

Lot #346. Worth *Sans Adieu* ['Without Farewell'] brilliant emerald green glass bottle and stopper of columnar shape, 2.6" [6.6 cm], the stopper molded as a series of six rings [the last one is the lip of the bottle], probably a first size of this model, empty, no label, signed *R. Lalique* in the mold. Utt #W-8. Est. $500.00-$600.00.

Lot #347. Raphael *Réplique* frosted glass bottle in the shape of an acorn with silver colored screw-on cap and red ribbon, 1.8" [4.6 cm], signed *Lalique* in black enamel under cap, in its original box with label on bottom, superb unused condition; designed by Marc Lalique. Utt #R-101. Est. $250.00-$350.00.

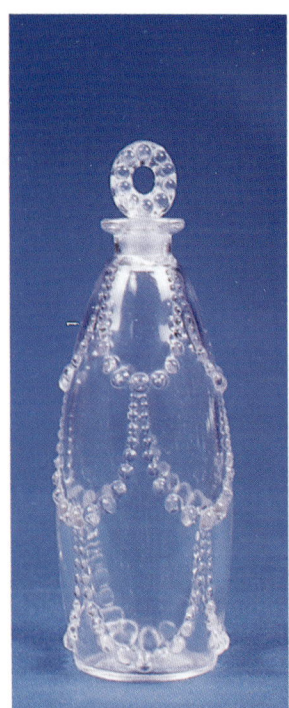 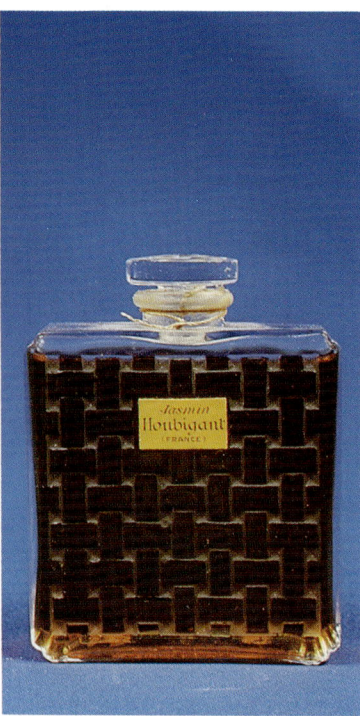 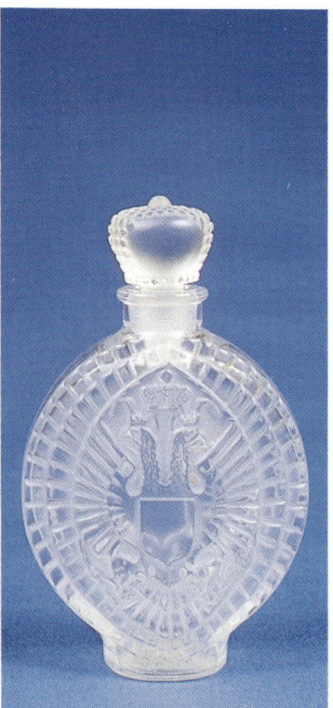 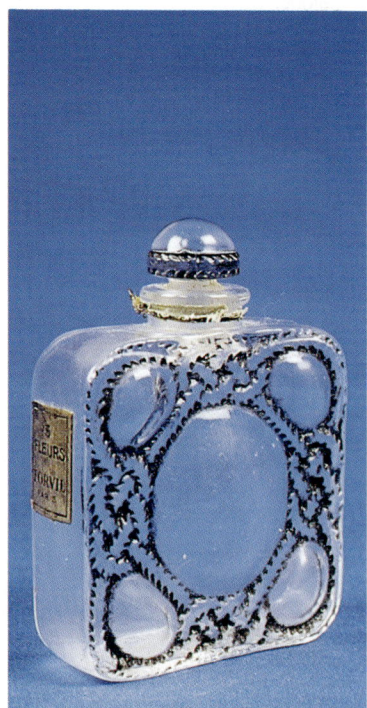

Lot #348. Maison Lalique *Palerme* clear glass bottle and stopper, 4.6" [11.7 cm], the teardrop shaped bottle molded with strands of pearls in three rows, stopper also similarly molded and with a tiny open part, bottom molded *R. Lalique*. Utt #ML-518. Est. $700.00-$850.00.

Lot #349. Houbigant *Jasmin* clear and frosted glass bottle and stopper, 3.2" [8.1 cm], of square shape with a basketweave motif on front and on stopper, near full, with its label, signed in the mold *R. Lalique*. Utt #H-6 [1922]. Est. $700.00-$850.00.

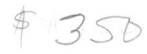

Lot #350. Lengyel *Parfum Impérial* clear and frosted glass bottle and stopper, 3.4" [8.6 cm], the bottle molded with the Russian Imperial double eagle on both sides, the stopper shaped as a crown in the Russian style, empty, label lacking, bottom signed *R. Lalique* in the mold. Utt #Len-1. Est. $800.00-$1,000.00.

Lot #351. Forvil *Cinq Fleurs* ['Five Flowers'] clear and frosted glass bottle and stopper, 2.7" [16 cm], a diminutive size for this perfume, a molded design of rope tied in elaborate knots around five cabochons, recesses with black enamel, gold metallic label on side of bottle, empty, molded signature *R. Lalique*. Utt #F-6. Est. $1,200.00-$1,500.00.

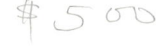

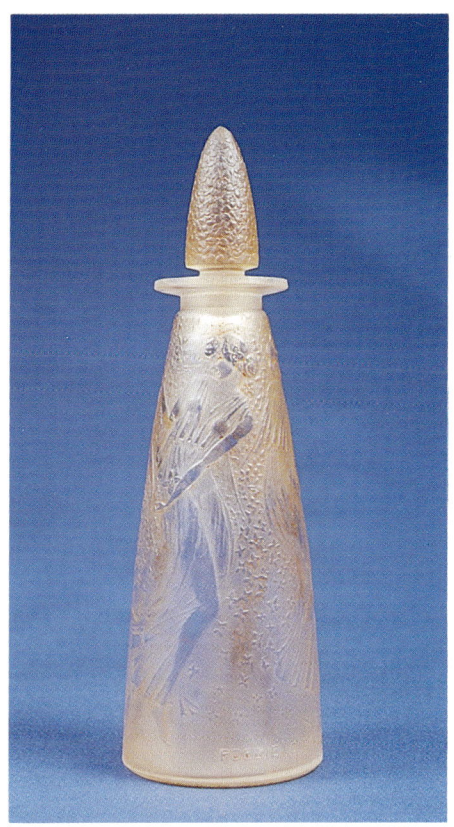

Lot #352. D'Orsay *Poésie d'Orsay* frosted glass bottle and stopper both of cone shape, 5.9" [15 cm], molded with a freize of classical maidens in diaphanous gowns dancing amid a background of flowers, same flowers also on stopper, names molded near bottom, rich amber patina, molded *R. Lalique*. Utt #DO-7. Est. $2,000.00-$2,500.00.

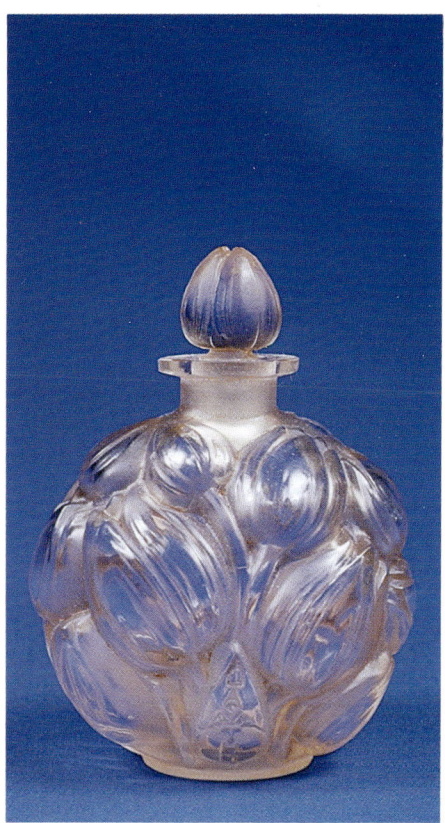

Lot #353. Jay Thorpe & Co. *Jaytho* clear and frosted glass bottle and stopper, 3.9" [10 cm], the entire bottle molded as a bouquet of tulips and the stopper as a bud, rich amber patina, the word *Jaytho* molded vertically in front, bottom molded *R. Lalique*. Utt #JT-1. Est. $1,200.00-$1,500.00.

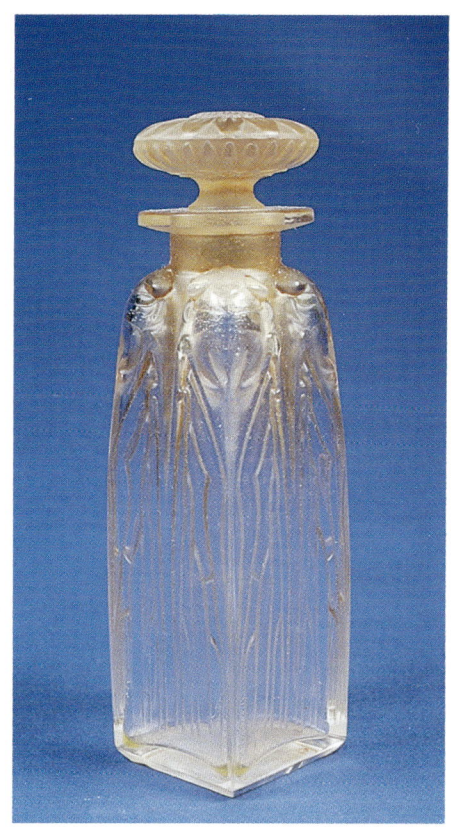

Lot #354. Maison Lalique *Cigales* ['Cicadas'] clear and frosted glass bottle and stopper, 5.5" [14 cm], the bottle designed with four huge cicadas facing upward toward the neck, the stopper molded as a flower, amber patina, side signed *R. Lalique* in script. Utt #ML-475. Est. $3,000.00-$3,500.00.

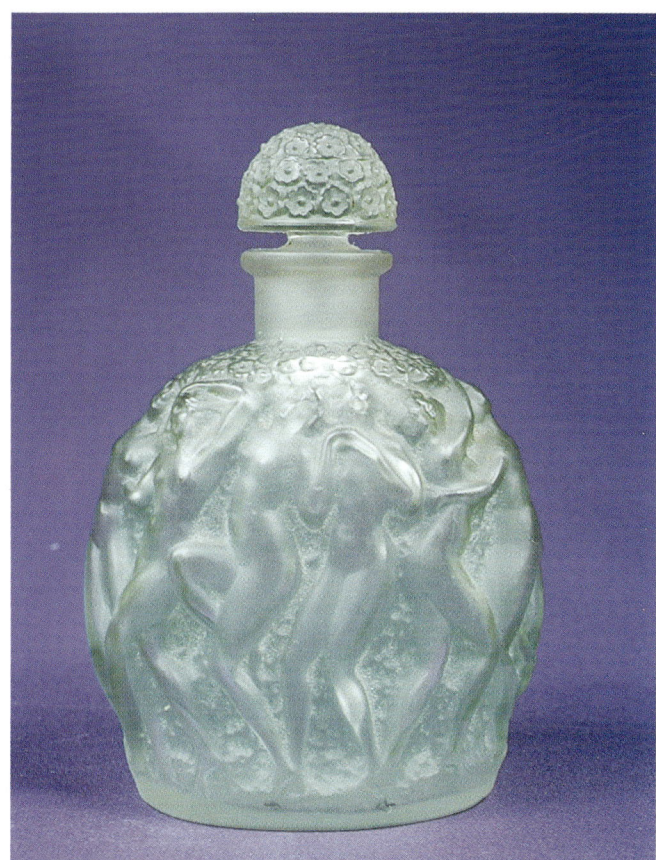

Lot #355. Molinard *Calendale* frosted glass bottle and stopper of beehive form, 4.5" [11.4 cm], the stopper molded with flowers, the bottle deeply molded with a design of cavorting nymphs, green patina, empty, bottom signed *Molinard Lalique* in script. Utt #M-101. Est. $2,000.00-$2,500.00.

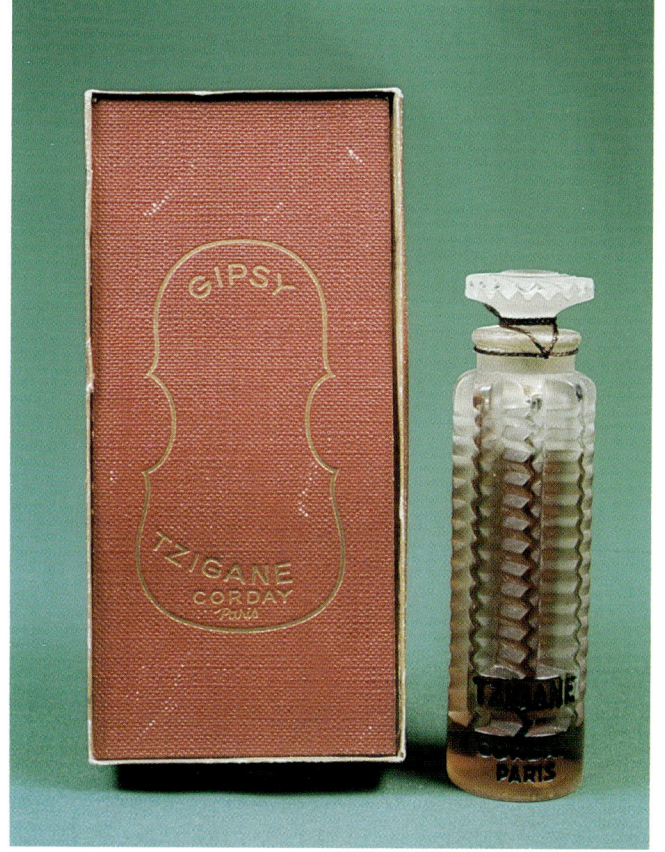

Lot #356. Corday *Tzigane* ['Gypsy'] clear and frosted bottle and stopper, 3.8" [9.7 cm], a column with an indented zigzag design, names enameled in black at base, full and sealed, molded signature *R. Lalique;* in its red box with the outline of a violin. Utt #Cor-1. Est. $1,000.00-$1,250.00.

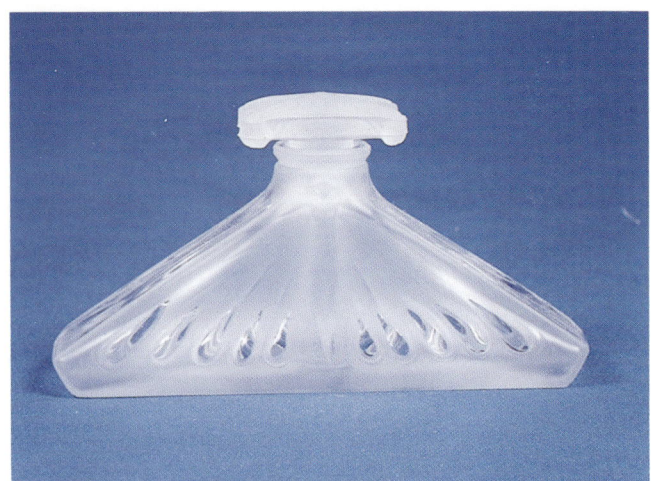

Lot #357. Clamy *Femmes Aillées* ['Wingèd Ladies'] frosted and clear glass bottle and stopper of flattened triangular shape, 2.5" [6.4 cm], molded front and back with the image of a woman against giant wings; the original of this bottle was designed in 1913 by L. Gaillard, this example was produced in 1986 by the Verreries Brosse, and is so marked on the bottom as well © MMA [New York Metropolitan Museum of Art]. Est. $75.00-$150.00.

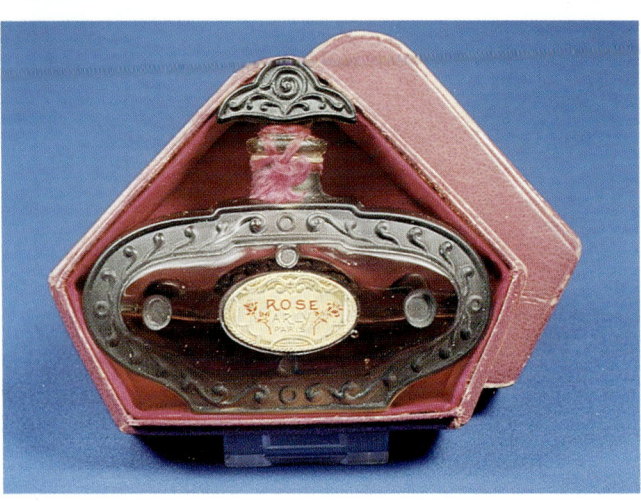

Lot #358. Arly *Rose* clear and frosted glass bottle and stopper, 3" [7.6 cm], of oblong oval shape, elaborate scroll design molded on front and back, dark gray patina, with perfume and sealed, in its rose colored box lined with brilliant red silk; possibly by Dépinoix, unsigned. Est. $700.00-$850.00.

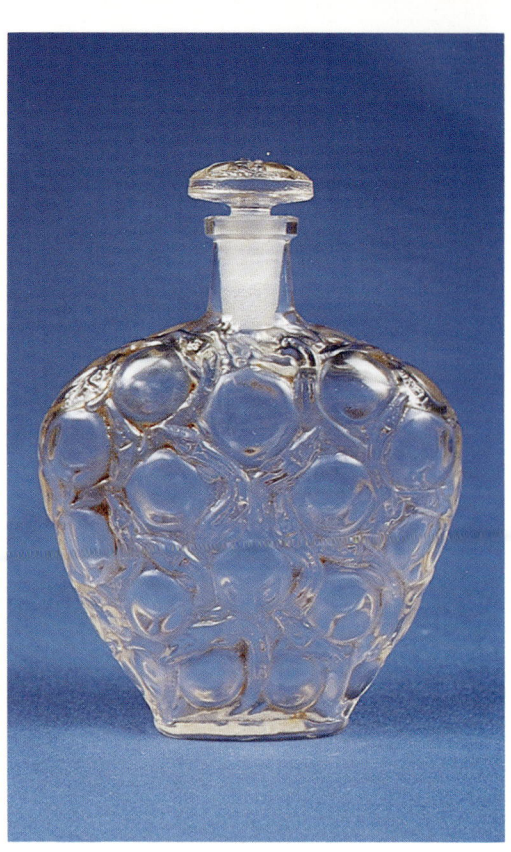

Lot #359. Maison Lalique *Salamandres* clear and frosted glass bottle and stopper, 3.7" [9.5 cm], the design on both bottle and stopper molded with a pattern of salamanders encircling cabochons of various sizes, rich amber patina, bottom signed *Lalique* in block letters. Utt #ML-491. Est. $1,500.00-$1,750.00.

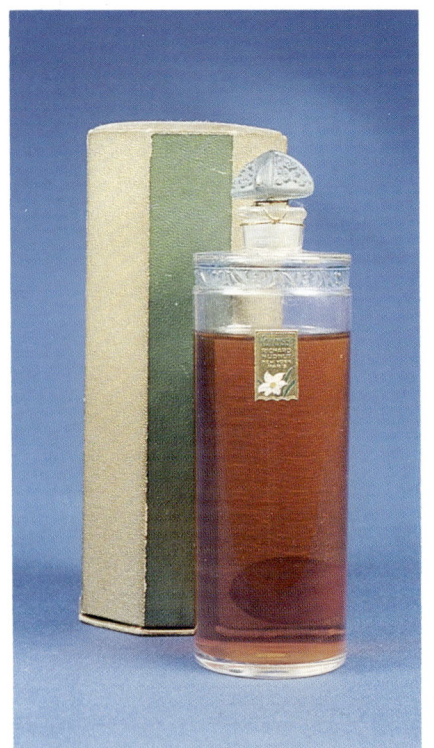

Lot #360. Richard Hudnut *Narcisse* clear glass bottle and frosted glass stopper, 5.5" [14 cm], of columnar shape with frosted glass flowers near the top, the stopper also molded with flowers, aqua patina, full and sealed, label on front, bottom signed with the Hudnut emblem, in its green and gold box. Est. $600.00-$750.00.

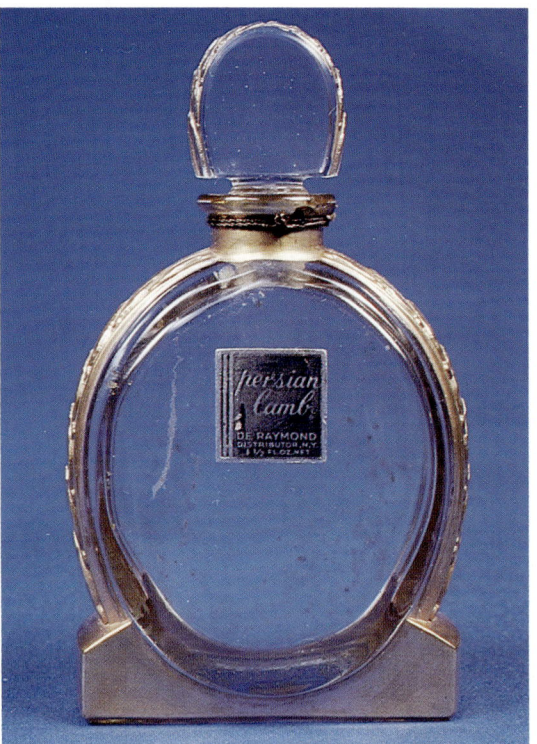

Lot #361. De Raymond *Persian Lamb* fine quality clear glass bottle, 4" [10.2 cm], the bottle shaped as a clear oval window with a rectangular pedestal base, the sides of the bottle molded with overlapping acanthus leaves and enameled in gold, stopper with conforming design, empty, silver and black label on front, possibly by A. Jollivet, unsigned. This bottle is not pictured in existing literature. Est. $600.00-$750.00.

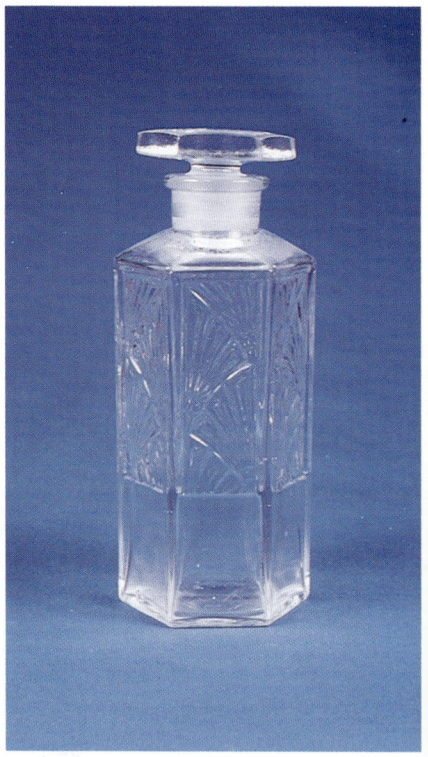

Lot #362. De Raymond *Mimzy* very large size clear glass bottle and stopper, 6.1" [15.5 cm], of hexagonal form with a stylized fan motif in each of six panels and on stopper, empty, no label, signed in the mold *A. Jollivet*. Est. $100.00-$200.00.

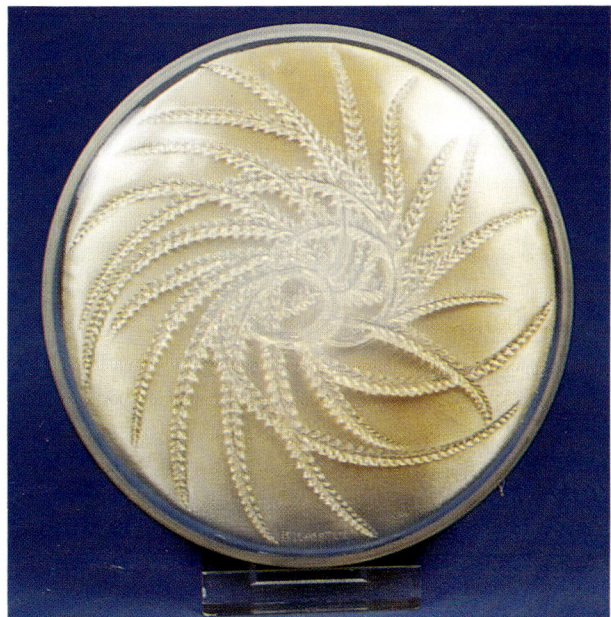

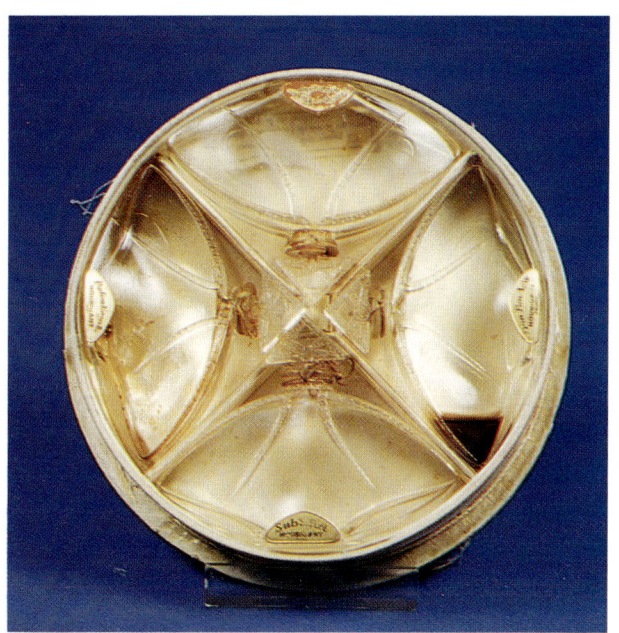

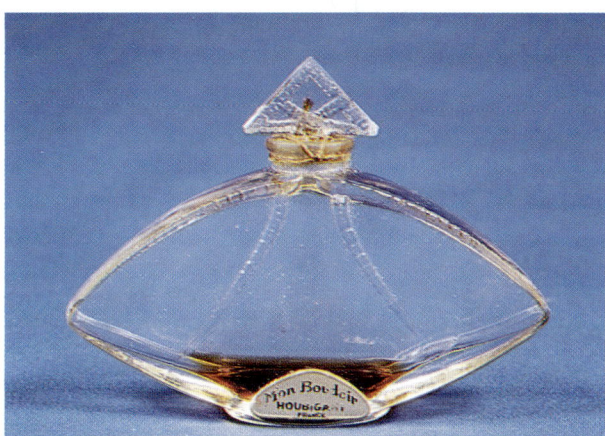

An example of one bottle from Lot #363.

Lot #363. Houbigant *Mon Boudoir, Quelques Fleurs, Parfum d'Argeville,* and *Subtilité,* set of 4 clear glass bottles of fan shape, each 2.4" [6 cm], with stoppers of triangular form, both bottles and stoppers decorated with molded bands of flowers, gold labels [one label worn], three empty, one unopened but perfume evaporated, in a lavish presentation box of opalescent glass molded with swirling leaves, all bottles and box signed in the mold *R. Lalique.* Utt #H-3. Est. $4,000.00-$4,500.00.

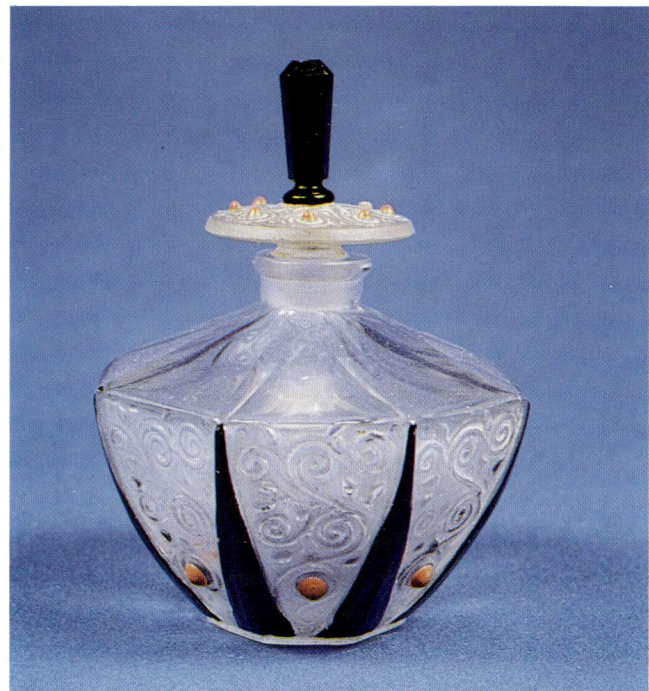

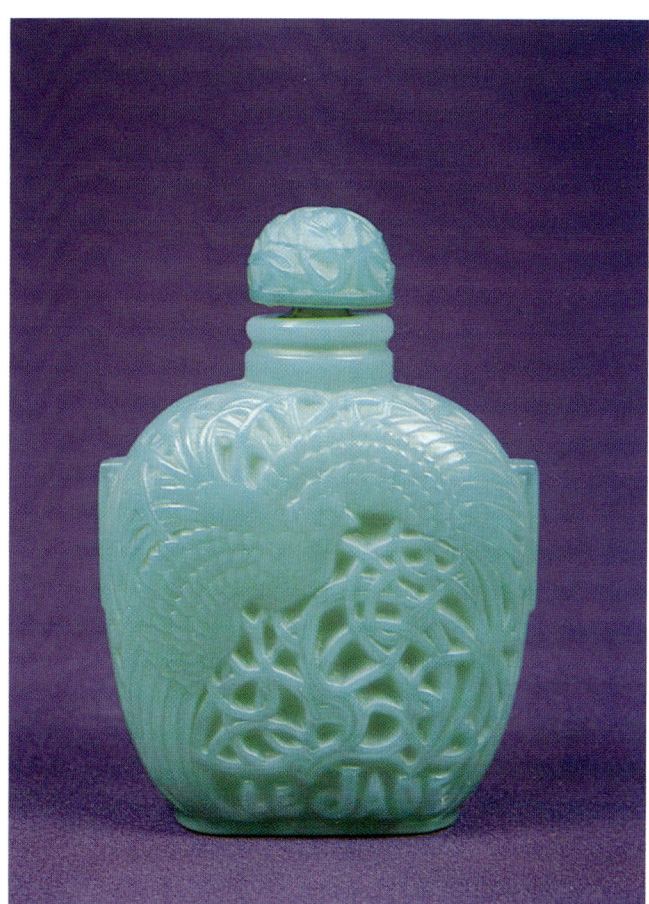

Lot #364. Unidentified perfumer and fragrance clear and frosted glass bottle and stopper with a black top, 3" [7.6 cm], of rounded octagonal form, the sides molded with scrolls and decorated with black and coral enamel, the stopper similarly decorated [one coral enamel dot with a tiny flake], unsigned. Est. $600.00-$750.00.

Lot #365. Roger and Gallet *Le Jade* fine quality semi-opaque green glass bottle and stopper, 3.2" [8.2 cm], the bottle designed to resemble an oriental snuff bottle, molded on one side with a bird with open wings amid vines and the words *Le Jade* as part of the design, and molded on the other side with intricate vines and the words *Roger et Gallet Paris,* signed *R. L.* on the base in the mold, empty. This example has beautiful, deep translucent color. Est. $2,500.00-$3,000.00.

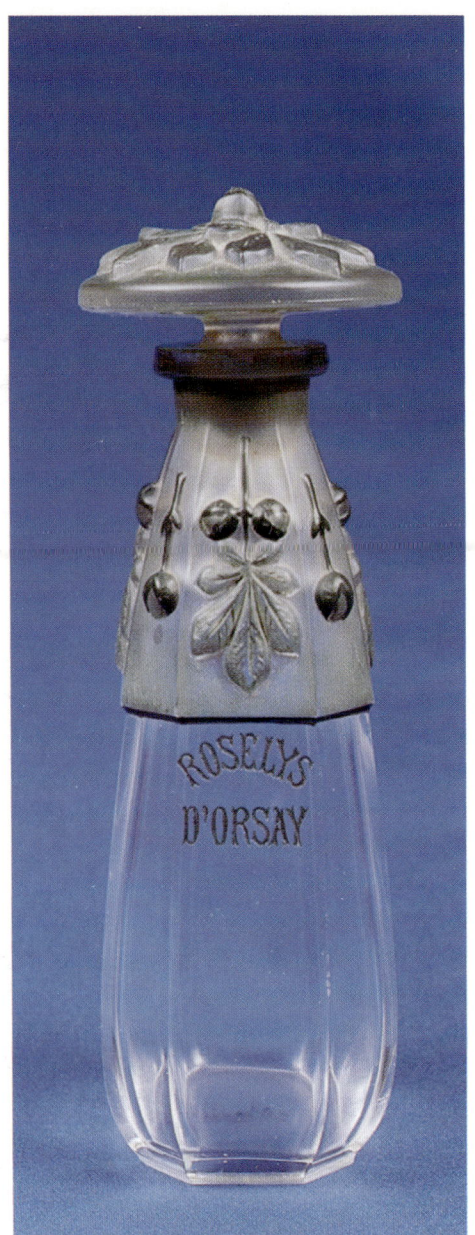

Lot #366. D'Orsay *Roselys* very rare clear and frosted glass bottle, 5.4" [13.7 cm], the slender bottle molded with vertical facets, the top part of the bottle molded with chestnuts and their leaves, conforming design on stopper, the design embellished with green patina and black enamel, names molded onto the front, signed *Daillet* on the bottom. This bottle is not seen in existing reference works. A picture of the signature is shown just below the lot photograph. Est. $1,500.00-$2,000.00.

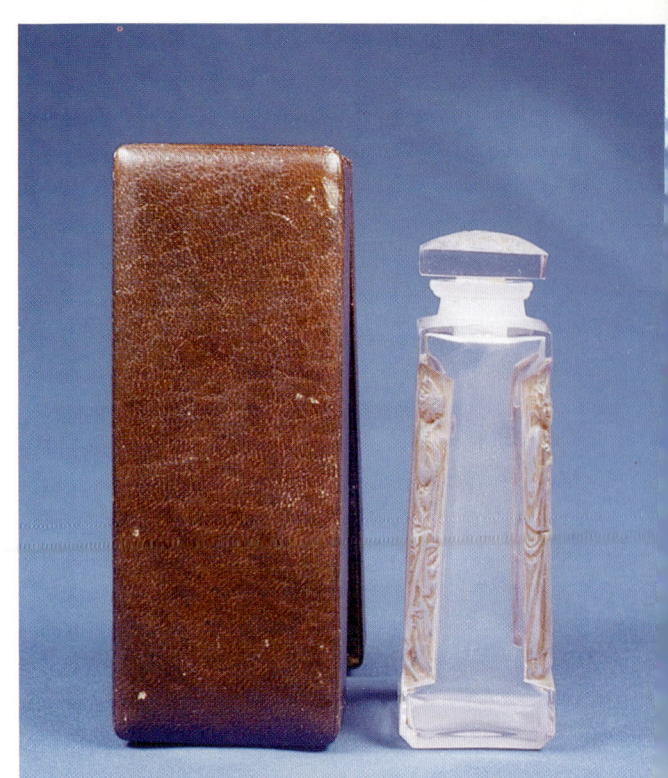

Lot #367. D'Orsay *Ambre d'Orsay* clear glass bottle and stopper, 5.2 [13.2 cm], the bottle of tall rectangular form with classical maidens molde into the four corners and appearing as caryatids, stopper molded wit flowers, amber patina on the designs, bottom edge signed *Lalique* in th mold and opposite edge molded *Ambre d'Orsay*, empty, in its brown leathe box with gold silk lining marked *D'Orsay, 17 rue de la Paix*. Utt #DO- Est. $3,000.00-$3,500.00.

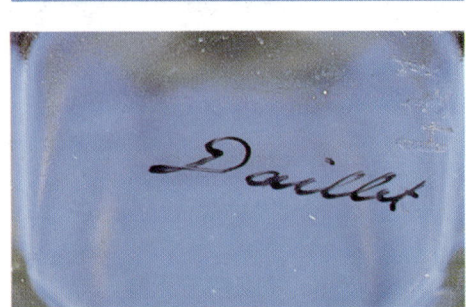

Lot #366, close-up of the signature.

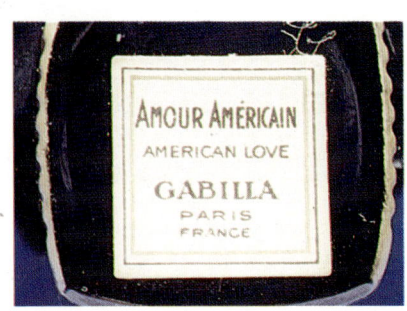

Lot #368, close-up of the label.

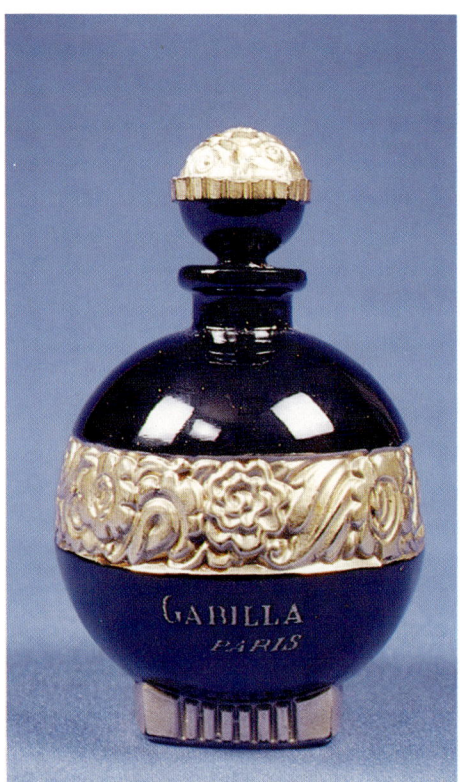

Lot #368. Gabilla *Amour Américain* ['American Love'] rare black glass bottle and stopper, 3.3" [8.4 cm], the round bottle on a short pedestal base, the center molded with a band of flowers in the Art Deco manner and brilliantly enameled in gold, stopper with conforming design, names in gold, paper label on bottom, empty, unsigned, by J. Viard. The overall condition is superb. Est. $1,750.00-$2,250.00.

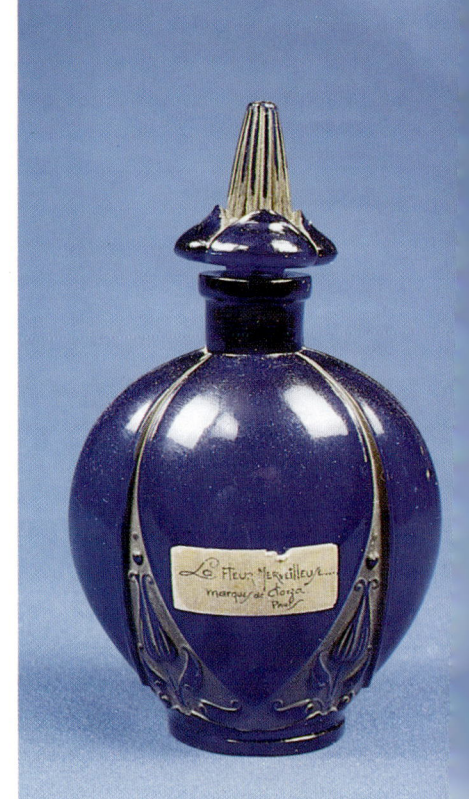

Lot #369. Marques de Elorza *La Fleur Merveilleu* ['The Marvelous Flower'], cobalt blue glass bot and stopper, 4.1" [10.4 cm], the bottle molded w flowers and with a gray patina, empty, label on fro small chip on the bottom of the bottle, signed *Ma in France* in a circle. Est. $800.00-$950.00.

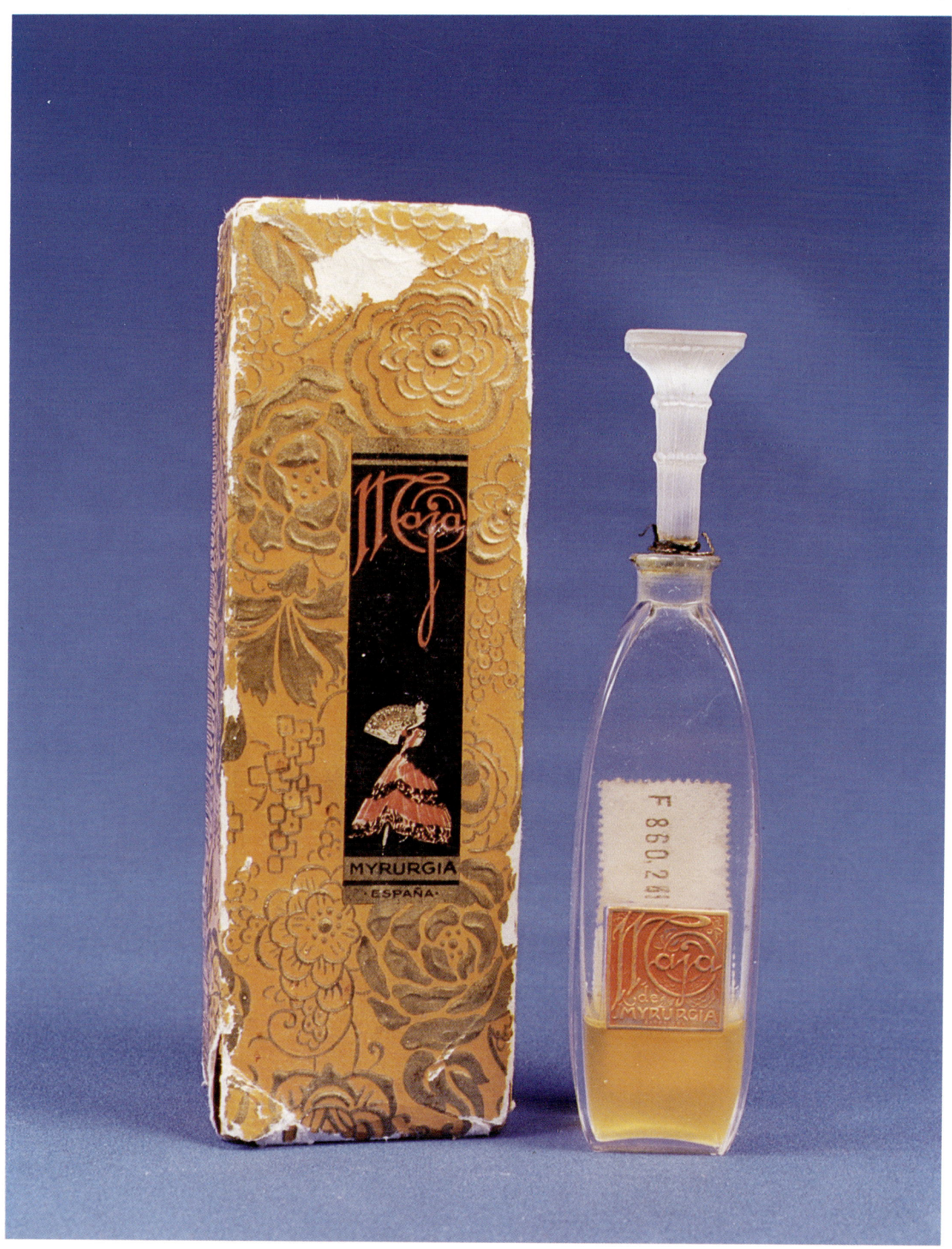

Lot #370. Myrurgia *Maja* rare clear glass bottle and frosted glass stopper, 5.4" [13.7 cm], the stopper designed as an architectural column, red and gold label, some perfume, Spanish tax stamps on the reverse side, in its beautiful but very worn box; written on the sides of the box in stylized letters are the words *En un solo perfume todas las flores de España* ['In one perfume all the flowers of Spain'], unsigned. This bottle is not pictured or catalogued in published sources. Est. $1,500.00-$2,000.00.

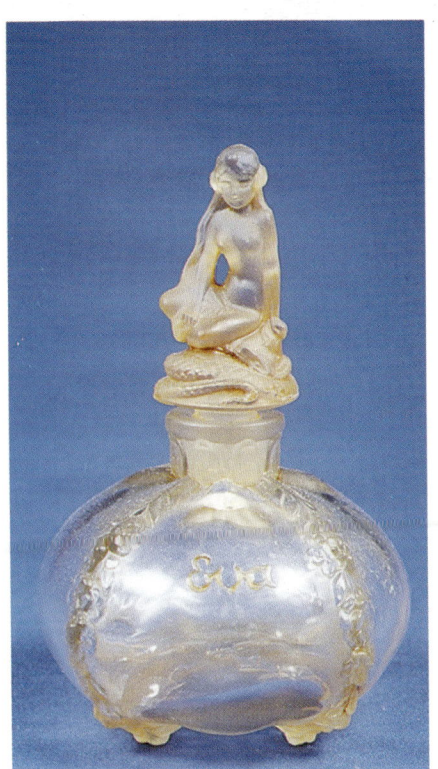

Lot #371. Lubin *Eva* clear and frosted glass bottle and stopper, 3.7" [9.4 cm], the cushion-form bottle with garlands of flowers molded down the sides and which form four feet at the base, the stopper molded as Eve crouched atop a coiled snake, amber patina, empty, unsigned, by J. Viard. Est. $2,000.00-$2,500.00.

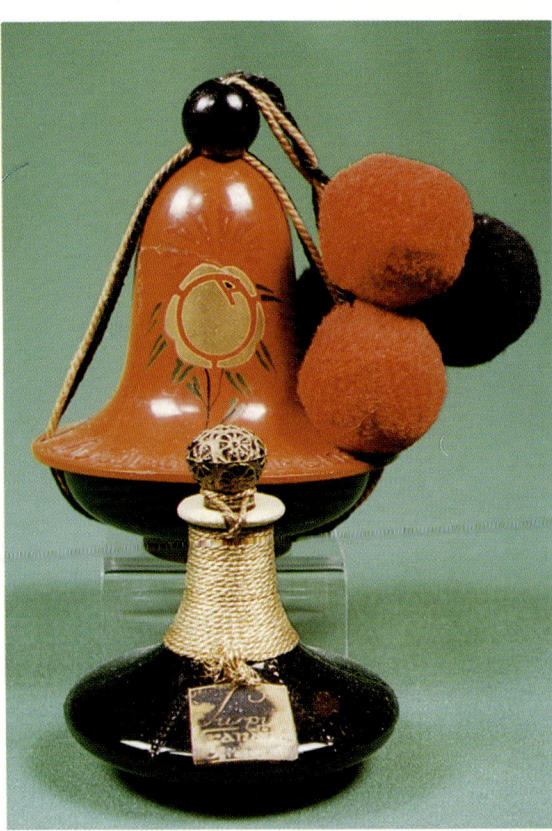

Lot #372. Myrurgia *Suspiro de Granada* ['Sigh of Grenada'] black glass bottle and stopper of bell form, 2.4" [6.1 cm], the stopper molded with flowers and gilded in the recesses, empty, label [worn] on front and with its elaborate gold cord still intact, in its red and black bakelite container [cracked] and decorative red and black pompoms, designed by J. Viard, unsigned. Cf. Lefkowith, p. 138. Est. $600.00-$750.00.

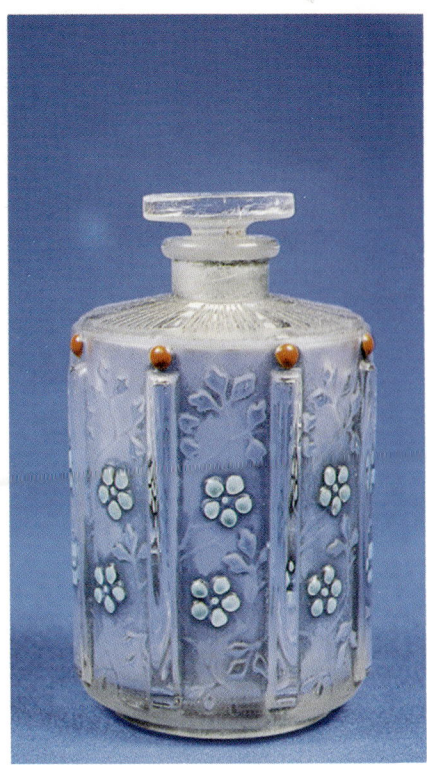

Lot #373. Isabey *Bleu de Chine* ['China Blue'] clear and frosted glass bottle and stopper, 2.9" [7.4 cm], the bottle molded with eight panels of flowers and leaves, narrow clear glass vertical windows, stopper with conforming design, the designs embellished with blue and orange enamel, bottom signed *J. Viard* in the mold. Est. $1,200.00-$1,500.00.

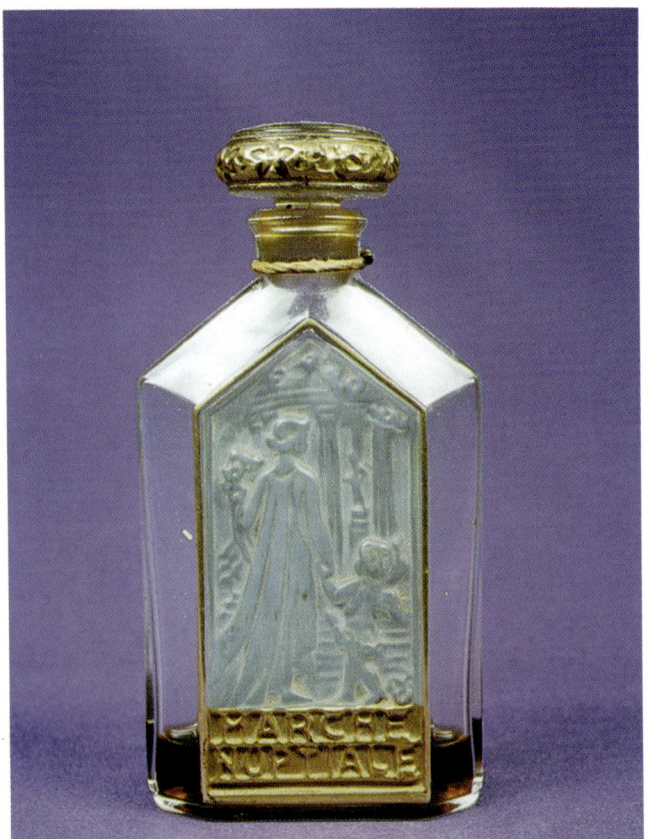

Lot #374. Marques de Elorza *Marche Nuptiale* ['Wedding March'] rare clear and frosted glass bottle and stopper, 4.1" [10.4 cm], the front with a molded tableau of Cupid leading a bride to the altar, light green patina with the name in gold enamel, the stopper molded *Marques de Elorza*, by J. Viard, unsigned. Cf. Lefkowith, p. 100. Est. $2,500.00-$3,000.00.

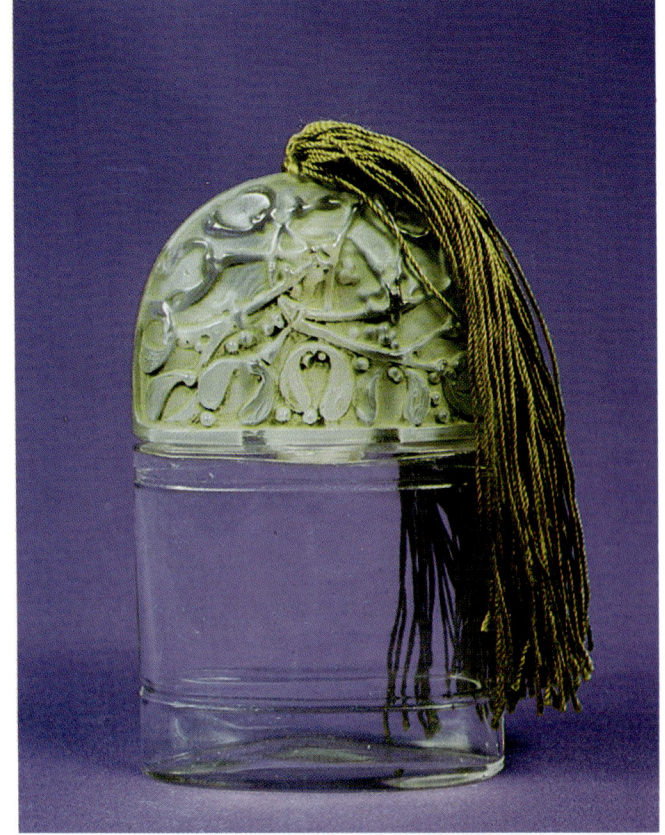

Lot #375. Jean de Parys *Sous le Gui* ['Under the Mistletoe'], rare clear glass perfume bottle with inner stopper and heavy frosted glass overcap, 4" [10.2 cm], in the shape of a Japanese inro, overcap molded with mistletoe, empty, no label, the overcap entirely patinated in green and with a green tassel, unsigned. Utt #JP-2. Est. $2,000.00-$2,500.00.

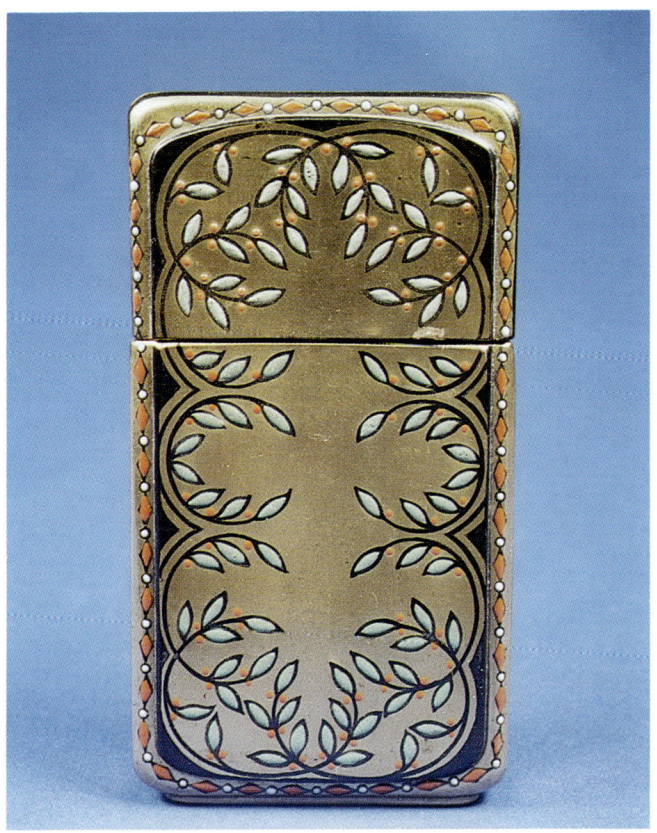

Lot #376. Babani *Abdulla* very rare clear glass bottle with inner stopper and black glass overcap, 4.9" [12.5 cm], in the shape of a Japanese inro, enameled in gold with a design of leaves and berries in green, orange and black, empty, [the gold generally in good condition, but with one worn spot on the side of cap and one very small wear spot on front]; bottom marked *Abdulla Babani Paris,* by Dépinoix. Probably made for the French market, note the spelling without a final *h;* cf. Monsen & Baer 1994, lot #281, Lefkowith, p. 90. Est. $2,500.000-$3,500.00.

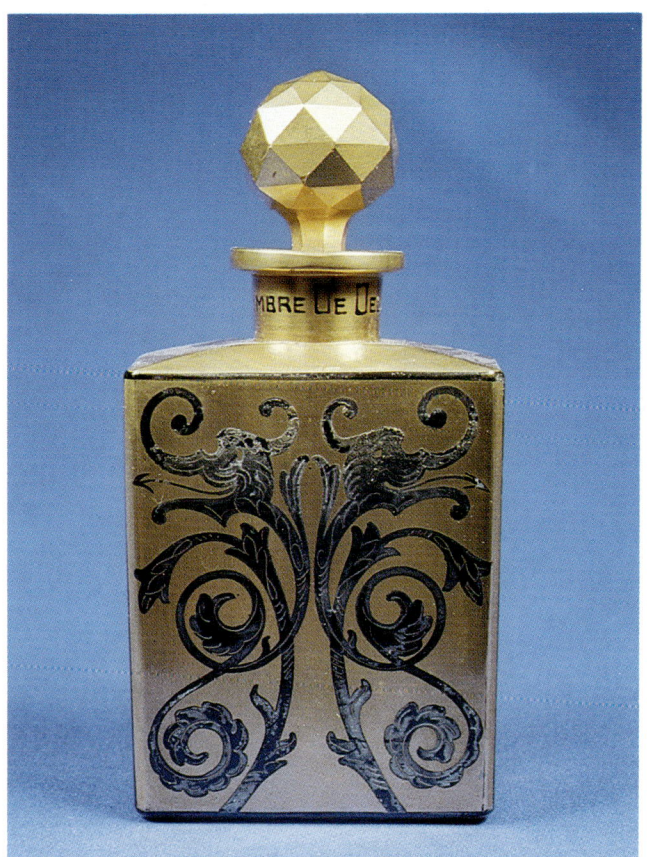

Lot #377. Babani *Ambre de Delhi* clear glass bottle and stopper, 5.2" [13.2 cm], the rectangular bottle and its ball-shaped stopper with triangular facets enameled in gold with a beautiful design of leaves and scrolls in black enamel, empty, names in black enamel around neck, bottom molded *Babani deposé Paris France;* designed by Dépinoix circa 1919, cf. Lefkowith, pl. 80. Est. $2,500.00-$3,500.00.

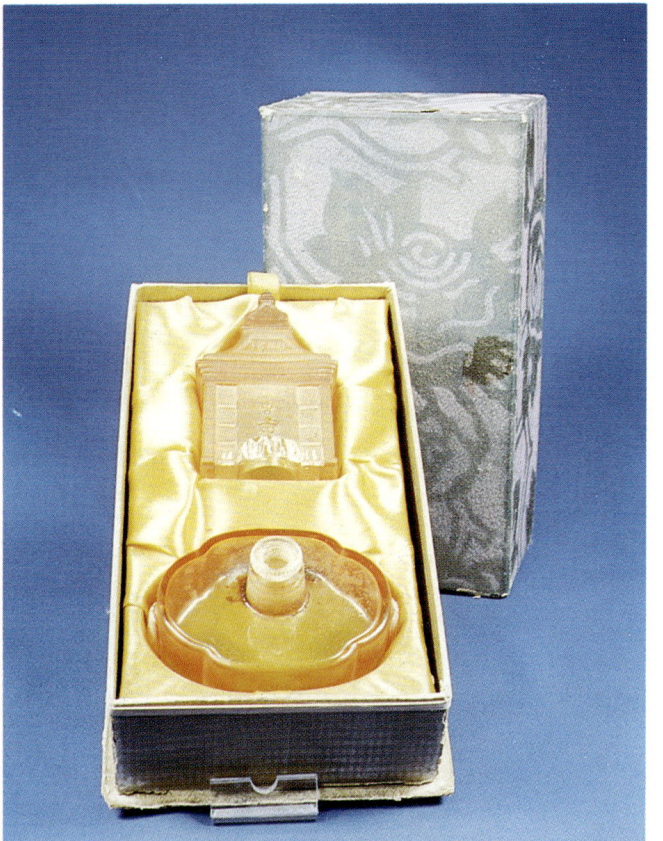

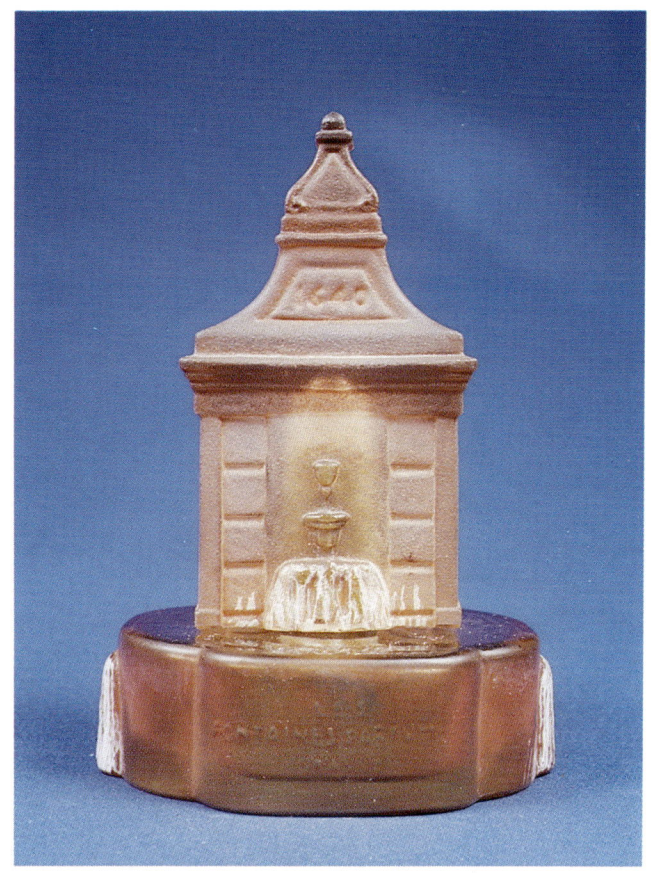

Lot #378. Pélissier-Aragon [Grasse] *Les Fontaines Parfumées* clear and frosted glass figural bottle, inner stopper and heavy overcap, 5" [12.7 cm], the bottle designed as the pool of the fountain with its upper surface in clear glass, the overcap designed as the fountain itself, amber patina overall with the jets of water enameled in white, in its box covered with blue and purple flowers and lined with yellow gold satin, by M. Dépinoix, unsigned. This is a very rare and unusual bottle. Est. $3,500.00-$4,500.00.

CZECHOSLOVAKIAN PERFUME BOTTLES

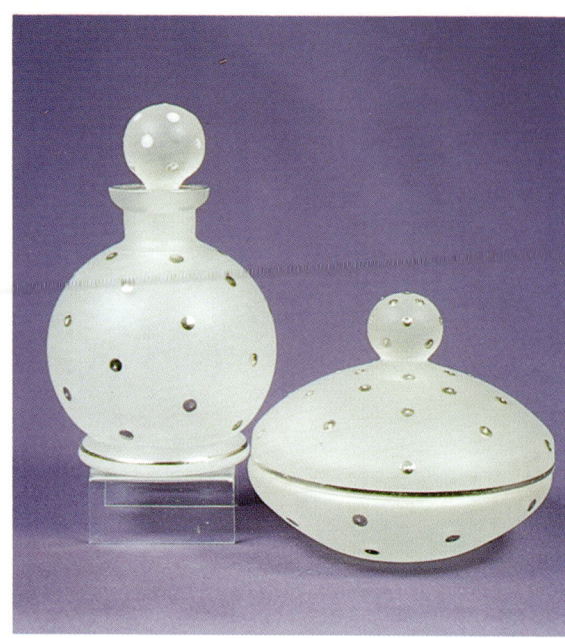

Lot #380. Frosted glass dresser set: perfume bottle and stopper, 5" [12.7 cm], of ball shape with a short pedestal base, decorated with silver-covered white enamel dots; powder box and cover, 3.5" [8.9 cm], similar design and decoration, small chip to edge of cover, both items signed *Czechoslovakia* in white enamel on the bottom. Est. $75.00-$125.00.

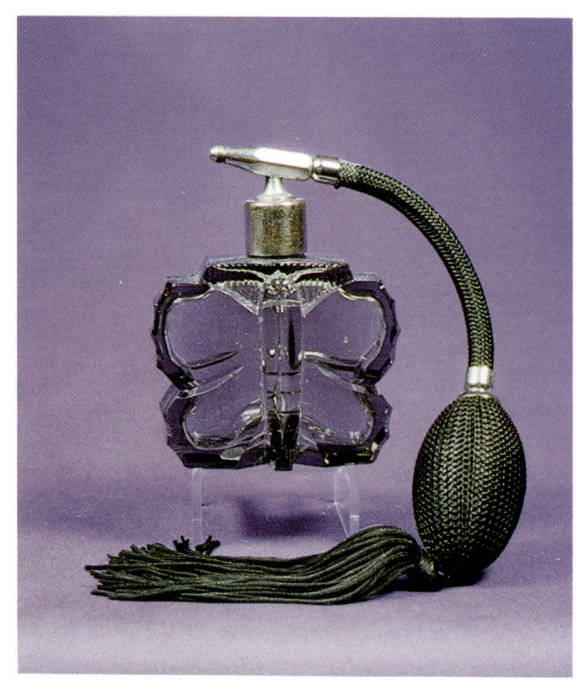

Lot #379. Lubin *Au Soleil* ['To the Sun'] frosted glass bottle and stopper, 5.6" [14.2 cm], an unusual bottle of trumpet shape molded with a salamander in relief making his way up a brick wall toward a fly perched on the side of the stopper, enameled in dark green and gold with gray patina, empty, name in gold enamel on front, bottom signed *Lubin Paris,* by M. Dépinoix, unsigned, circa 1909-1912. Est. $2,500.00-$3,000.00.

Lot #381. Smoke-colored crystal bottle with chrome atomizer attachment, 3.6" [9.1 cm], the bottle molded in the shape of a butterfly, new ball and tassel, bottom signed *Czechoslovakia* in a line. Est. $200.00-$300.00.

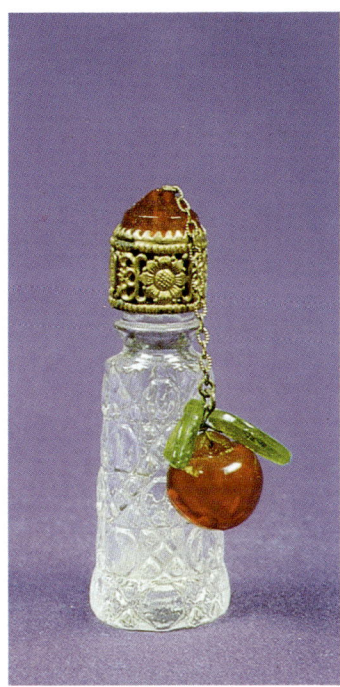

Lot #382. Clear glass perfume bottle with gold metal filagree cap, 2.6" [6.6 cm], the cap mounted with a red glass stone and a glass dauber, a red glass apple with green glass leaves hangs by a chain from the cap, signed *Czechoslovakia* on the metal cap. Est. $100.00-$150.00.

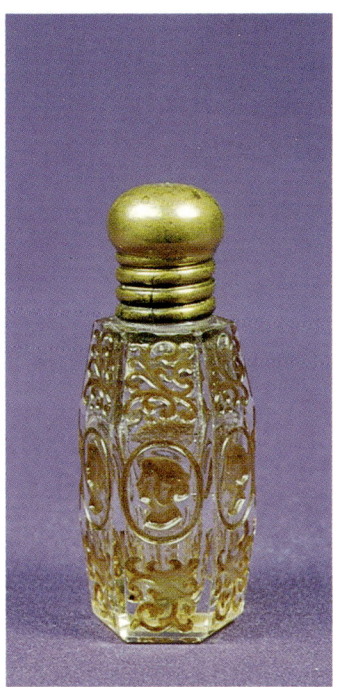

Lot #383. Clear crystal bottle with round brass cap, 2.5" [6.4 cm], of hexagonal shape with a cameo of a woman's head intaglio cut on each side, amber patina, unsigned. Est. $100.00-$150.00.

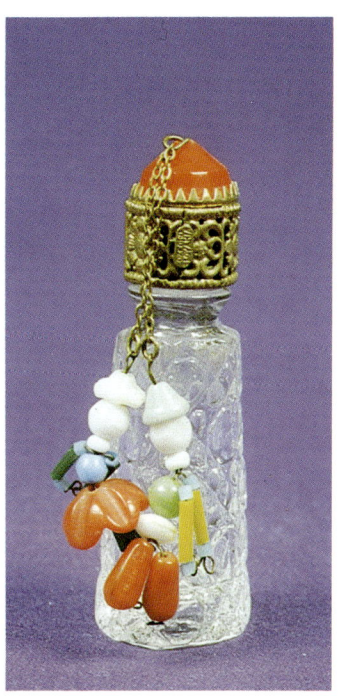

Lot #384. Clear glass bottle and and metal filigree cap, 2.5" [6.4 cm], metal cap with glass dauber and topped with an opaque red stone; two dancers fashioned out of beads are attached with a small chain at the top of the cap, signed *Czechoslovakia* on a metal tag on cap. Est. $125.00-$150.00.

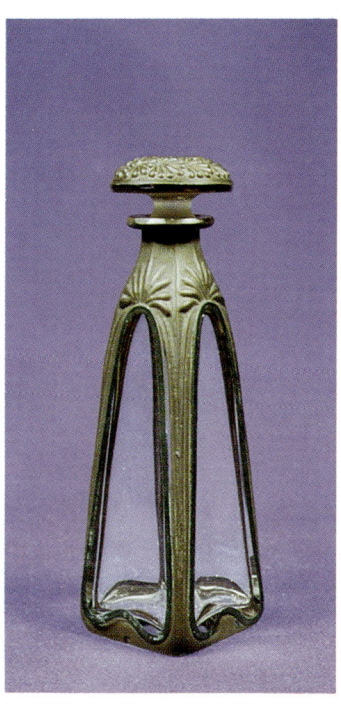

Lot #385. Clear crystal bottle and stopper, 4.4" [11.2 cm], the bottle with four clear windows and molded with a leaf motif, stopper with conforming design, parts of the bottle covered with brown and black enamel, unsigned, undoubtedly for a commercial perfume. Est. $150.00-$250.00.

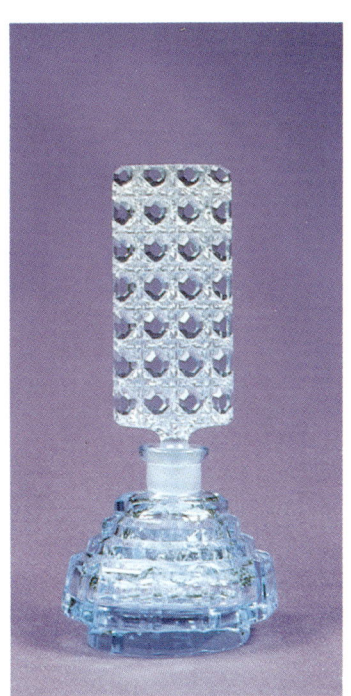

Lot #386. Blue crystal bottle and stopper, 5.9" [15 cm], the large rectangular stopper cut in the Russian pattern giving a jewel-like appearance, the bottle molded with a step motif and highly cut, with its dauber, signed *Czechoslovakia* in an oval. Est. $175.00-$250.00.

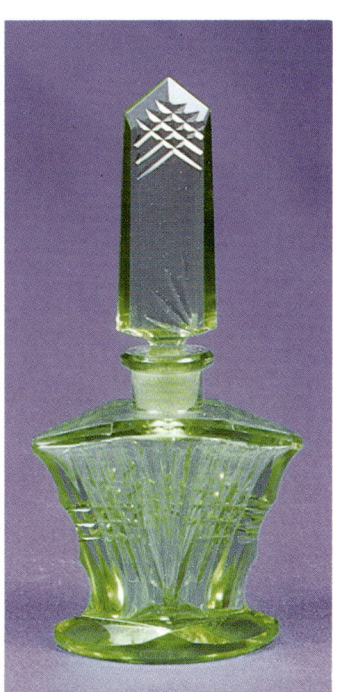

Lot #387. Green crystal bottle and stopper, 5.8" [14.7 cm], the urn-shaped bottle cut with vertical facets and then with three horizontal ones, the stopper shaped as a flat prism and with facets conforming to those of the bottle, with its dauber, signed *Czechoslovakia* in an oval. Est. $150.00-$225.00.

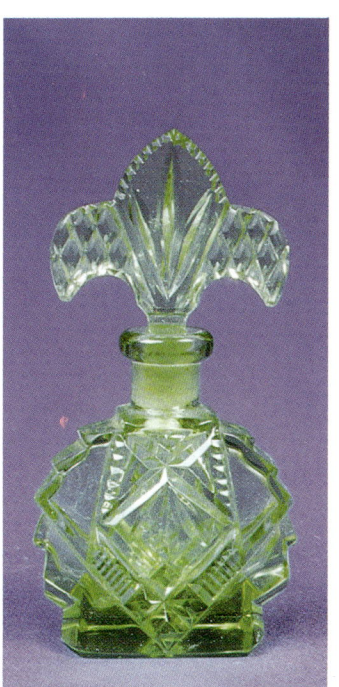

Lot #388. Green crystal bottle and stopper, 5" [12.6 cm], the stopper of unusual leaf-form shape, both bottle and stopper cut with leaf-form and geometric facets, with its dauber, unsigned. Est. $150.00-$225.00.

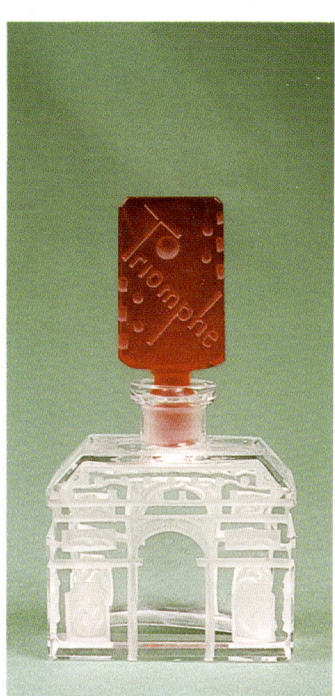

Lot #389. Leon Laraine *Triomphe* clear and frosted crystal bottle and red crystal stopper in the form of the Arc de Triomphe, 5.2" [13.2 cm], empty, name intaglio cut into stopper, signed *Czechoslovakia* in an oval. Cf. North #821. Est. $175.00-$250.00.

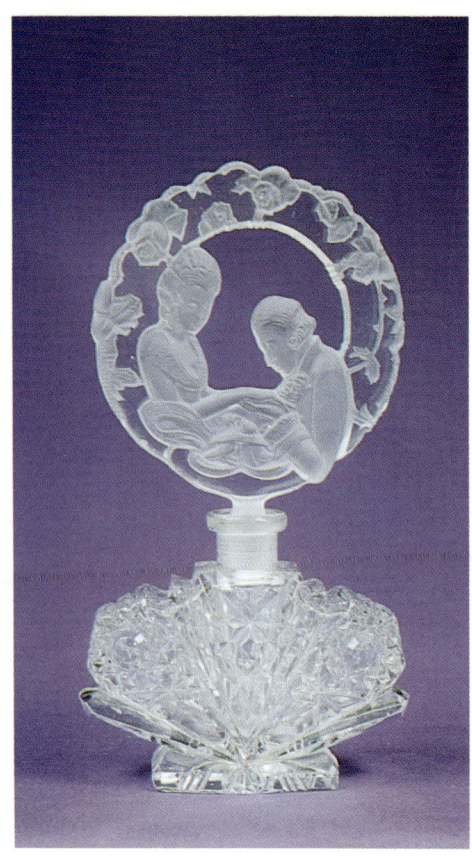
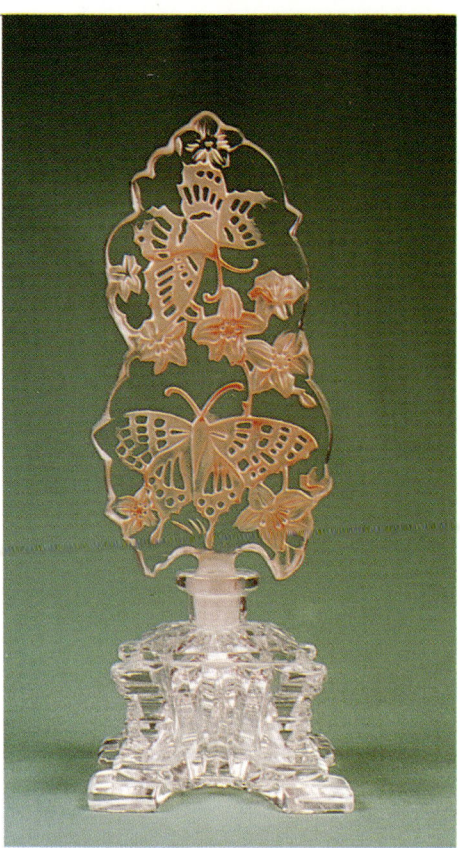
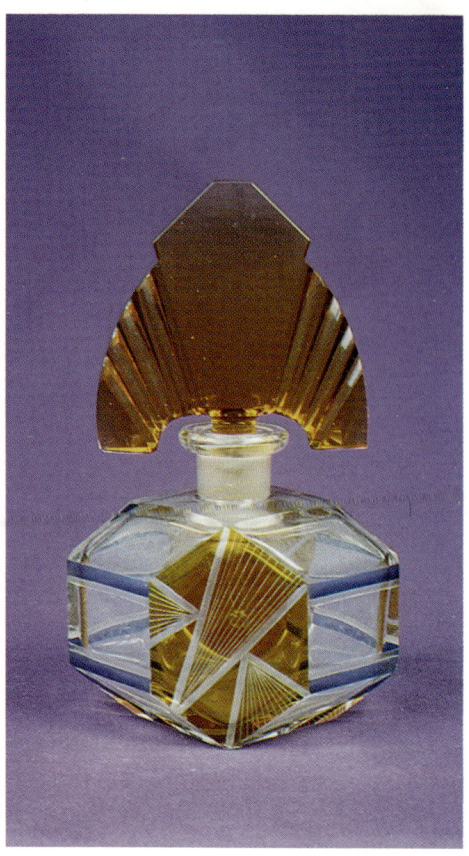

Lot #390. Statuesque clear crystal perfume bottle and stopper, 8" [20.3 cm], heavily cut base, stopper molded with a gentleman caressing a lady's hand in a ring of flowers, no dauber, bottom with *Premier* silver label and signed *Czechoslovakia* in a line. North #304 [stopper]. Est. $400.00-$500.00.

Lot #391. Very large clear crystal bottle and stopper, 8.5" [21.6 cm], the base designed with four feet and multiple facets, the huge stopper intaglio cut with butterflies and flowers which bear a reddish patina, dauber lacking, signed *Czechoslovakia* in an oval. Est. $450.00-$550.00.

Lot #392. Clear crystal bottle with amber and blue overlay, amber crystal stopper, 6" [15.2 cm], the base of the bottle wheel cut to create an Art Deco sunray motif, with its dauber, apparently unsigned. Est. $300.00-$400.00.

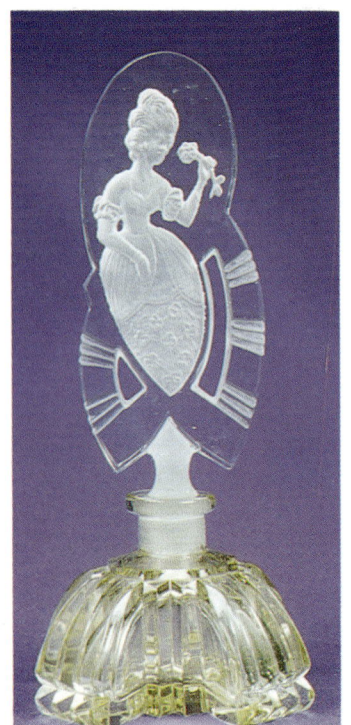
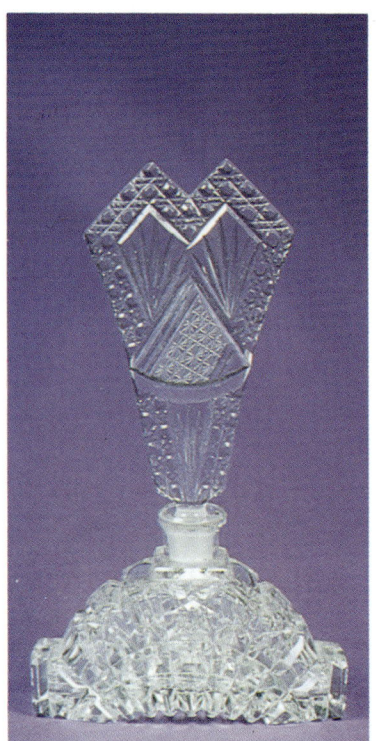
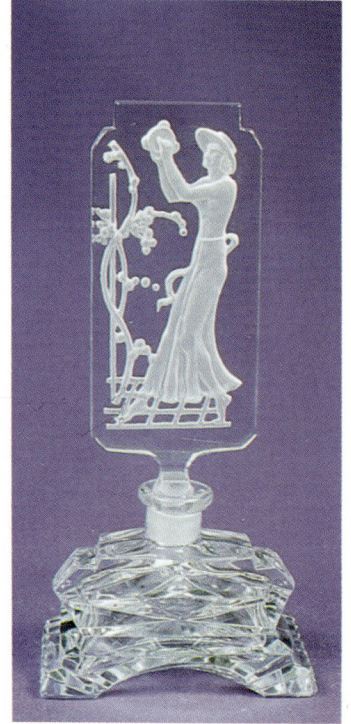
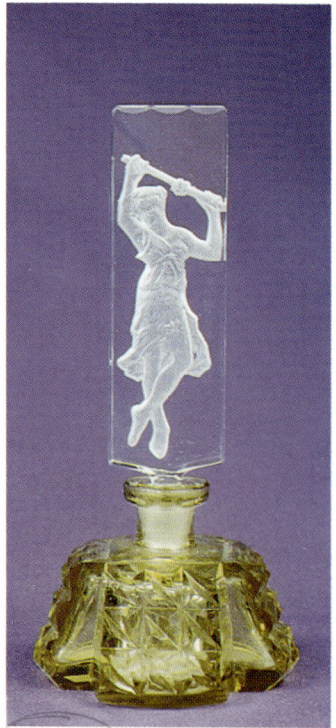

Lot #393. Yellow crystal bottle and clear crystal stopper, 7.3" [18.5 cm], the bottle molded with four feet and with vertical facets, the stopper intaglio cut with a maiden holding a rose, the stopper also with cut out parts, dauber lacking, signed *Czechoslovakia* in a line. Est. $400.00-$500.00.

Lot #394. Large clear crystal bottle and stopper, 7.9" [20.1 cm], the bottle of fan shape and cut with elaborate intersecting facets, the stopper also highly cut, dauber lacking, bottom signed *Czechoslovakia* in a small circle and also in an unusual much larger circle. Est. $200.00-$300.00.

Lot #395. Clear crystal bottle and stopper, 6.8" [17.3 cm], the bottle with highly cut facets, the stopper intaglio cut with a tambourine dancer, corners of stopper faceted at an angle, dauber lacking, signed *Czechoslovakia* in a circle. Cf. North #402; Monsen & Baer 1992 lot #273. Est. $350.00-$450.00.

Lot #396. Yellow crystal bottle and clear crystal stopper, 5.5" [14 cm], the stopper intaglio cut with a baton dancer dressed *à la grecque,* dauber lacking, apparently unsigned. Cf. North #49. Est. $250.00-$350.00.

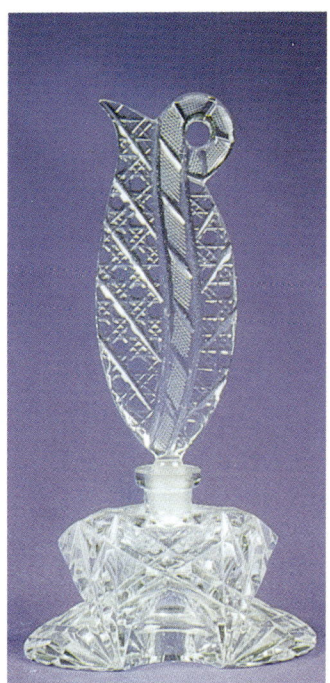

Lot #397. Clear crystal bottle and stopper, 7.6" [19.3 cm], the bottle of oblong shape and cut with deep facets, the stopper shaped as a leaf with an additional abstract motif and cut in an elaborate design, dauber lacking, bottom signed *Czechoslovakia* in an oval and with *Sico* silver label. Est. $250.00-$350.00.

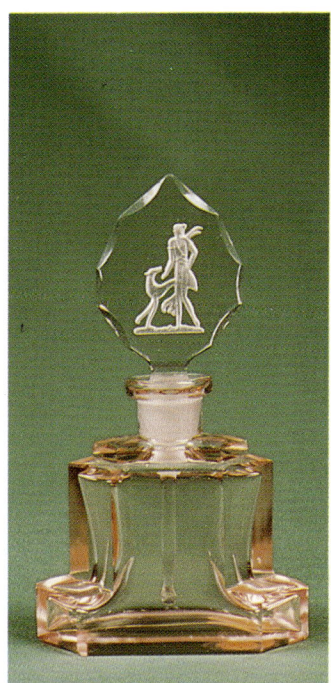

Lot #398. Pink crystal bottle and clear crystal stopper, 4.8" [12.2 cm], the base of flattened hexagonal form, the stopper with scalloped edges and intaglio cut with a woman and a dog, with its dauber, signed *Czechoslovakia* in an oval and with silver *Morlee* label. Cf. Forsythe II, #845. Est. $200.00-$275.00.

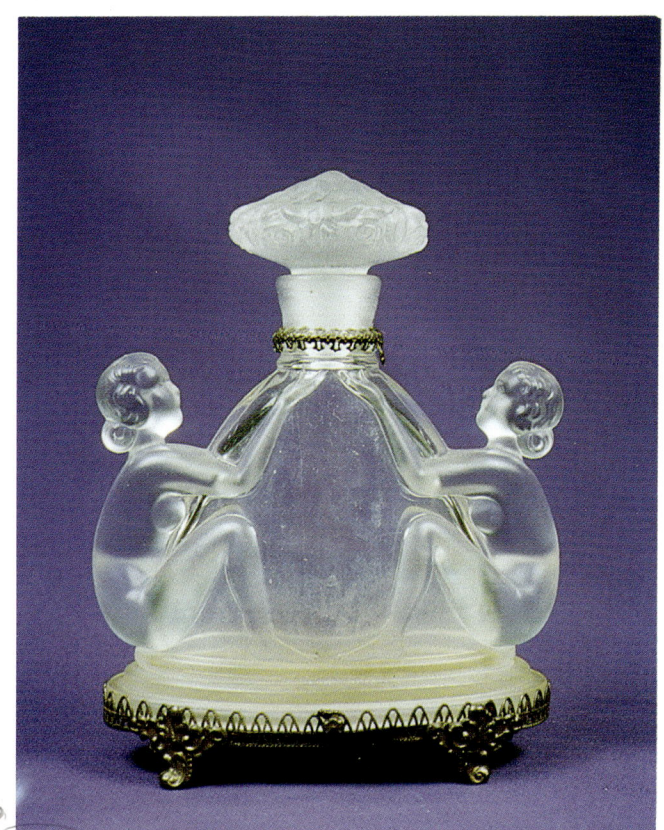

Lot #399. Rare clear crystal bottle and stopper, 5.2" [13.2 cm], designed as two nudes encircling an urn, metalwork band around neck and on a metal plinth, stopper, without dauber, molded as a bouquet of flowers, unsigned. North #590; Forsythe II #727. Est. $500.00-$750.00.

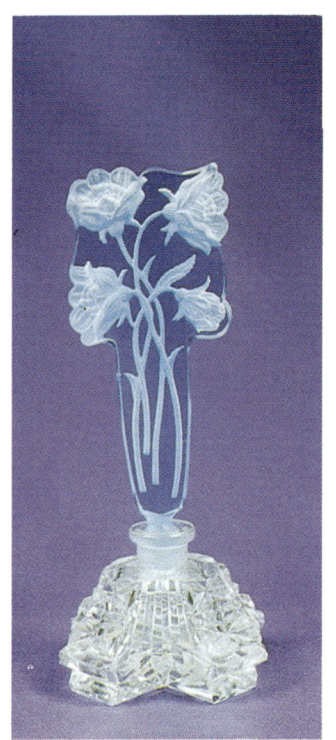

Lot #400. Clear crystal bottle and blue crystal stopper, 6.4" [16.3 cm], the bottle designed with four sides, all heavily faceted, the stopper intaglio cut with roses, with its dauber, original I.Rice label, signed *Czechoslovakia* in a circle. Est. $150.00-$200.00.

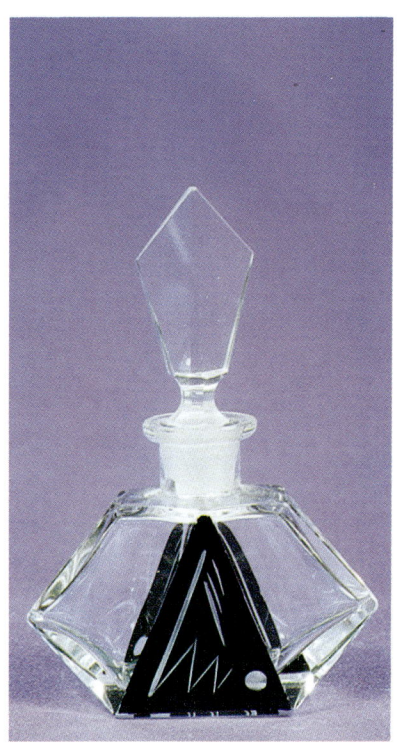

Lot #401. Clear crystal bottle and stopper, 3.7" [9.4 cm], the front and back with triangular facets enameled with an Art Deco design, with its dauber, signed *Czechoslovakia* in a circle. Est. $100.00-$150.00.

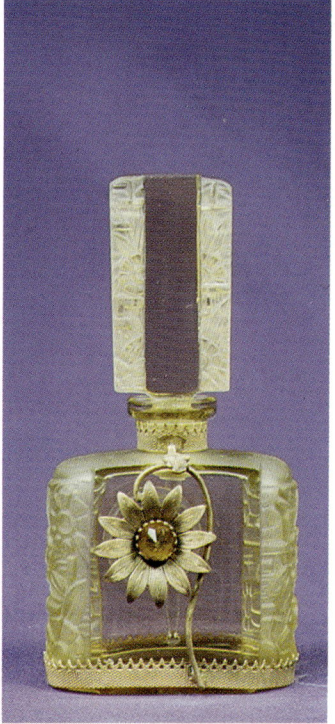

Lot #402. Yellow crystal bottle and stopper, 5.3" [13.5 cm], with stylized Art Deco flowers on both sides of the bottle and on the stopper, with its dauber, mounted with a metal jeweled flower attached to a metal band around the neck and around the base of the bottle, signed *Czechoslovakia* in a circle. Est. $350.00-$450.00.

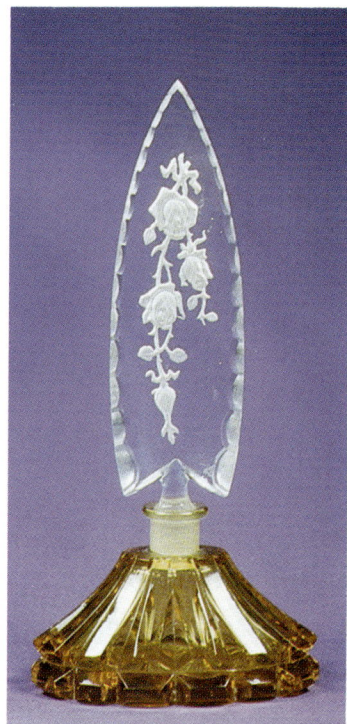

Lot #403. Very large amber crystal bottle and clear crystal stopper, 8.8" [22.4 cm], the oval base cut with facets all around, the stopper intaglio cut with a spray of roses, with its dauber, signed *Czechoslovakia* in a line. Est. $450.00-$550.00.

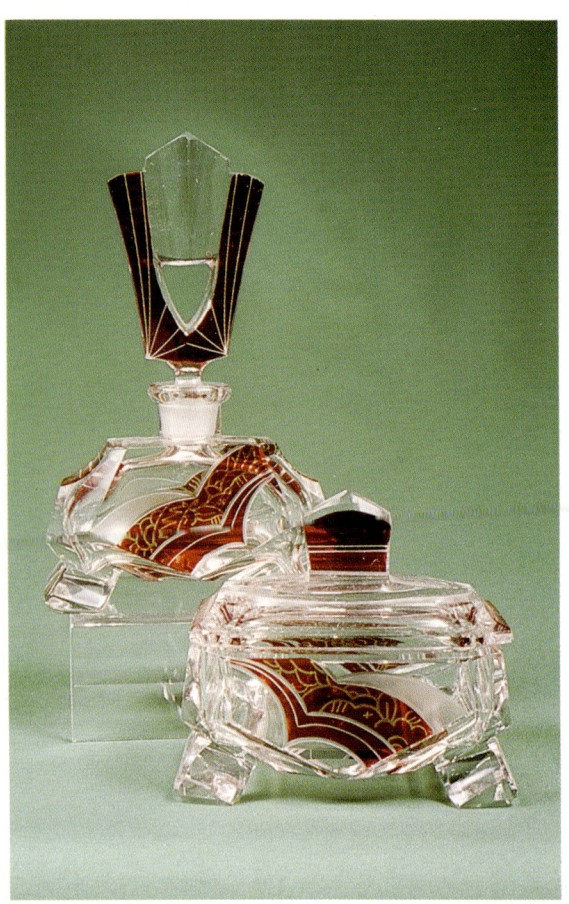

Lot #404. Clear crystal bottle and stopper, 5.9" [15 cm], the bottle resting on two feet with multiple angular facets, the stopper with a cut out triangle, parts enameled in translucent scarlet and then wheel-cut in an Art Deco leaf design; clear crystal covered powder box of identical design, 3" [7.6 cm], both unsigned. Two items. Est. $300.00-$400.00.

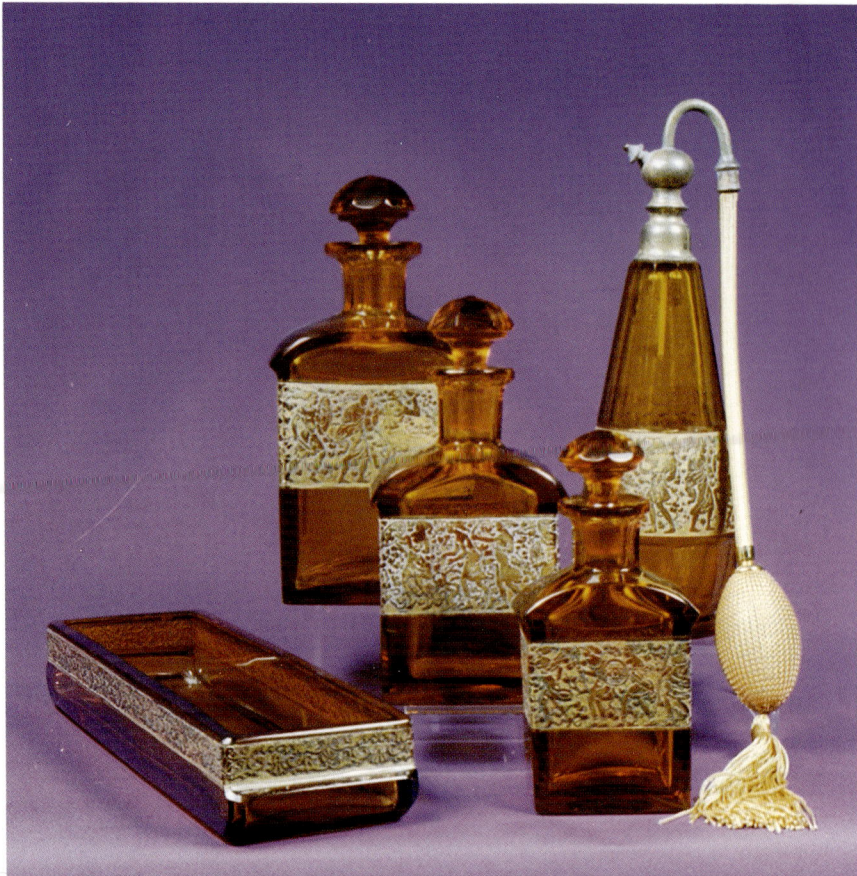

Lot #405. Moser sumptuous dresser set of five items in amber crystal, all with decorative gilded friezes: large cologne bottle and stopper, 6.7" [17 cm], molded with a frieze of Centaurs and warriors; middle cologne bottle, 6" [15.2 cm], molded with a frieze of female warriors; perfume bottle and stopper, 5.2" [13.2 cm], with a frieze of female warriors; comb tray, 9" long [22.9 cm], with a band of scrolls; bottle with atomizer attachment, new ball and tassel, with a frieze of Centaurs and warriors; each piece is signed *Moser Carlsbad Made in Cecko-Slovakia*. Five items. Est. $1,500.00-$2,000.00.

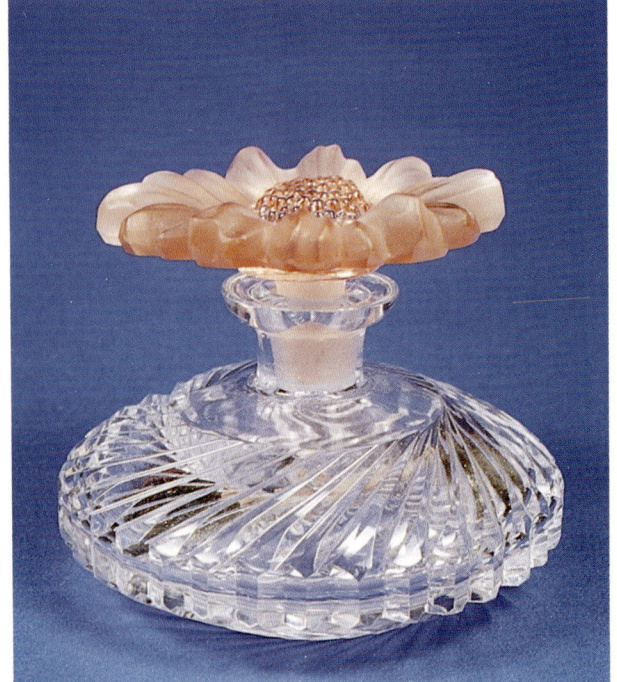

Lot #406. Clear crystal bottle and frosted peach-colored stopper, 2.8" [7.1 cm], the round flattened bottle cut entirely with facets, the stopper in the shape of an open flower, no dauber, signed *Czechoslovakia* in a line. Est. $250.00-$350.00.

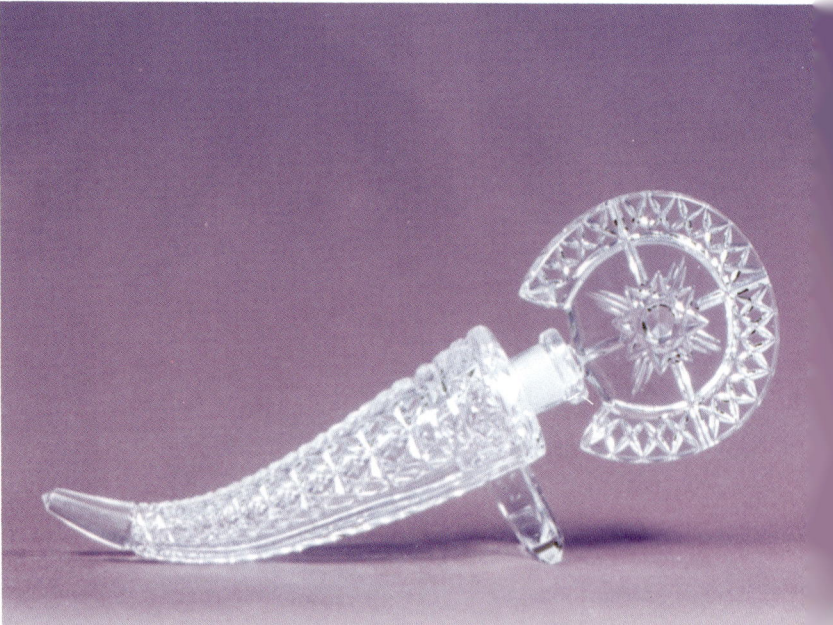

Lot #407. Clear crystal bottle and stopper, 9.5" long and 4.3" tall [24 x 10.9 cm], the bottle of scimitar form and resting on a single foot, both bottle and stopper with a star-form motif, dauber lacking, signed *Czechoslovakia* in a circle. Est. $300.00-$400.00.

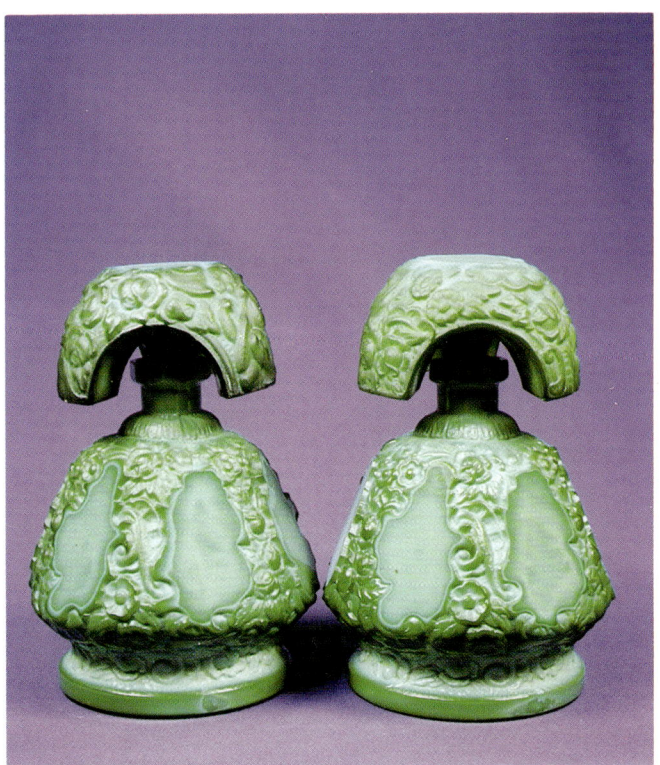

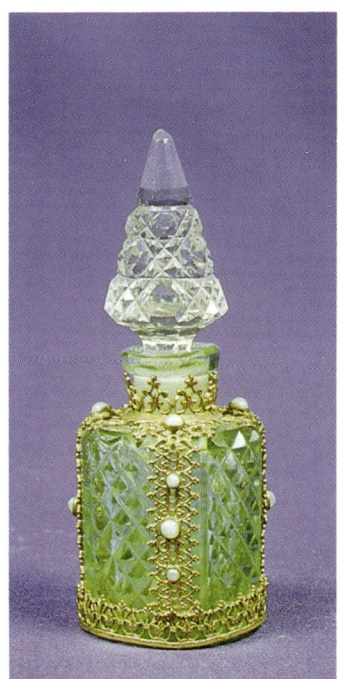

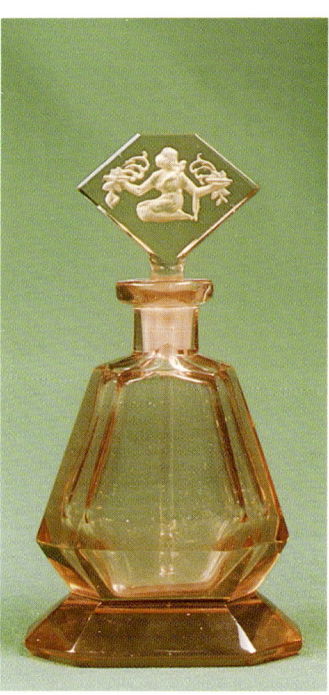

Lot #408. Stunning pair of malachite glass bottles and stoppers, 6" [15.2 cm], the stoppers designed in a tiara form with three parts, a cupid amid branches and flowers is molded on the stopper and its top is highly polished to show the variegated malachite colors; the bottles are molded with flowers and cut with polished facets on six sides, both unsigned. Two items. Est. $1,000.00-$1,200.00.

Lot #409. Green crystal bottle and clear crystal stopper, 3.9" [9.9 cm], the bottle cut with a diamond motif, the stopper shaped as a spire and also with facets, dauber lacking, covered with metalwork and opalescent green jewels, bottom signed *Czechoslovakia* in a circle, metal signed *Tchecoslovakie* on a tag. Est. $150.00-$225.00.

Lot #410. Peach crystal bottle and stopper, 5.4" [13.7 cm], the bottle designed with a large faceted base, the stopper intaglio cut with a kneeling maiden holding flowers in both hands, with its dauber, signed *Czechoslovakia* in an oval. Est. $200.00-$250.00.

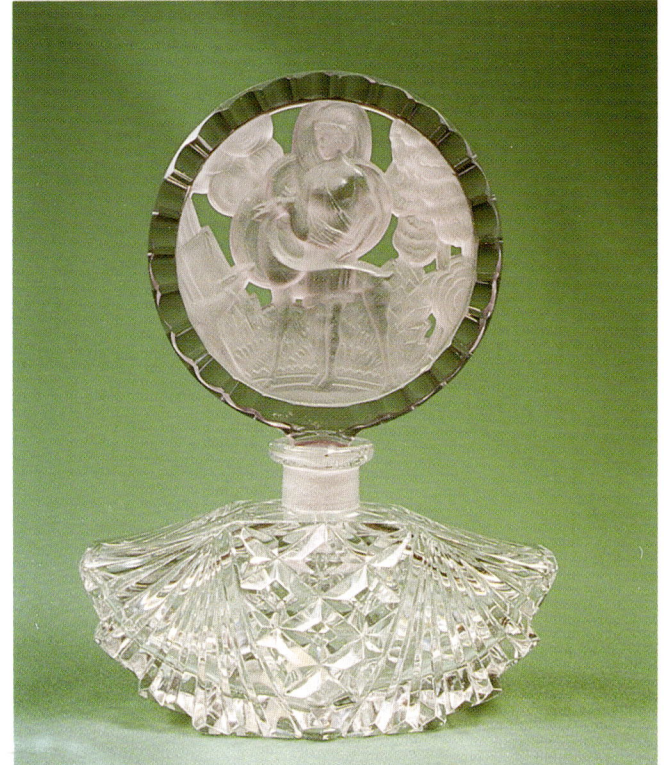

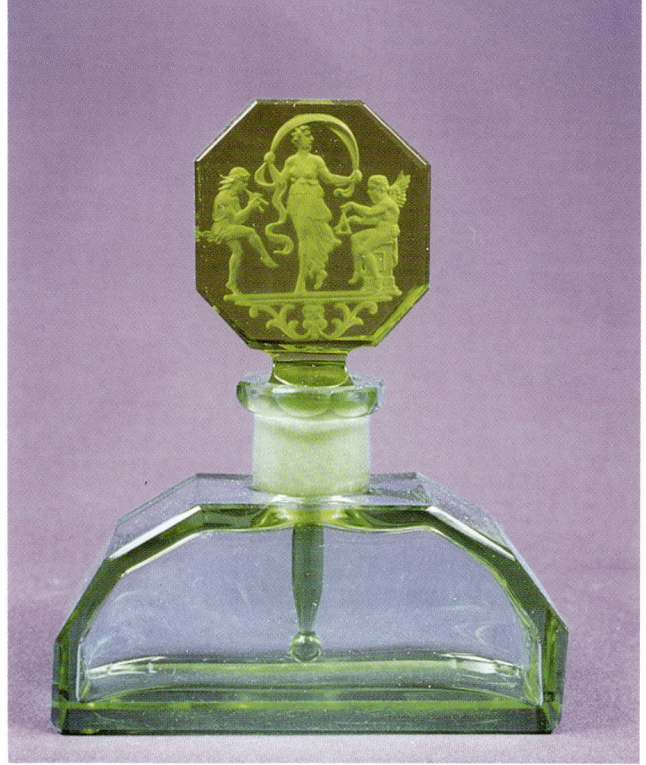

Lot #411. Rare clear crystal bottle and heather-colored stopper, 6.3" [16 cm], the bottle of boat shape with facets in a fan and diamond motif, the stopper intricately molded on both sides with a classical youth feeding a deer and her fawn against a background of flowers and leaves, part of dauber remaining, bottom signed *Czechoslovakia* in an oval and with *Morlee* paper label; the intricate cut-out parts of the stopper and its rare pinkish-violet color make it very exceptional. Cf. Forsythe II, #689. Est. $650.00-$800.00.

Lot #412. Emerald green crystal bottle and stopper, 4" [10.2 cm], the bottle with a rectangular shape at the bottom and rounded in facets over the top, the stopper depicting a lady in classical dress with two cupids playing the Pan flute and the triangle, with its original green dauber, by Hoffman, signed *Czechoslovakia* in a line. Cf. North #812. Est. $300.00-$400.00.

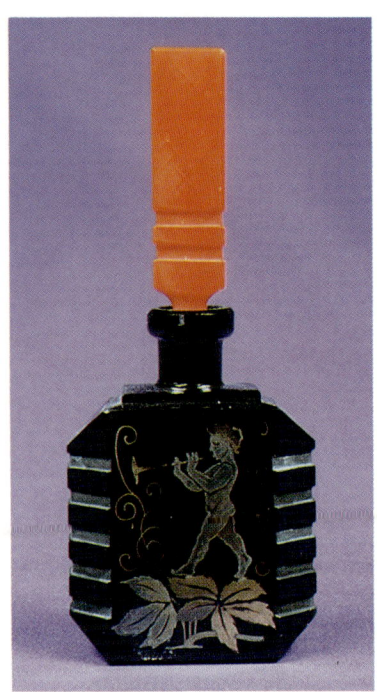

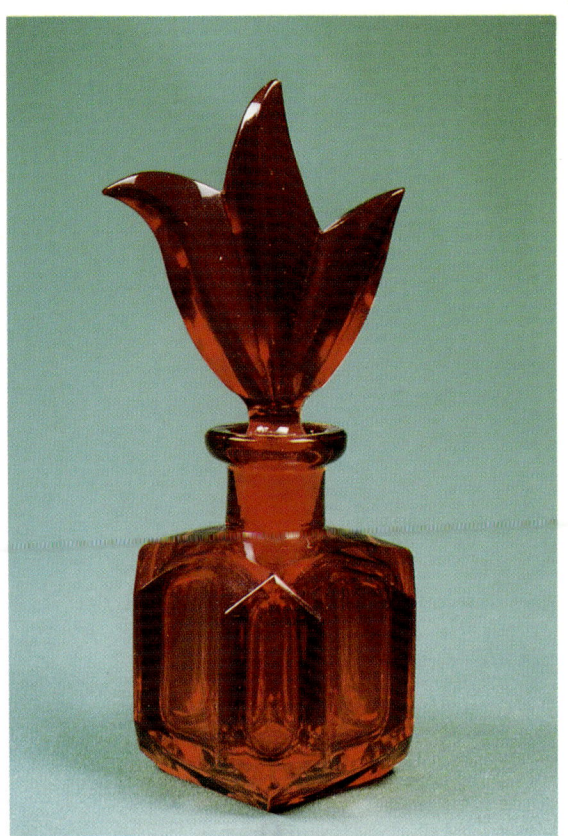

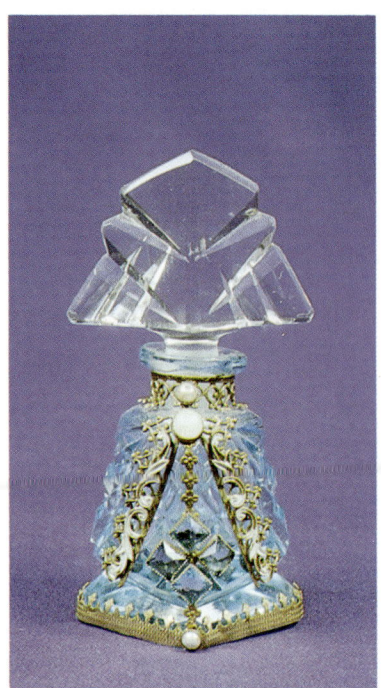

Lot #413. Black crystal bottle and red crystal stopper, 5.8" [14.7 cm], the sides of the bottle cut with rectangular indented bars which are frosted, the stopper also designed with the same bars [dauber lacking], the front of the bottle enameled in gold with a cupid playing a horn among leaves and scrolls, unsigned. Est. $400.00-$500.00.

Lot #414. Rare red crystal bottle and stopper, 5.6" [14.2 cm], the square-shaped bottle with indented sides, the stopper molded as stylized leaves, no dauber, unsigned; the use of red crystal for both bottle and stopper is extremely rare among Czechoslovakian perfume bottles. Est. $600.00-$850.00.

Lot #415. Blue crystal bottle and clear crystal stopper, 3.8" [9.7 cm], both bottle and stopper highly cut with facets in a similar motif, the front of the bottle covered in metalwork with pearls and blue stones, with its dauber, silver *Morlee* label, signed *Czechoslovakia* in oval. Est. $375.00-$475.00.

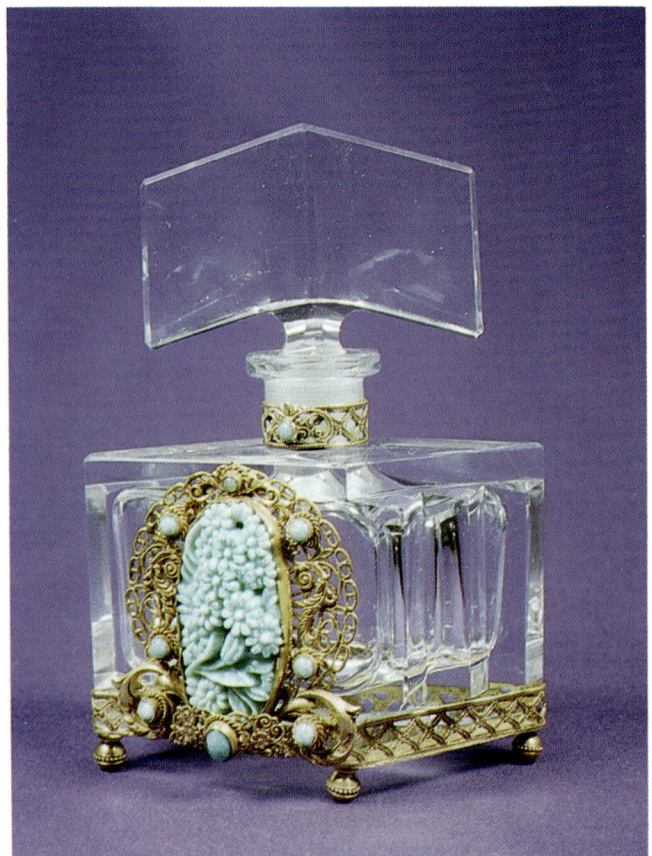

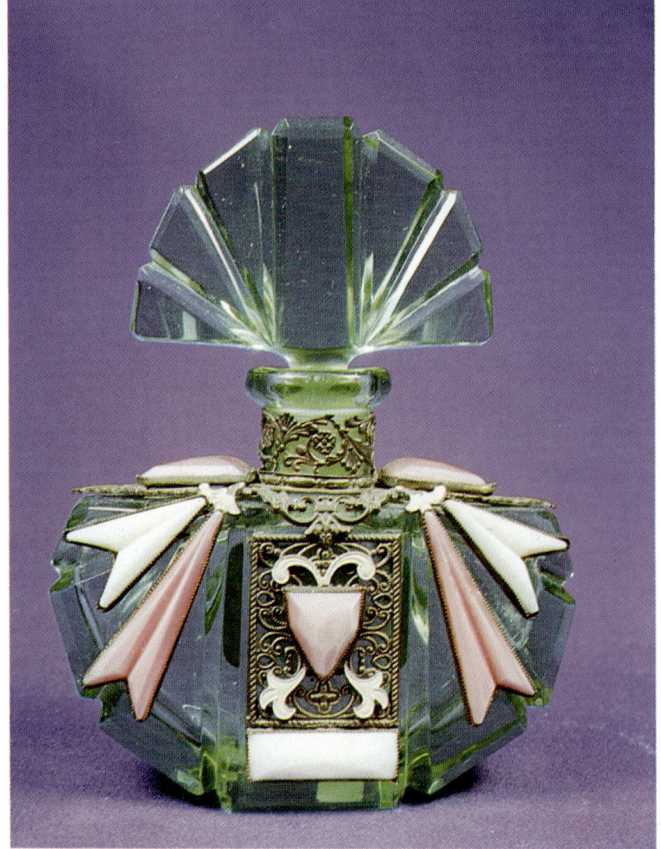

Lot #416. Clear crystal bottle and stopper, 5.3" [13.5 cm], the bottle of diamond form with large triangular facets cut on two opposite sides, in a gold metal framework with jade glass cabochons and a large jade glass medallion of flowers, dauber lacking, signed *Czechoslovakia* in a line. Cf. Forsythe II, #1001. Est. $375.00-$475.00.

Lot #417. Green crystal bottle and stopper, 4.4" [11.2 cm], designed with fan-shaped facets, beautifully jeweled with pink and white stones cut in chevron shapes on the front and shoulders of the bottle, no dauber, silver *Morlee* label, bottom signed *Czechoslovakia* in a circle and metalwork also stamped *Czechoslovakia*. Est. $500.00-$650.00.

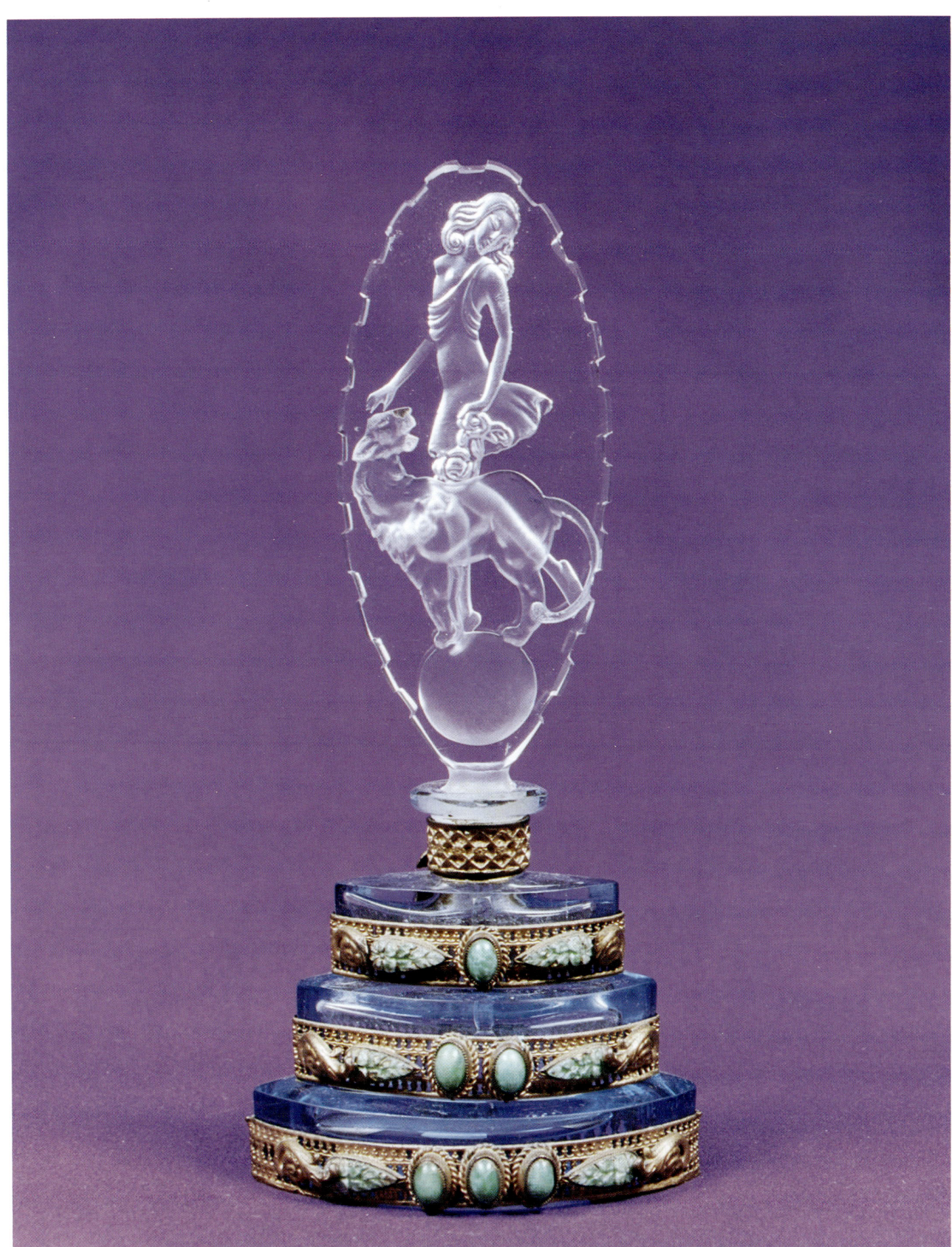

Lot #418. Blue crystal bottle and clear crystal stopper, 6.9" [17.5 cm], the bottle designed in a step motif and wrapped with a metal band with green glass stones, the stopper intaglio-cut on both sides with the figure of a woman with a garland of roses on one side and a panther on the other; the edges of the stopper cut with rectangular indentations, with its dauber, signed *Czechoslovakia* in a line. Est. $1,000.00-$1,250.00.

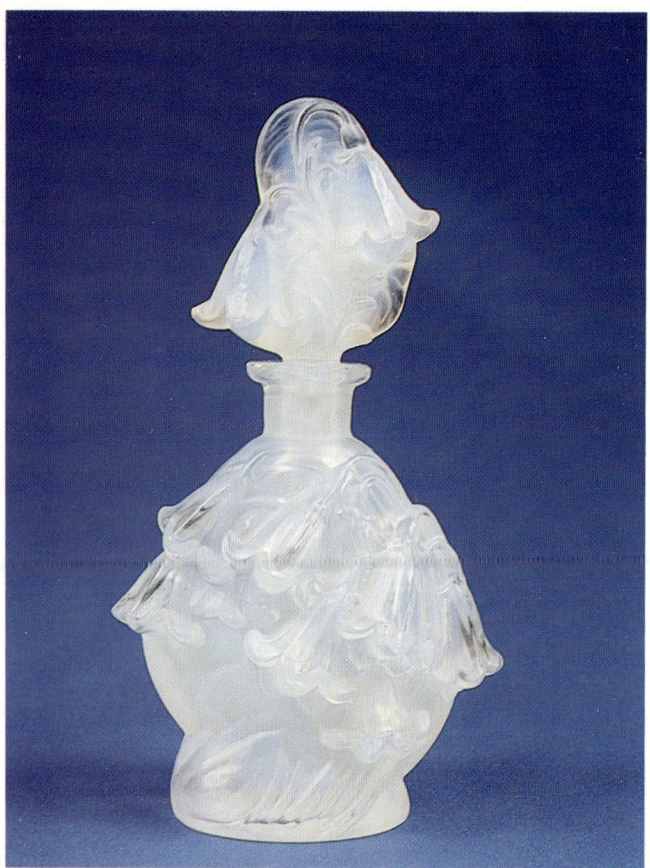

Lot #419. Opalescent crystal bottle and stopper, 6.6" [16.8 cm], the bottle and stopper molded with large bluebells, with its long dauber intact, by Ingrid, apparently unsigned. Est. $800.00-$1,000.00.

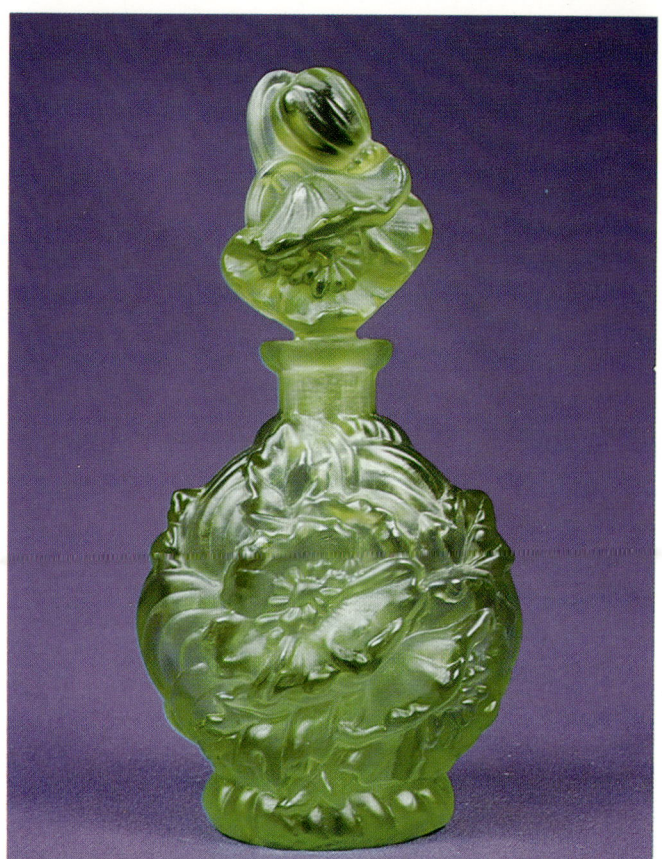

Lot #420. Rare translucent green glass perfume bottle and stopper, 6.6" [16.8 cm], the bottle molded completely with oriental poppies in full bloom, the stopper molded as a poppy seed pod and blossom, with its dauber, signed *Ingrid Czechoslovakia*. Est. $900.00-$1,100.00.

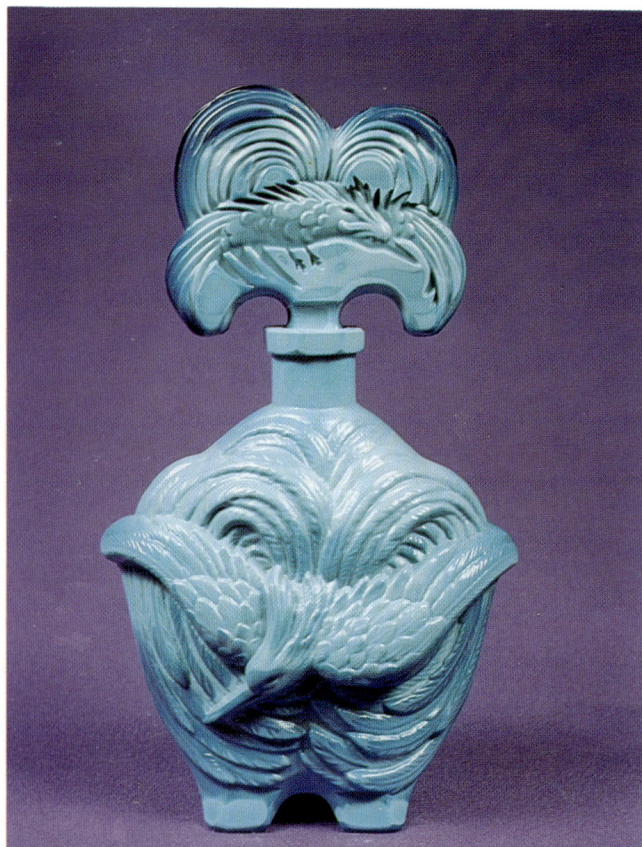

Lot #421. Ingrid very fine opaque blue crystal bottle and stopper, 6.8" [17.3 cm], the bottle with four feet, molded on both sides with a large bird whose feathers in swirls cover the entire surface of the bottle, the stopper also molded with a plumed bird, with its very long dauber, signed *Ingrid Czechoslovakia* on one foot. Cf. North #200; Monsen and Baer 1997, lot #418. Est. $1,200.00-$1,500.00.

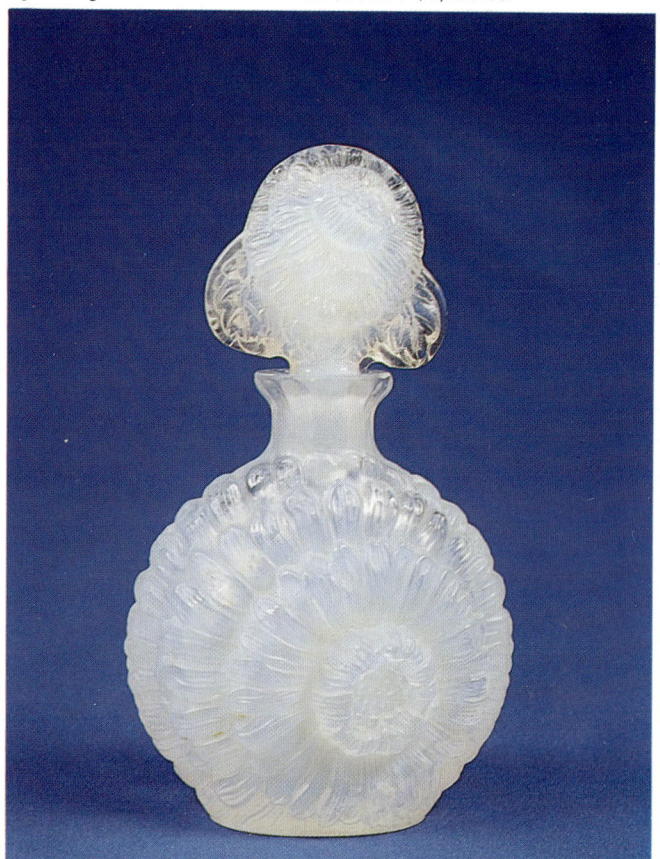

Lot #422. Opalescent crystal bottle and stopper, 5" [14.2 cm], the bottle molded on both sides as a single open chrysanthemum, the stopper with the same design on a smaller scale, with its long dauber, by Ingrid, unsigned. Est. $800.00-$1,000.00.

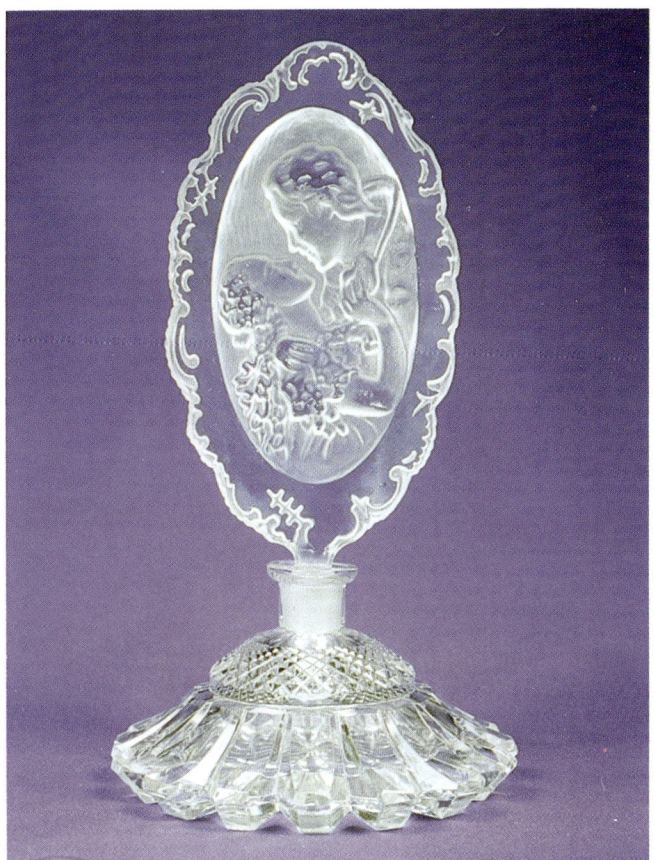

Lot #423. Rare and very fine clear crystal bottle and stopper of very large proportions, 8.7" [22 cm], the bottle shaped as an star form with sixteen points, the stopper molded as two lovers [thought by many collectors to be Rhett and Scarlet] in an embrace, dauber lacking, unsigned, bottom of bottle also faceted. Cf. Forsythe II, #682. Est. $600.00-$750.00.

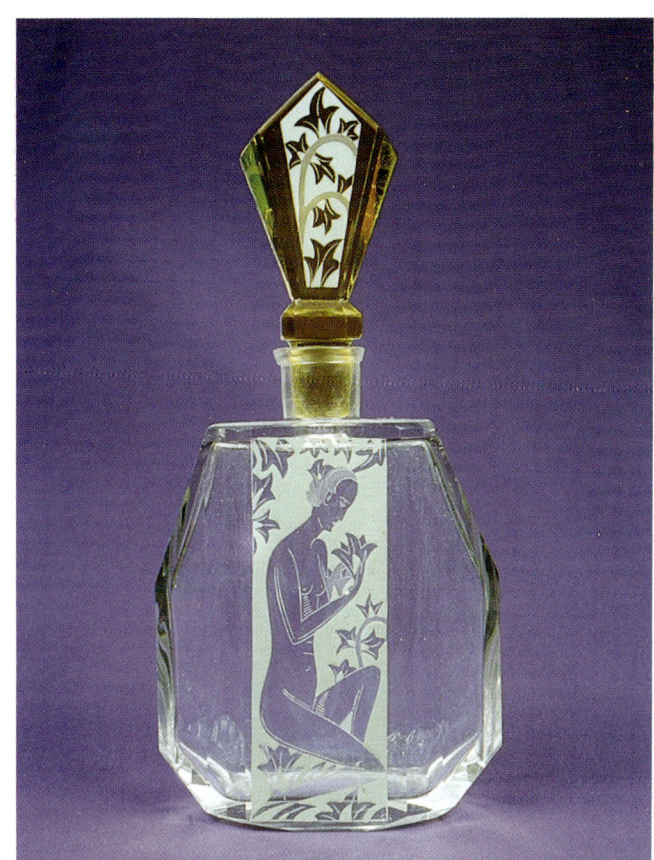

Lot #424. Very large clear crystal decanter bottle for cologne or cordials with yellow crystal stopper, 11.6" [29.5 cm], the bottle designed with large geometric facets, the front of the bottle enameled in green with a nude woman caressing flowers, the stopper also enameled with a conforming design, bottom signed *Czechoslovakia* in a line. Est. $500.00-$600.00.

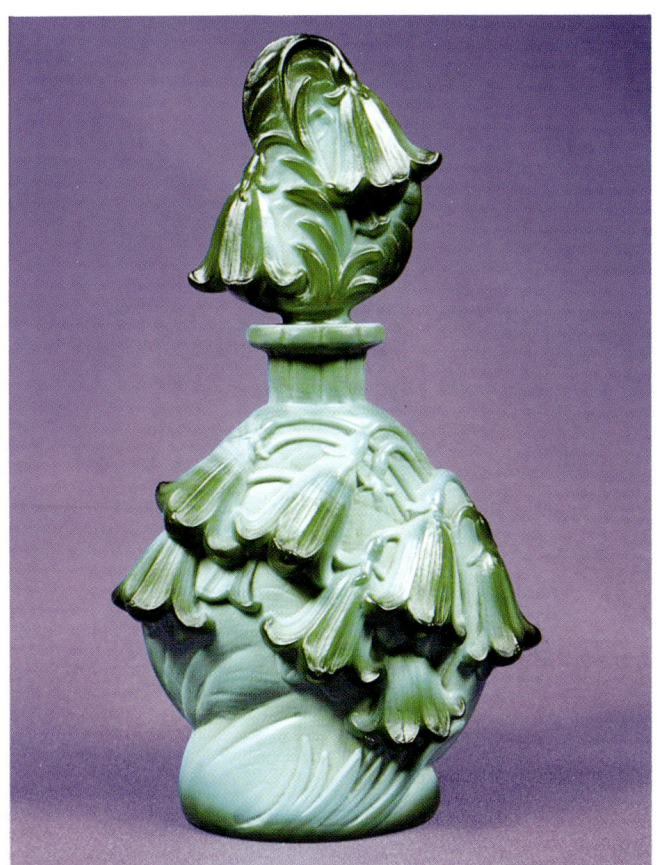

Lot #425. Malachite crystal bottle and stopper, 6.8" [17.3 cm], the bottle and stopper molded with large bluebells, dauber lacking, bottom signed *Ingrid Czechoslovakia*. Est. $500.00-$600.00.

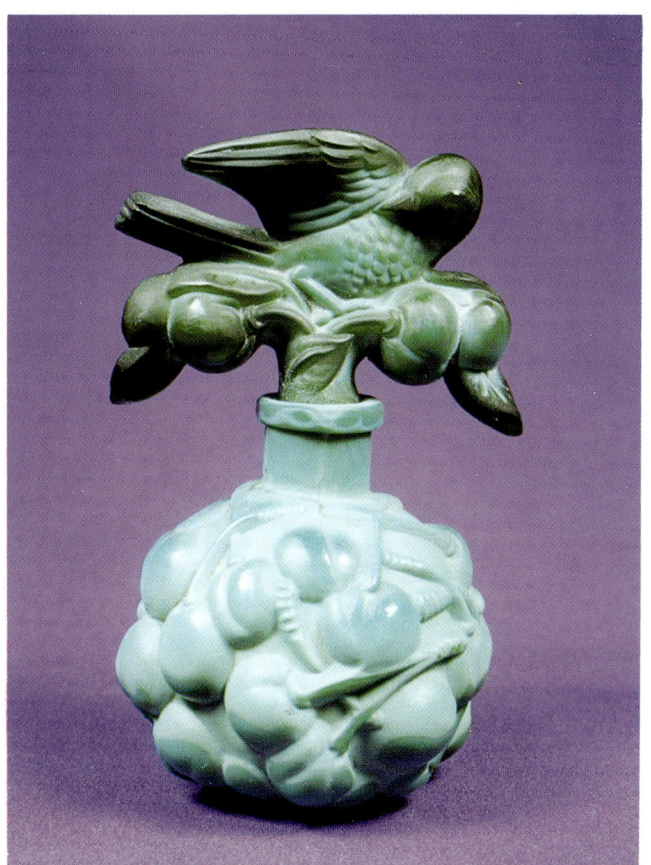

Lot #426. Malachite glass perfume bottle and stopper, 4.5" [11.4 cm], a rare design in which the bottle is molded with cherries and the stopper is a bird perched amid a cherry branch, part of its original green glass dauber is present, unsigned, by Ingrid. Est. $700.00-$850.00.

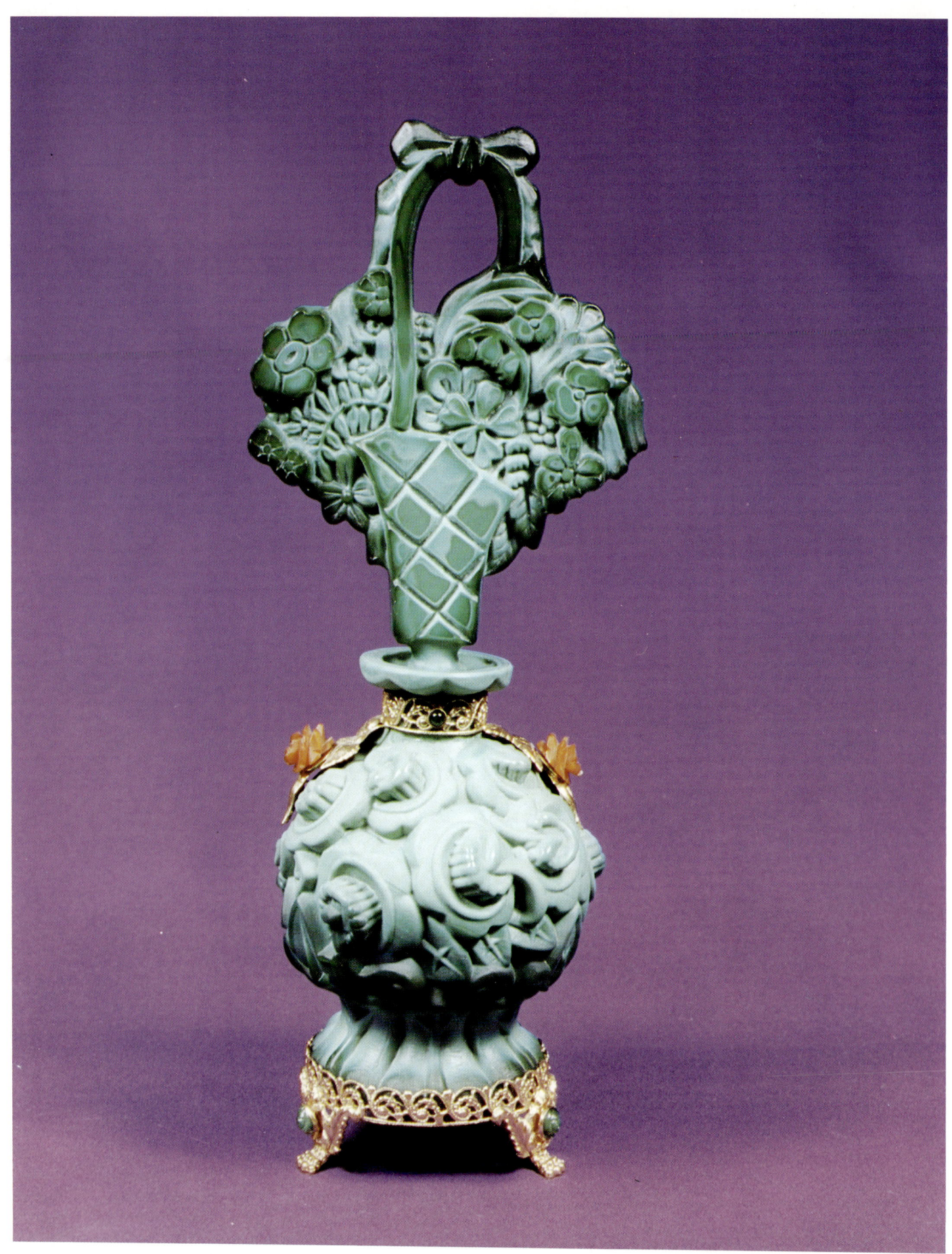

Lot #427. Very rare and desirable malachite glass perfume bottle and stopper on a metal base, 9" [22.9 cm], the bottle molded as a cluster of stylized flowers and leaves, the stopper as a basket overflowing with flowers, dauber lacking, gold metalwork base with three feet decorated with small carved green glass jewels, the neck also with gold metalwork and amber glass carved roses, bottom signed *Ingrid Czechoslovakia*. Cf. Forsythe II, #795. Est. $1,500.00-$2,000.00.